Veröffentlichungen aus der
Geomedizinischen Forschungsstelle
(Leiter: Professor Dr. Dres. h. c. G. Schettler)
der Heidelberger Akademie der Wissenschaften

Supplement zu den Sitzungsberichten der
Mathematisch-naturwissenschaftlichen Klasse
Jahrgang 1988

International Society and Federation of Cardiology
Société et Fédération Internationale de Cardiologie
Sociedad y Federación Internacional de Cardiología

Proceedings of the Joint Meeting of the Heidelberger Akademie der Wissenschaften and the International Society and Federation of Cardiology, Scientific Board "Possibilities to Improve and Reconstruct Occluded Coronary Vessels", Heidelberg, 15–17 September 1987

G. Schettler R. B. Jennings E. Rapaport
N. K. Wenger R. Bernhardt (Eds.)

Reperfusion and Revascularization in Acute Myocardial Infarction

With 66 Figures and 43 Tables

Springer-Verlag
Berlin Heidelberg New York
London Paris Tokyo

Prof. Dr. Dr. h.c. mult. Gotthard Schettler
Präsident der Heidelberger Akademie der Wissenschaften
Karlstrasse 4, 6900 Heidelberg, FRG

Dr Robert B. Jennings
Duke University Medical Center, Department of Pathology
P.O. Box 3712, Durham, NC 27710, USA

Dr. Elliot Rapaport
San Francisco General Hospital, R.5 GI
1001 Potrero Street, San Francisco, CA 94110, USA

Dr. Nanette K. Wenger
Department of Medicine (Cardiology)
Emory University School of Medicine
69 Butler Street S.E., Atlanta, GA 30303, USA

Dr. Ralph Bernhardt
Heidelberger Akademie der Wissenschaften
Geomedizinische Forschungsstelle
Karlstrasse 4, 6900 Heidelberg, FRG

ISBN-13:978-3-642-83546-9 e-ISBN-13:978-3-642-83544-5
DOI: 10.1007/978-3-642-83544-5

Library of Congress Cataloging-in-Publication Data
Reperfusion and revascularization in acute myocardial infarction / [edited by] G. Schettler, R.B. Jennings, E. Rapaport, N.K. Wenger, R. Bernhardt
p. cm. – (Veröffentlichungen aus der Geomedizinischen Forschungsstelle der Heidelberger Akademie der Wissenschaften) (Supplement zu den Sitzungsberichten der Mathematisch-naturwissenschaftlichen Klasse; Jahrg. 1988)
"Proceedings of the joint meeting of the Heidelberger Akademie der Wissenschaften and the International Society and Federation of Cardiology, Scientific Board ... Heidelberg, 15–17 September 1987" – T.p. verso.
ISBN-13:978-3-642-83546-9 (U.S.)
1. Heart – Infarction – Surgery – Congresses. 2. Myocardial revascularization – Congresses. 3. Heart – Infarction – Chemotherapy – Congresses. I. Schettler, Gotthard. II. Jennings, Robert B., 1926– . III. Rapaport, Elliot, 1924– . IV. Wenger, Nanette K. V. Bernhardt, Ralph. VI. Heidelberger Akademie der Wissenschaften. VII. International Society and Federation of Cardiology. Scientific Board. VIII. Series. IX. Series: Supplement zu den Sitzungsberichten der Mathematisch-naturwissenschaftlichen Klasse; Jahrg. 1988.
[DNLM: 1. Coronary Circulation – congresses. 2. Myocardial Infarction – surgery – congresses. 3. Myocardial Revascularization – congresses. WG 300 R425 1987]
RD598.R46 1988 617'.412–dc 19 DNLM/DLC 88-24950

Softcover reprint of the hardcover 1st edition 1988

2125/3140-543210 – Printed on acid-free paper

Contents

List of Authors

Applebaum, D.,
Department Medicine B, Hadassah University Hospital
P.O. Box 12000, 91120 Jerusalem, Israel

Bardos, P.,
Kardiologische Abteilung, Universitätsklinikum
5100 Aachen, FRG

Berra, P.,
Cattedra di Cardiologia, Universita degli Study di Brescia
c/o Spedali Civili, P. le Spedali Civili 1, Brescia 25100
Italy

Bigham, H. J.
Section of Cardiology, Yale University School of Medicine
333 Cedar Street, 87 L.M.P., New Haven, CT 06519, USA

Bleifeld, W.
Abteilung Kardiologie, Medizinische Klinik
Universitäts-Krankenhaus Eppendorf
Martinistr. 52, 2000 Hamburg 20, FRG

Boden, Ch.
Medizinische Klinik III
Bergheimerstr. 58, 6900 Heidelberg, FRG

Boskis, B.
Argentine Heart Foundation
Azcuenaga 980/86, Buenos Aires 1115, Argentina

Broustet, J. P.
Hopital Cardiologique du Haut Leveque
Avenue de Magellan, 33604 Pessac, France

Ceconi, C.
Cattedra di Cardiologia, Universita degli Study di Brescia
c/o Spedali Civili, P. le Spedali Civili 1, Brescia 25100
Italy

Ciampalini, G.
Cattedra di Cardiologia, Universita degli Study di Brescia
c/o Spedali Civili, P. le Spedali Civili 1, Brescia 25100
Italy

Curello, S.
Cattedra di Cardiologia, Universita degli Study di Brescia
c/o Spedali Civili, P. le Spedali Civili 1, Brescia 25100
Italy

Douard, H.
Hopital Cardiologique du Haut Leveque
Avenue de Magellan, 33604 Pessac, France

Dussel, R.
Innere Medizin III, Kardiologie,
Bergheimerstr. 58, 6900 Heidelberg, FRG

Effert, S.
Kardiologische Abteilung, Universitätsklinikum
5100 Aachen, FRG

Erbel, E.
Klinikum der Johannes Gutenberg-Universität
II. Medizinische Klinik und Poliklinik
Langenbeckstr. 1, 6500 Mainz, FRG

Ferrari, R.
Cattedra di Cardiologia, Universita degli Study di Brescia
c/o Spedali Civili, P. le Spedali Civili 1, Brescia 25100
Italy

Ganote, C. E.
Department of Pathology, Ward Memorial Building
303 East Chicago Avenue, Chicago, Illinois 60611, USA

Gotsman, M. S.
Department Medicine B, Hadassah University Hospital
P.O. Box 12000, 91120 Jerusalem, Israel

Hugenholtz, P. G.
Thoraxcenter BD 408, Erasmus University
P.O. Box 1738, 3000 DR Rotterdam, The Netherlands

Jennings R. B.
Duke University Medical Center
Department of Pathology
P.O. Box 3712, Durham, North Carolina 27710, USA

Kellermann, J. J.
Chaim Sheba Med CTR, Inst. Cardiac Rehab
Tel Hashomer 52621, Israel

König, K.
Fachklinik für Herz-Kreislauf-Erkrankungen
Kandelstr. 41, 7808 Waldkirch bei Freiburg, FRG

Kübler, W.
Innere Medizin III, Kardiologie,
Bergheimerstr. 58, 6900 Heidelberg, FRG

Kusuoka, H.
First Department of Medicine
Osaka University School of Medicine
Osaka, Japan

Leinberger, H.
Innere Medizin III, Kardiologie,
Bergheimerstr. 58, 6900 Heidelberg, FRG

Lichtlen, P.
Abteilung Kardiologie MHH
Postfach 610180, 3000 Hannover 61, FRG

Lotan, C.
Department Medicine B, Hadassah University Hospital
P.O. Box 12000, 91120 Jerusalem, Israel

Marban, E.
Cardiology, Department of Medicine
Johns Hopkins Hospital, Baltimore, Maryland 21205
USA

Markwardt, F.
Medizinische Akademie Erfurt,
Inst. für Pharmakologie und Toxikologie
Nordhäuser Str. 74, 5060 Erfurt, DDR

Mathey, D. G.
Abteilung Kardiologie, Medizinische Klinik
Universitäts-Krankenhaus Eppendorf
Martinistr. 52, 2000 Hamburg 20, FRG

Messmer, B. J.
Kardiologische Abteilung, Universitätsklinikum
5100 Aachen, FRG

Meyer, J.
Klinikum der Johannes Gutenberg-Universität
II. Medizinische Klinik und Poliklinik
Langenbeckstr. 1, 6500 Mainz, FRG

Minale, C.
Kardiologische Abteilung, Universitätsklinikum
5100 Aachen, FRG

Mora, B.
Hopital Cardiologique du Haut Leveque
Avenue de Magellan, 33604 Pessac, France

Neuhaus, K. L.
Städtisches Klinikum Kassel, Medizinische Klinik II
Mönchebergstr. 41/43, 3500 Kassel, FRG

Neumann, F.-J.
Innere Medizin III, Kardiologie,
Bergheimerstr. 58, 6900 Heidelberg, FRG

O'Neill, W.
Cardiology Service, University Hospital
Ann Arbor, Michigan 48109, USA

O'Rourke, R.
Division of Cardiology, Department of Medicine
University of Texas, Science Centre at San Antonio
7703 Floyd Curl Drive, San Antonio, TX 78284, USA

Parekh, N.
Innere Medizin III, Kardiologie,
Bergheimerstr. 58, 6900 Heidelberg, FRG

Pitt, B.
Cardiology Service, University Hospital
Ann Arbor, Michigan 48109, USA

Pop, T.
Klinikum der Johannes Gutenberg-Universität
II. Medizinische Klinik und Poliklinik
Langenbeckstr. 1, 6500 Mainz, FRG

Porterfield, J. K.
Cardiology, Department of Medicine
Johns Hopkins Hospital, Baltimore, Maryland 21205, USA

Rapaport, E.
San Francisco General Hospital, R.5GI
1001 Potrero Street, San Francisco, CA 94110, USA

Reimer, K. A.
Department of Pathology
Duke University Medical Center
Durham, NC 27710, USA

Rosenheck, S.
Department Medicine B, Hadassah University Hospital
P.O. Box 12000, 91120 Jerusalem, Israel

Sanne, H.
Dept. of Phys. Med and Rehabilitation
Sahlgrenska Hospital, 41345 Göteborg, Sweden

Sapoznikov, D.
Department Medicine B, Hadassah University Hospital
P.O. Box 12000, 91120 Jerusalem, Israel

Schmutzler, H.
Abteilung Innere Medizin, – Kardiologie –
Klinikum Westend
Spandauer Damm 130, 1000 Berlin 19, FRG

Schettler, G., Prof. Dr. Dr. h.c. mult.
Geomedizinische Forschungsstelle der
Heidelberger Akademie der Wissenschaften
Karlstr. 4, 6900 Heidelberg, FRG

Schönermark, S.
Medizinische Klinik III
Bergheimerstr. 58, 6900 Heidelberg, FRG

Schofer, J.
Abteilung Kardiologie, Medizinische Klinik
Universitäts-Krankenhaus Eppendorf
Martinistr. 52, 2000 Hamburg 20, FRG

Schröder, R. K.
Universität Steglitz, Med. Klinik und Poliklinik
Hindenburgdamm 30, 1000 Berlin 45, FRG

Schuler, G.
Medizinische Klinik III
Bergheimerstr. 58, 6900 Heidelberg, FRG

Schwarz, F.
Abt. Kardiologie, Rotes Kreuz Krankenhaus
Königswarterstr. 16, 6000 Frankfurt am Main 1, FRG

Seidel, D.
Lehrstuhl für klinische Chemie
Universitätsklinik Göttingen
Robert-Koch-Str. 40, 3400 Göttingen, FRG

Simanek, H.-G.
Medizinische Klinik III
Bergheimerstr. 58, 6900 Heidelberg, FRG

Simoons, M. L.
Thoraxcenter BD 408, Erasmus University
P.O. Box 1738, 3000 DR Rotterdam, The Netherlands

Steenbergen, Ch.
Duke University Medical Center
Department of Pathology
P.O. Box 3712, Durham, North Carolina 27710, USA

Steinhausen, M.
Innere Medizin III, Kardiologie
Bergheimerstr. 58, 6900 Heidelberg, FRG

Suryapranta, H.
Thoraxcenter BD 408, Erasmus University
P.O. Box 1738, 3000 DR Rotterdam, The Netherlands

Topol, E.
Cardiology Service, University Hospital
Ann Arbor, Michigan 48109, USA

Tillmanns, H.
Innere Medizin III, Kardiologie
Bergheimerstr. 58, 6900 Heidelberg, FRG

Uebis, R.
Kardiologische Abteilung, Universitätsklinikum
5100 Aachen, FRG

Vander Heide, S.
Department of Pathology, Ward Memorial Building
303 East Chicago Avenue, Chicago, Illinois 60611, USA

Varnauskas, E.
Sahlgrenska Hospital, Cardiology
41345 Göteborg, Sweden

Vermeer, F.
Thoraxcenter BD 408, Erasmus University
P.O. Box 1738, 3000 DR Rotterdam, The Netherlands

Verstraete, M.
Katholieke Universiteit Leuven, Department of Medical Research, Center for Thrombosis and Vascular Research
Herestraat 49, 3000 Leuven, Belgium

Visioli, O.
Cattedra di Cardiologia, Universita degli Study di Brescia
c/o Spedali Civili, P. le Spedali Civili 1, Brescia 25100
Italy

Welber, S.
Department Medicine B, Hadassah University Hospital
P.O. Box 12000, 91120 Jerusalem, Israel

Weiss, A. T.
Department Medicine B, Hadassah University Hospital
P.O. Box 12000, 91120 Jerusalem, Israel

Walter, P.J.
Dept. Cardiovascular Surgery
University Hospital Antwerp
Wilrijkstraat 10, 2520 Edegem, Belgium

Wenger, N. K.
Department of Medicine (Cardiology), Emory University School of Medicine
69 Butler Street, S.E. Atlanta, Georgia 30303, USA

Zaret, B.L.
Section of Cardiology
Yale University School of Medicine
333 Cedar Street, 87 L.M.P., New Haven, CT 06519
USA

Zimmermann, R.
Innere Medizin III, Kardiologie
Bergheimerstr. 58, 6900 Heidelberg, FRG

List of Discussion Participants

Augustin, J.
Bereich Medizin, Merckle GmbH
Postfach 1780, 7900 Ulm-Donautal

Ganten, D.
Pharmakol. Institut der Universität
Im Neuenheimer Feld 366, 6900 Heidelberg, FRG

Lucchesi, B. R.
Dept. of Pharmacology, M6322 Medical Science Building
The University of Michigan, Ann Arbor, Michigan 48109
USA

Olsen, E.
Department of Histopathology, National Heart Hospital
Westmoreland Street, London W1M 8BA, Great Britain

Opening Address

G. Schettler

The Heidelberg Academy for the Humanities and Sciences welcomes all of you to this symposium. It has been planned at the suggestion of a member of Council Chairpersons and is being held under the auspices of the International Society and Federation of Cardiology.

The Heidelberg Academy is certainly the right place for a meeting such as this. It was founded in 1763 and due to the initiative of Voltaire. It has served at all times for interdisciplinary cooperation, including that beyond national frontiers. Academies have been and still are autonomous institutions. The Heidelberg Academy consists of a scientific and a historical section. At the moment each section has 35 members who are elected by the Academy itself. In addition, there is double this number of corresponding members who, in contrast to the regular members, do not necessarily come from the state of Baden-Württemberg and they include scientists from around the world.

The Academy carries out independent scientific projects, mainly in arts subjects. However, science subjects such as mathematics, physics, chemistry, biology, and medicine are increasingly becoming integral parts of our work. Organizing and holding symposia is an important task of the Academy. So far, under my chairmanship we have held three international symposia concerned with molecular biology. In cooperation with the German Cancer Research Center, the European Molecular Biology Laboratory, the Department of Molecular Biology of the University of Heidelberg, and the Max Planck Institute for Molecular Biology, we plan to concentrate our future work on molecular biology.

Our present subject of discussion, the reperfusion of occluded coronary vessels, will also have to be increasingly concerned with molecular biology. Prophylaxis and therapy are, of course, closely related to pathogenesis. The complex process of arterial occlusion must therefore be elucidated from different points of view. An occlusion can be initiated by changes in the vessel wall itself, such as the formation of atheromas in their different stages. The process can also be initiated by ulcerations, with subsequent thrombosis, and by intramural subendothelial thrombi. The development of atheromas must be understood on a humoral as well as on a cellular level. Of special importance is the endothelial barrier. The interaction between circulating blood and the vessel wall is influenced by rheological factors in particular. Therefore, it is indicated initially to discuss the etiologic and pathogenetic basis of cardiovascular diseases. Epidemiological and case-control studies have shown that certain risk constellations promote arterial occlusion. Any preventive approach must therefore consider these factors. There have been a number of recent findings in the field of lipid research which have also influenced therapeutic concepts. The whole range of lipid-lowering measures is a subject of discussion. Circulatory factors had been neglected for some time, but these are increasingly coming under consideration. Noninvasive procedures are being complemented by mechanical and physical measures.

All these procedures must be discussed, and it should be noted that there are successful combinations of procedures, e.g., with PTCA and fibrinolytic measures. Collaboration with cardiovascular surgeons is important, as are subsequent measures for permanent optimization of coronary circulation. Here we depend on experts in the field of coagulation, who have made great progress in recent years. The results will help to make the life of coronary patients easier, give them pain-free years of life, and prevent recurring occlusions. Besides curative procedures, preventive measures are playing an ever more important role. Thus, the worldwide occurrence of arterial occlusions can be tackled by a new strategy. We know from observations made in times of starvation that regression of even advanced coronary alterations is possible and that the development of coronary thromboses and coronary events is practically prevented. Without a doubt, diet plays a special role in this context. Recent results obtained in the People's Republic of China show the advantages of a "prudent diet" such as that which has been fixed by the Consensus Conferences of United States and European Cardiological Societies as a basis of all preventive and curative measures. We hope our symposium will provide to a clear summary of all procedures available. This would accomplish one goal of the International Society and Federation of Cardiology.

I wish to thank all those who have helped to organize this symposium, especially the Chairpersons of the Scientific Councils, our office in Geneva, and our local assistants.

Session I
Pathophysiology of Salvage of Ischemic Myocardium by Reperfusion

Chairman: R. B. Jennings

Acute Regional Ischemia*

R. B. Jennings, K. A. Reimer, and C. Steenbergen, Jr.

A series of changes are initiated in the myocardium following the sudden onset of ischemia in vivo, which, by the time 60 min of ischemia have passed, result in the death of virtually all of the severely ischemic myocytes. However, results of studies of the effect of reperfusion of arterial blood after 15 min of ischemia have shown that the myocytes, though badly damaged, are still alive. Thus, between 15 and 60 min, an event or series of events occurs in the myocytes which causes them to pass the "point of no return," i.e., to be unsalvageable even though successfully reperfused [1]. The change or changes which cause the injury to become lethal remain unknown; at present, sarcolemmal disruption is the prime candidate for the lethal event [2, 3].

Biology of Acute Ischemia. Figure 1 summarizes the major changes which occur when a major branch of a coronary artery is occluded near its origin in the dog heart. Arterial flow to the myocardium supplied by the vessel is depressed to the level provided by collateral arterial flow. After occlusion of the circumflex artery, the flow is reduced to less than 5% of control (severe or low-flow ischemia) in the subendocardial myocardium. The mid- and subepicardial layers generally receive greater quantities of collateral flow.

The studies reviewed in this paper were made on low-flow ischemic tissue because (a) the injury is uniformly severe in such tissue and (b) the damaged tissue can be identified through the use of thioflavine S [2]. Also, some experiments have been performed on left ventricular tissue subjected to total ischemia in vitro, i.e., to tissue receiving no arterial flow. The metabolic changes of ischemia are identical in both models. However, the changes occur more quickly in low-flow ischemia in vivo than in total ischemia in vitro.

The depressed arterial flow of ischemia limits the amount of oxygen available to the tissue. Within 8 – 10 s of the onset, the pO_2 falls to low levels. Aerobic metabolism ceases and anaerobic glycolysis begins at a high rate. Effective contraction ceases at about the same time and electrocardiographic changes appear [2].

The chief consequences of ischemia fall into two broad categories: the consequences of the osmolar load and the consequences of energy deficiency (Fig. 1).

---

* Supported in part by NIH grants HL23138, HL27416, and HL01337.

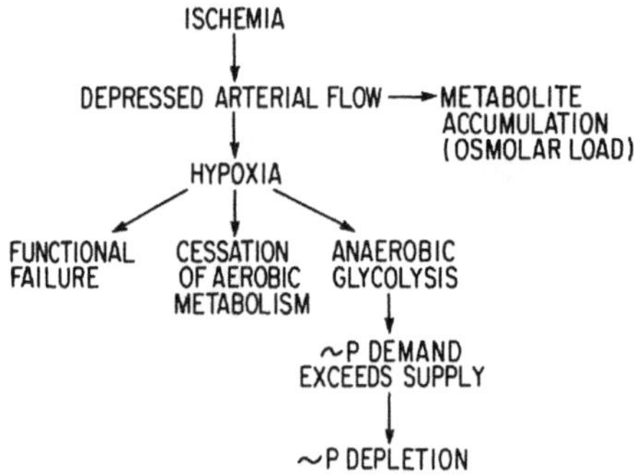

Fig. 1. Principal consequences of ischemia. Metabolites are produced intracellularly by hypoxic metabolism where they accumulate (the osmolar load) and equilibrate to a variable extent with the extracellular fluid. Since the demand of the tissue for HEP exceeds the supply, the net level of ATP falls until it is virtually zero in zones of low-flow ischemia. (Reproduced with permission, from [4])

Creatine phosphate is broken down within 10 – 20 s of the onset to creatine and phosphate, both of which are retained intracellularly. The products of anaerobic glycolysis, chiefly lactate, accumulate in the myocytes along with other intermediates, principally glucose-6-phosphate and α-glycerol phosphate. Because there is little or no arterial flow, most of these metabolites are retained in the tissue along with other products of ischemic metabolism. These intracellular products increase the osmolality of the intracellular water. As a consequence, the myocytes quickly become edematous and exhibit a volume dependent loss of K^+. The latter change is associated with alterations in the membrane potential and the appearance of electrocardiographic abnormalities. All of these changes occur within seconds of the onset of ischemia [2].

Glycolysis is inhibited by reduced nicotinamide adenine dinucleotide (NADH), lactate, H^+, and perhaps other intermediates [5, 6]. Moreover, if glycolysis continued its initial high rate, the glycogen supply would be exhausted after only 5 – 10 minutes of ischemia. Since reserves of HEP are low and since the demand of the tissue for HEP exceeds the supply, adenosine triphosphate (ATP) falls quickly to low levels. Accumulation of phosphate and H^+ are directly related to nucleotide and creatine phosphate (CP) breakdown and lactate accumulation.

Myocardial Energy Production. Myocardium is virtually totally dependent on aerobic (mitochondrial) respiration to produce the large quantity of HEP required to support the continued contraction of the heart. Effective myocardial contractions cease a few seconds after the onset of ischemia. Once the aerobic to anaerobic transition has occurred, the demand of the myocardium for HEP exceeds the supply. Among the reactions producing demand for HEP are: (a) continued ineffective contractile efforts secondary to the ongoing electrical stimuli from the AV node, (b) activity of ATPases including the Na/K and Ca ATPases of the sarcolemma and the Ca ATPase of the sarcoplasmic reticulum, and (c) minor reactions such as acetyl-CoA synthetase, adenyl cyclase, and other phosphorylating reactions occurring in the myocyte. The supply side effectively has only two components, anaerobic glycolysis, and the preexisting pool of CP and ATP (see [2] for details). Detailed analyses have shown that about 80% of the HEP produced and utilized during an episode of severe or total ischemia

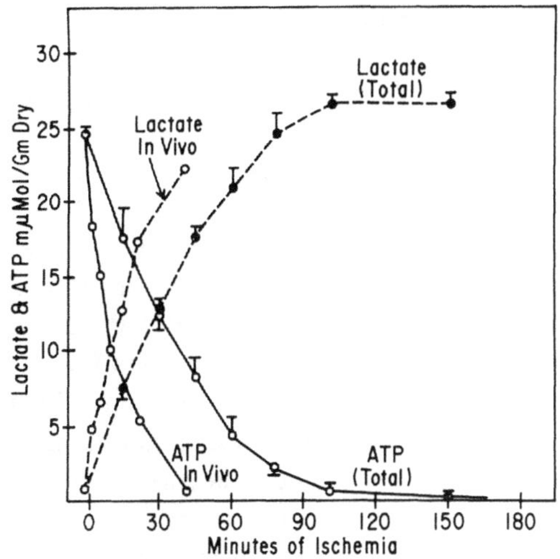

Fig. 2. The inverse relationship between the ATP and lactate of the subendocardial tissue of canine left ventricle after varying periods of total ischemia in vitro at 37 °C (total). The in vitro data are from Jones et al. [11]. For comparison, the ATP and lactate of severely ischemic left ventricular myocardium of the circumflex bed (in vivo) is plotted. The severe ischemia was induced by occlusion of the circumflex coronary artery in the pentobarbital-anesthetized open-chest dogs ($n = 4 - 6$). A different group of dogs was used for each time point on the in vivo curves. Note that even though there is no flow in the totally ischemic tissue, both ATP depletion and lactate accumulation develop much more quickly in vivo than in vitro. Most of the in vivo data is from [2, 12, and 13]. (Reproduced with permission, from [4])

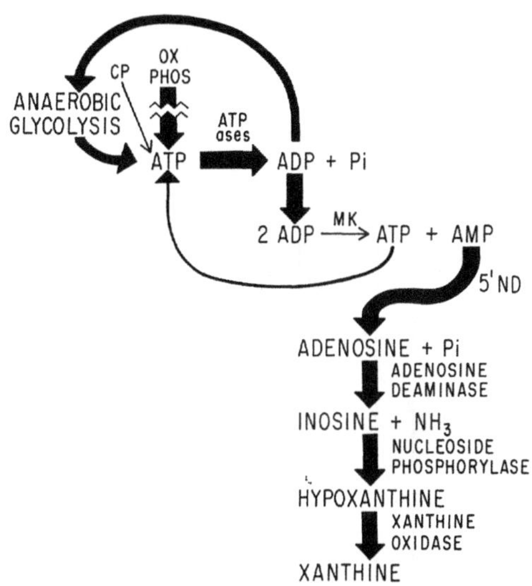

Fig. 3. Summary of the pathways through which the adenine nucleotide pool is destroyed in ischemia. The inadequate production of ATP of the ischemic tissue leads to elevated ADP. The high energy phosphate of ADP is salvaged via the action of adenylate kinase (MK) with the production of an ATP and an AMP from two molecules of ADP. This AMP is dephosphorylated with 5′ nucleotidase (5′ ND) to adenosine plus inorganic phosphate. Adenosine is deaminated via adenosine deaminase to inosine plus ammonia. Inosine is further degraded via nucleoside phosphorylase and xanthine oxidase.

comes from glycolysis and 20% from depleting the pools of CP, ATP, and adenosine diphosphate (ADP) [4].

ATP depletion is virtually complete after 40 min of ischemia have passed and is accompanied by the accumulation of enormous quantities of lactate (Fig. 2). According to the lactate accumulation curve, by the time 40 – 60 min of ischemia have passed, anaerobic glycolysis has ceased.

In addition to depletion of HEP, the adenine nucleotide pool is destroyed. The reactions involved are summarized in Fig. 3. The critical reaction involves adenylate kinase (myokinase), a reaction in which two ADP molecules are converted into one ATP which is utilized and one AMP which is degraded to adenosine. In contrast to the nucleotides, adenosine and its deaminated catabolite, inosine, can diffuse from the myocyte. Once they enter the extracellular space, they are lost and cannot be used for salvage resynthesis of the pool if the tissue is reperfused with arterial blood. The consequences of these reactions are shown in Fig. 4.

Reversible and Irreversible Injury. Injury during the first 15 – 18 minutes of in vivo low-flow ischemia is considered to be *reversible.* Removing the cause of injury by restoring arterial flow prevents the cell death which inevitably would develop in the zone of low-flow ischemia if the tissue was allowed to remain ischemic.

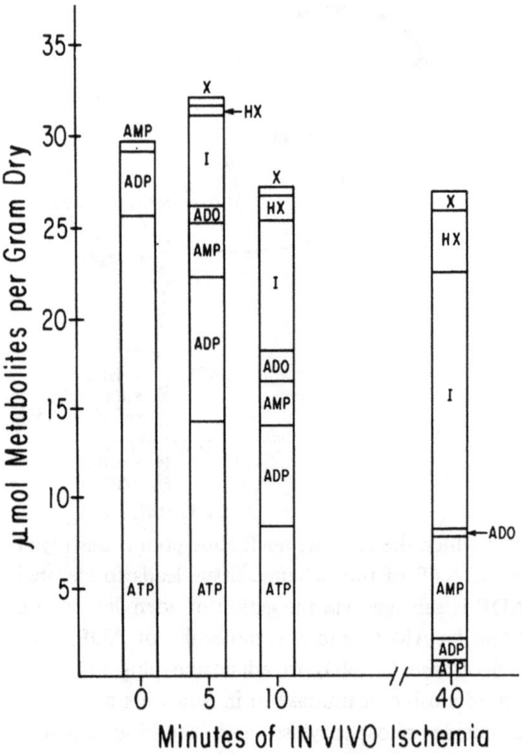

Fig. 4. Total adenine nucleotide (*TAN*) pool of ischemic left ventricular tissue is compared with nonischemic myocardium in groups of hearts subjected to varying periods of ischemia. *ADO*, Adenosine; *I*, inosine; *HX*, hypoxanthine; *X*, xanthine. The TAN pool is ATP + ADP + AMP. (Reproduced with permission, from [13])

If the ischemia is allowed to persist for 20–25 min, a few myocytes cannot be salvaged by reperfusion. These myocytes are termed *irreversibly injured.* By the time 60 min of low-flow ischemia have passed, virtually all of the myocytes in the zone of low-flow ischemia are dead. These definitions with respect to viability are reviewed in detail elsewhere [2].

Ultrastructural Changes of Ischemia. During the early phase of ischemia, few ultrastructural changes are detectable. Edema is noted as an increase in the sarcoplasmic space. Also, fewer glycogen particles are found. Some margination of nuclear chromatin occurs and a rare mitochondrion is swollen.

Early in the phase of irreversible injury, the myocytes exhibit all of the changes seen in the reversible phase plus a dramatic series of changes, including (a) mitochondrial swelling, (b) the appearance of amorphous matrix densities in the mitochondria, and (c) focal areas of disruption of the sarcolemma. The mitochondrial and sarcolemmal changes are characteristic of the irreversible phase of injury. Sarcolemmal disruption is considered to be the most likely cause of the transition to irreversibility.

The capillaries in the center of the zone of severe ischemia become necrotic about 30–60 min after myocyte injury becomes irreversible. After this time, reperfusion is impossible. Such tissue exhibits the so-called no-reflow phenomenon [7].

Biochemical and Structural Features of the Reversible and Early Irreversible Phases. The changes developing in a zone of low-flow ischemia appear quickly and develop continuously until the myocyte dies. No sudden metabolic change which signifies that the myocyte has passed the point of no return has been identified. Gradually developing subcellular changes include [8]: (a) depletion of ATP and high-energy phosphate, (b) utilization of glycogen, (c) increasing acidity, (d) accumulation of glycolytic intermediates including lactate, glucose-6-phosphate, and α-glycerol phosphate, (e) accumulation of other metabolites including AMP, phosphate, adenosine, inosine, creatine, and NH_4, (f) increasing intracellular osmolarity, (g) myocyte edema, (h) depression followed by cessation of macromolecular synthesis, (i) a decrease in the K^+, Cl^-, and Na^+ ion gradients, (j) a gradual decrease in the adenylate charge, (k) mild ultrastructural changes, and (l) a variety of other changes.

The transition to irreversibility of a significant number of myocytes in a sample of ischemic myocardium is characterized by: (a) ATP < 2 μmol/g dry, i.e., less than 8% of control, (b) a low adenine nucleotide pool consisting chiefly of AMP, (c) virtual cessation of anaerobic glycolysis, (d) low glycogen, (e) high inosine and hypoxanthine, (f) ultrastructural and functional evidence of disruption of the plasmalemma of the sarcolemma. The latter change is considered to be an unequivocal sign that the myocyte is dead and therefore cannot be salvaged by reperfusion.

Effects of Reperfusion with Arterial Blood. Successful reperfusion is associated with the prompt development of reactive hyperemia. Arterial flow increases by 600% or more. The myocardium blushes bright red compared to adjacent control myocardium. At about the same time that reactive hyperemia appears, the electrocardiographic changes return toward control. Successful reperfusion early in the irreversible phase is followed by the prompt development of contraction-band necrosis. This form of massive contraction develops presumably because of the entry through the defective sarcolemma of large amounts of extracellular Ca^{2+} from the plasma reperfusing the tissue [8]. The entry of Ca^{2+} also is associated with accumulation of Ca phosphate in the mitochondria. The latter change requires active oxidative metabolism and an intact electron transport chain.

Reversibly injured myocardium responds to reperfusion by a brief period of increased mitochondrial swelling followed by restoration of the myocyte architecture to an appearance generally indistinguishable from control. The mitochondrial swelling phase is obvious at 3 min, but the tissue is back to control after 20 min of reperfusion [9]. However, a small fraction of mitochondria remain badly damaged and exhibit swelling, plus in some cases, amorphous matrix densities. These still are detectable 4 days after the tissue is reperfused.

The adenylate charge of the ischemic myocytes is restored to control levels after 3 min of reperfusion [9]. However, the pool itself requires more than 4 days to be restored to control levels [10]. Resynthesis is slow because phosphoribosyl pyrophosphate synthesis is slow in myocardium.

Summary. The dynamic state of acutely ischemic myocardium is reviewed with respect to the metabolic and ultrastructural changes which develop during ischemia. The probable event or series of events which causes the injury to become irreversible is postulated to be sarcolemmal disruption. Except for sarcolemmal disruption, no sudden change has been identified which is correlated with the development of irreversible injury. However, the metabolic conditions associated with irreversibility now are well established and include: (a) cessation of anaerobic glycolysis, (b) virtual total depletion of high-energy phosphates, and (c) a large osmolar load of intracellular metabolites including lactate, phosphate, creatine, glucose-6-phosphate, and α-glycerol phosphate.

References

1. Jennings RB, Reimer KA, Steenbergen C Jr (1986) Myocardial ischemia revisited. The osmolar load, membrane damage, and reperfusion (Editorial). J Mol Cell Cardiol 18:769–780
2. Jennings RB, Reimer KA (1981) Lethal myocardial ischemic injury. Am J Pathol 102:241–255
3. Steenbergen C, Hill ML, Jennings RB (1987) Cytoskeletal damage during myocardial ischemia: changes in vinculin immunofluorescence staining during total in vitro ischemia in canine heart. Circ Res 60:478–486

4. Jennings RB, Reimer KA, Steenbergen C, Murry CE (1987) Energy metabolism in myocardial ischemia and reperfusion. In: Dhalla NS, Innes IR, Beamish RE (eds) Myocardial ischemia. Martinus Nijhoff, Leiden, pp 185 – 198
5. Neely JR, Liedtke AJ, Whitmer JT, Rovetto MJ (1975) Relationship between coronary flow and adenosine triphosphate production from glycolysis and oxidative metabolism. In: Roy PE, Harris P (eds) Recent advances in studies on cardiac structure and metabolism, vol. 8. The cardiac sarcoplasm, University Park Press, Baltimore, pp 301 – 321
6. Neely JR, Rovetto MJ, Whitmer JT (1976) Rate-limiting steps of carbohydrate and fatty acid metabolism in ischemic hearts. Acta Med Scand [Suppl] 587:9 – 13
7. Kloner RA, Ganote CE, Jennings RB (1974) The "no-reflow" phenomenon after temporary coronary occlusion in the dog. J Clin Invest 54:1496 – 1508
8. Jennings RB, Reimer KA, Steenbergen C Jr (1985) Myocardial ischemia and reperfusion. Role of calcium. In: Parratt JR (ed) Control and manipulation of calcium movement. Raven, New York, pp 273 – 302
9. Jennings RB, Schaper J, Hill ML, Steenbergen C, Reimer KA (1985) Effect of reperfusion late in the phase of reversible ischemic injury: changes in metabolism and ultrastructure. Circ Res 546:262 – 278
10. Reimer KA, Hill ML, Jennings RB (1981) Prolonged depletion of ATP and of the adenine nucleotide pool due to delayed resynthesis of adenine nucleotides following reversible myocardial ischemic injury in dogs. J Mol Cell Cardiol 13:229 – 239
11. Jones RN, Reimer KA, Hill ML, Jennings RB (1982) Effect of hypothermia on changes in high energy phosphate production and utilization in total ischemia. J Mol Cell Cardiol 14 [Suppl 3]:123 – 130
12. Jennings RB, Hawkins HK, Lowe JE, Hill ML, Klotman S, Reimer KA (1978) Relation between high energy phosphate and lethal injury in myocardial ischemia in the dog. Am J Pathol 92:187 – 214
13. Jennings RB, Murry CE, Steenbergen C, Reimer KA (1988) The acute phase of regional ischemia. In: Cox RH (ed) Acute myocardial infarction: emerging concepts of pathogenesis and treatment. Praeger Scientific, New York
14. Jennings RB, Reimer KA, Jones RN, Peyton RB (1983) High energy phosphates, anaerobic glycolysis and irreversibility in ischemia. In: Spitzer JJ (ed) Myocardial ischemia. Plenum, New York, pp 403 – 419

The Role of Free Radical Scavengers in Reperfusion

R. Ferrari, C. Ceconi, S. Curello, G. Ciampalini, P. Berra, and O. Visioli

Introduction

Recently, oxygen radicals have been implicated in the pathogenesis of many diseases. This is reflected in the many conferences devoted to this topic and in the numerous books that cover the field in a systematic manner [1, 2, 3, 4, 5, 6]. Much attention is currently focused on a role for oxygen radicals in heart and blood-vessel abnormalities and in myocardial changes secondary to antitumour anthracyclines [7], alcohol [8] and iron overload [9]. Oxygen radical reactions probably contribute to the production of ischaemic and reperfusion myocardial injury [10, 16]. However, with the exception of specific instances in which oxygen radicals have been proved to be important (for example, hyperoxia and iron overload), their involvement in many disease processes is still a controversial topic [17, 18].

Often the evidence is based on experimental data indicating increased rates of lipid peroxidation in diseased tissue, the ameliorating effect of anti-oxidants, or both. Such studies often use experimental end points of cell and tissue damage that may not reflect the human disease process, and these should be interpreted cautiously. Whereas end products of lipid peroxidation certainly may be harmful to the cell, lipid peroxidation can occur as a consequence of tissue damage [19], and it is not necessarily related to the primary mechanism of tissue injury. Lipid peroxidation may result in amplification of the original injury through a chain reaction, through a disruption of cellular metabolism, such as glutathione depletion, or through generation of toxic aldehydes capable of causing cell damage at some distance from their source. Thus, oxygen radicals can be implicated in almost all disease processes in which cell injury occurs.

In addition, enzymatic production of lipid peroxides, such as during the arachidonic acid cascades, are not necessarily harmful. It follows that the finding of lipid peroxidation end products may be significant, but it does not necessarily convey information about the primary process of cell injury. For these reasons, in the present study we have determined the occurrence of oxidative stress as an index of oxygen-free radical damage. Oxidative stress is a condition in which, because of an increased production of radicals or altered metabolism the redox state of the cell is shifted towards oxidation. Oxidative stress is reflected in an oxidation of lable thiols of proteins and small molecules and is a prerequisite for major cellular alterations; it can be accurately detected by simultaneously measuring tissue formation and rate of release of oxidized glutathione.

The objective of this paper is to summarize the evidence in favour of a role for oxygen-free radicals in the pathogenesis of myocardial reperfusion injury which we have accumulated in our laboratories. Four topics are considered in detail: the source of free radicals in the ischaemic and reperfused myocardium; the effects of ischaemia on the defence mechanism against oxygen-free radicals; the occurrence of oxidative stress during reperfusion in isolated heart preparations and in man during surgically induced cardiac arrest; and the possibility of reducing ischaemic and reperfusion damage with interventions able to protect against oxygen-free radicals. Some of the data presented here have already been published [10, 11, 12, 13, 14, 15, 16].

Oxygen Toxicity and Source of Free Radicals During Myocardial Ischaemia and Reperfusion

It is well-known that oxygen supplied at concentrations greater than those in normal air might damage plants, animals and aerobic bacteria. There is a considerable body of evidence that as much as 21% O_2 has slowly manifested damaging effects [20]. These effects vary considerably with the type of organism used, its age and diet.

The inherent nature of the oxygen molecule makes it susceptible to univalent reduction reactions in the cell to form superoxide anions ($O_2^{\dot{-}}$), a highly reactive free radical [21]. A free radical is any substance which has one or more unpaired electrons. Oxygen itself is actually a biradical, but it is not a very reactive radical even though it has two unpaired electrons. This is because oxygen has a strong property of the electrons both spinning in the same direction. Other reactive products of oxygen metabolism can be formed from subsequent intracellular reduction of $O_2^{\dot{-}}$, including oxygen peroxide (H_2O_2) and the hydroxyl radical ($^{\cdot}OH$). The hydroxyl radical lasts for about a billionth of a second. It is the most dangerous radical in biological systems and is the most potent oxidizing agent known.

In a cell this destructive radical becomes free to attack unsaturated fatty-acid side chains by abstracting a hydrogen and leaving a carbon radical. The lipid radical subsequently rearranges to produce a conjugated diene and, in the presence of oxygen, results in formation of organic oxygen radicals [22] which abstract hydrogen from additional fatty-acid side chains resulting in an oxidative stress and in a chain reaction, with production of lipid peroxides. The rate of lipid peroxidation is increased in the presence of iron or copper salts and results in an increased fluidity, increasing permeability and loss of membrane integrity [22]. The ischaemic and reperfused cardiac cell appears to be a prime candidate for such a reaction sequence, which could explain the molecular mechanism underlying pathological events related to membrane dysfunction, such as enzyme release, alteration of mitochondrial function and of calcium homeostasis.

Free radicals may arise from a number of sources, and cellular mechanisms and their production occur under both normal and pathological circumstances. The mitochondria are one of the most important sources of oxygen-free radicals in the myocardium, and their production of $O_2^{\dot{-}}$ and H_2O_2 is enhanced under ischaemia and reperfusion, the electron transport chain being in the reduced state [23, 24].

The xanthine oxidase pathway is also an important site of free radical production, particularly during ischaemia, when cytosolic calcium increases, and ATP is broken down to AMP, which is ultimately metabolized to hypoxanthine. The concomitant elevation of cytosolic calcium concentration enhances the conversion of xanthine dehydrogenase, an enzyme localized in the endothelium of the capillaries of coronary arteries, to xanthine oxidase [25, 26]. According to this concept, when molecular oxygen is reintroduced to cells containing high concentrations of hypoxanthine, this enzyme causes the release of $O_2^{\dot{-}}$ and H_2O_2. Endoperoxide intermediates, resulting from the conversion of arachidonic acid also leads to the production of oxygen-free radicals by leukocytes and other cell types in the heart [27, 28].

Another possible mechanism of free radical generation are the neutrophils. The neutrophils accumulate in the vascular space of reperfused ischaemic myocardium, where they may adhere to the endothelium and release oxygen-free radicals [29]. Although there are multiple stimuli for neutrophil migration, one chemoattractant may arise from the interaction of plasma lipids with oxygen-free radicals derived from the activity of cyclo-oxygenase or xanthine oxidase on their respective substrates. Engler et al. [30] have proposed that capillary plugging by leukocytes contributes to the occurrence of "no reflow" after reperfusion of ischaemic myocardial tissue.

Finally, the auto-oxidation of catecholamines could provide another source of free radicals under ischaemic conditions [31, 32].

Defence Mechanisms Against Oxygen-Free Radicals and Occurrence of Oxidative Stress in Isolated and Perfused Rabbit Hearts

In the heart there are defence mechanisms which are able to protect the cell against the cytotoxic oxygen metabolites. These include the enzymes superoxide dismutase (SOD), catalase and glutathione peroxidase plus other endogenous antioxidants such as vitamin E, ascorbic acid and cysteine [33]. The basic premise for the involvement of oxygen in reperfusion damage is that ischaemia and reperfusion have altered the defence mechanisms against oxygen toxicity.

To investigate the possible role of oxygen in reperfusion injury, we have determined in isolated and perfused rabbit hearts the effects of ischaemia on the activity of mitochondrial and cytosolic SOD – the first line of defence against oxygen toxicity – and of glutathione peroxidase (GPD) and glutathione reductase (GRD) – the second lines of defence against oxygen-free radical

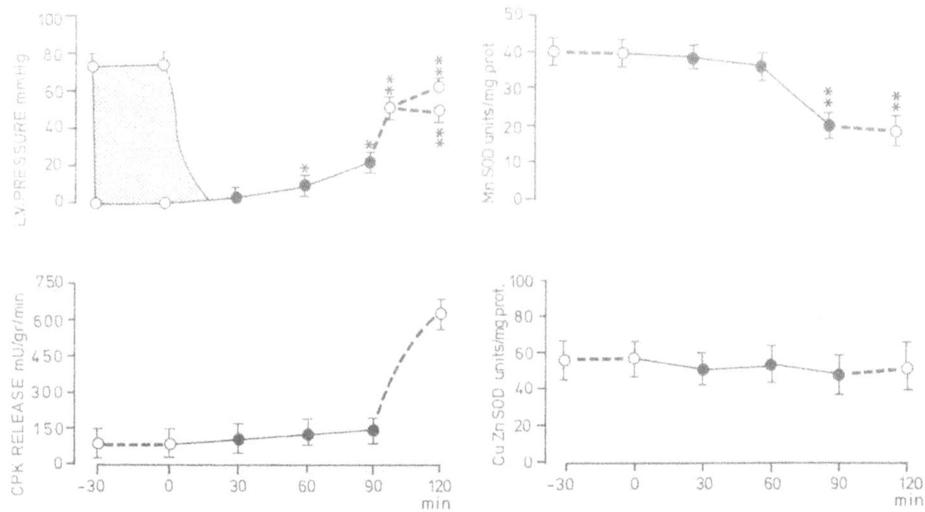

Fig. 1. Effects of ischaemia and reperfusion on mechanical function, creatine phosphokinase (*CPK*) release and superoxide dismutase activity of the isolated and perfused rabbits hearts. Determinations for superoxide dismutase (*SOD*) have been performed in the homogenate as described elsewhere [10]; *Mn*, mitochondrial; *Cu-Zn*, cytosolic. Results are given as mean ± standard error of six experiments. Significance (p) relates to the difference between values obtained after aerobic reperfusion and those obtained after ischaemia and reperfusion

production. The data on SOD are shown in Fig. 1. This enzyme catalyses the following reaction:

$$O_2^{\dot{-}} + O_2^{\dot{-}} + 2\,H^+ \rightarrow H_2O_2 + O_2 .$$

In Fig. 1, together with the changes on SOD the effects of ischaemia and reperfusion on left ventricular pressure and creatine phosphokinase (CPK) release are shown. Reduction of coronary flow to 1 ml/min induced a rapid decline of developed pressure, contractile activity ceasing completely 9 min after the onset of ischaemia. Resting pressure began to rise progressively 20 min after the onset of ischaemia. On reperfusion there was further increase of resting pressure, massive release of CPK and almost no recovery of developed pressure.

Figure 1 also shows that 90 min of ischaemia specifically reduced the activity of mitochondrial SOD, whilst the same period of ischaemia did not affect the activity of cytosolic SOD. Furthermore, re-admission of coronary flow did not significantly modify the SOD activities. Thus, these data suggest that prolonged ischaemia induces a significant and specific alteration of the mitochondrial SOD. This is remarkable when considering that the mitochondria are one of the most important sites of production of oxygen-free radicals in conditions of ischaemia and reperfusion.

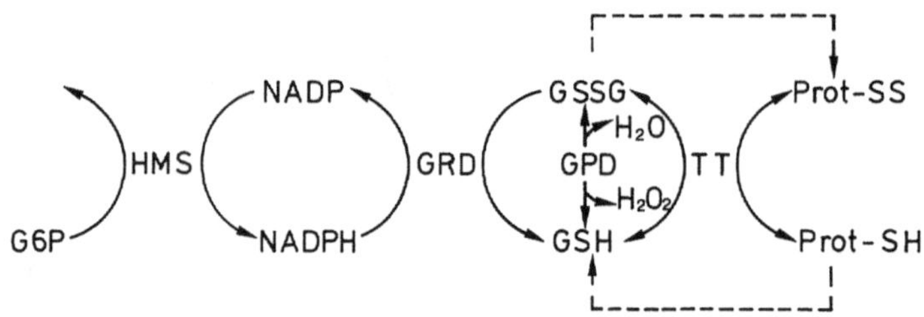

Fig. 2. Schematic representation of the glutathione system in the myocardium. *GRD,* Glutathione reductase; *GPD,* glutathione peroxidase; *HMS*, hexose monophosphate shunt; *TT*, thiol transferase

Therefore, under these conditions the second line of defence against oxygen toxicity, GPD, should be highly stimulated, causing an imbalance of the cellular glutathione status.

The schema illustrated in Fig. 2 represents the glutathione reduction-oxidation cycle in the heart. The hexose monophosphate shunt produces, from glucose-6-phosphate, the reducing equivalents (NADPH) for the action of GRD. Reduced glutathione (GSH) is then utilized by GSH peroxidase, but it is also in dynamic equilibrium with all cellular sulphhydryl groups. In fact, glutathione disulphides mixed with proteins constitutes an important part of total cellular glutathione, and the entire equilibrium is regulated by thiol transferases. Therefore, GSH, as a co-substrate of GPD plays an essential protective role against oxygen-free radicals and prevents peroxidation of membrane lipids. This protective mechanism results in an increased formation of intracellular oxidized glutathione (GSSG). It follows that the changes of glutathione status occurring during ischaemia and reperfusion provide important information regarding the cellular oxidative events, and a tissue accumulation and/or release of GSSG in the coronary effluent is a sensitive and accurate index of oxidative stress.

Figure 3 shows the effects of 90 min of ischaemia followed by 30 min of reperfusion on GPD and GRD activity as well as on GSH/GSSG, tissue content and release of GSH and GSSG of the isolated and perfused rabbit hearts. Reduction of coronary flow did not affect the activity of GPD or GRD. However, Fig. 3 shows that ischaemia induced a reduction in myocardial GSH/GSSG ratio. This was mainly due to a significant reduction of tissue content of GSH, GSSG being unchanged. Reperfusion did not modify GPD or GRD activity but further reduced the tissue content of GSH, which was concomitant with an important increase of tissue GSSG from the ischaemic value of 0.18 ± 0.04 to 0.60 ± 0.07 nmol/mg protein, resulting in a further decline of GSH/GSSG ratio. Figure 3 also shows that on reperfusion there was a sustained release of GSH and GSSG into the coronary effluent. This finding is of importance because during reperfusion there was a massive production and release of GSSG, indicating that the cellular content of this compound was increased at least five-fold [10, 11, 12, 13, 16].

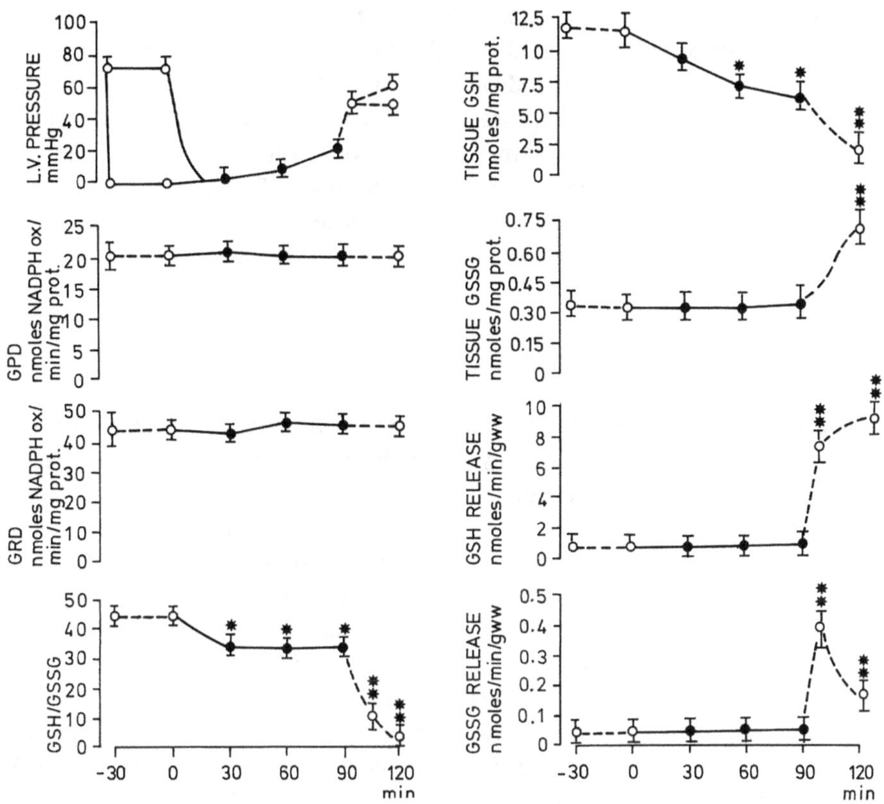

Fig. 3. Effects of ischaemia and reperfusion on glutathione peroxidase (GPD) and reductase (GRD) activity, tissue content and release of GSH and GSSG and on cellular GSH/GSSG. The determinations were performed as described previously [10]. Results are given as mean ± standard error of six experiments. Significance relates to the difference between values obtained after ischaemia and reperfusion and those obtained after aerobic perfusion

These results suggest that ischaemia induces metabolic alterations capable of reducing the defence mechanism against oxygen toxicity. The prime alteration seems to be at the level of mitochondrial SOD, its activity being reduced 50% after severe ischaemia. Under these conditions the re-admission of molecular oxygen is likely to stimulate the production of $O_2^{\dot{-}}$ radicals above the neutralizing capacity of mitochondrial SOD. Consequently, the second line of defence against oxygen toxicity, GPD, is likely to be highly stimulated. We found a severe alteration of the glutathione status, indicating that myocardial oxidative damage had occurred, and that it probably had been counteracted at this level. Therefore, the changes of glutathione status occurring during ischaemia and reperfusion which we found provide important information regarding the cellular oxidative events; the tissue accumulation and release of GSSG in the coronary effluent is a sensitive and accurate index of oxidative stress [10].

It is important to recall here that in animal studies the evidence of an oxidative stress on reperfusion is correlated with the duration of the ischaemic period [15]. Reperfusion after a short period of ischaemia (30 – 60 min) does not result in oxidative stress, probably because the defence mechanisms are still able to protect the myocardial cells against the burst of oxygen-free radicals generated by re-admission of oxygen with coronary flow. Reperfusion after more prolonged period of ischaemia, when the defence mechanisms are likely to be reduced, results in further damage with no recovery in function.

Occurrence of Oxidative Stress

Clinical evidence of the occurrence of oxidative stress in man is still very poor. This is partly due to the inadequacy of reliable indices able to detect in man the occurrence of oxidative damage.

In the present and in other studies [15, 46], we have attempted to resolve this problem by measuring the arterial and coronary sinus difference of GSH and GSSG of coronary artery disease (CAD) patients subjected to different periods of global ischaemia followed by reperfusion during coronary artery by-pass grafting. Because of the high rate of glutathione auto-oxidation and disappearance in the blood, we have determined plasma levels of GSH and GSSG with a method modified by us [46], treating the blood immediately after collection with thiol re-agents, dithionitrobenzoic acid (DTNB) for GSH and NEM for GSSG determination, respectively. In Figs. 4 and 5 are reported the arterial-coronary sinus differences for GSH and GSSG of seven CAD patients subjected to aortic clamping for 30 min (Fig. 4) and 60 min (Fig. 5) followed by 30 min of reperfusion.

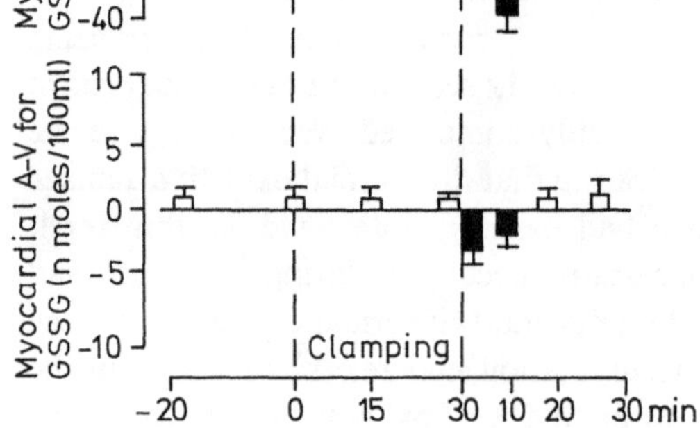

Fig. 4. Arterio-coronary sinus difference for GSH and GSSG during coronary artery by-pass grafting of the left anterior descending coronary artery. Data are means ± standard error of seven cases. Duration of the clamping period, 30 min

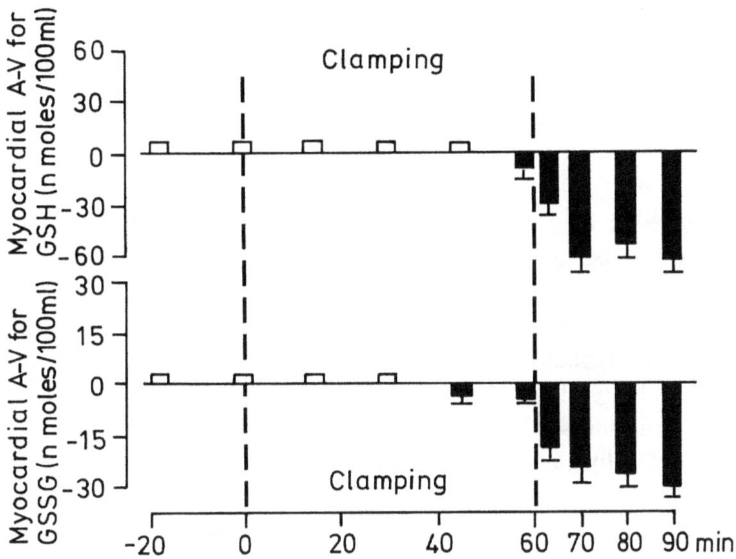

Fig. 5. Arterio-coronary sinus difference for GSH and GSSG during coronary artery bypass grafting of the left anterior descending coronary artery. Data are means ± standard error of seven cases. Duration of the clamping period, 60 min

Before clamping, in all patients there was a small positive arterio-venous (A-V) difference for GSH and GSSG. During the following 30 or 60 min of global ischaemia, the A-V difference for GSH remained constant except in one patient. In this case, 15 min after clamping, the concentration of GSH in the coronary sinus rose above the arterial levels, which did not change. Figures 4 and 5 also demonstrate that during global ischaemia there were no major changes in the A-V difference of GSSG except in two patients showing a small release of GSSG in the coronary sinus, one after 30 and one after 60 min of clamping. During reperfusion after 30 min of clamping there was a transient release of GSH and GSSG into the coronary sinus, reaching a peak 5 min after the onset of reperfusion. During the following 15 min the GSH and the GSSG concentrations in the coronary sinus declined and fell below the arterial values, reflected by the positive myocardial A-V difference (Fig. 4). However, reperfusion after 60 min of clamping resulted in a pronounced and sustained release of GSH and GSSG from the myocardium, and at the end of the procedure the concentration of GSH and GSSG in the coronary sinus greatly exceeded the arterial levels, leading to a negative A-V difference (Fig. 5).

Reperfusion reinstated after 60 min of ischaemia led to an important release of GSH and GSSG which was still continuing at the end of the procedure. This is similar to the effects of reperfusion after prolonged ischaemia in the isolated heart and presumably implies oxidative stress. We suggest that these cases illustrate some aspects of pathophysiology of reperfusion of the human heart. They indicate that reperfusion may induce oxidative damage after a prolonged period of ischaemia and suggest that oxygen-free radicals may be involved in reperfusion damage. These findings are of importance as they constitute the rationale for therapeutic interventions designed to improve the efficacy of myocardial reperfusion.

Importance of Reducing Cytotoxic Oxygen Metabolites in the Protection of the Ischaemic Myocardium

Indirect evidence that cytotoxic oxygen metabolites play an important role in the genesis of myocardial ischaemic and reperfusion damage comes from studies on the possibility of protecting heart muscle from ischaemic and reperfusion injury with substances able to interfere with oxygen metabolism. Depletion of neutrophils by administration of hydrourea [34] or neutrophil antiserum [35] has been found to limit the extent of canine myocardial injury after temporary coronary occlusion. However, the extent to which neutrophil-mediated myocardial damage is due to leukotrienes and lysosomal enzymes, rather than oxygen radicals, remains uncertain [36].

More direct evidence of oxygen radical induced myocardial damage is derived from the observation that treatment with SOD [36, 37] reduces the amount of myocardial damage in occlusion-reperfusion preparations of canine myocardial ischaemic injury. Accordingly, the effect of allopurinol, an inhibitor of xanthine oxidase, has been re-evaluated by several laboratories. Chambers et al. [38] measured infarct size in dogs in which the anterior descending coronary artery was occluded, followed by reperfusion. Animals pretreated with allopurinol 24 h before the induction of regional myocardial ischaemia had significantly smaller infarcts than those not treated. Similar experiments undertaken by Wernes et al. [39] confirmed these results. Reimer and Jennings [40], however, recently reported that allopurinol did not limit infarct size in canine hearts when the extent of tissue injury was quantitated 4 days after 40 min of ischaemia followed by reperfusion. We have demonstrated the efficacy of tocopherol, a typical anti-oxidant, in reducing re-oxygenation and reperfusion damage [13, 41, 42]. Other anti-oxidants shown to be able to reduce reperfusion damage are: tocopherol [42], *N*-2-mercaptopropionyl-glycine [43], dimethylthiourea and catalase [44].

We have investigated the role of *N*-acetyl-cysteine in the protection of the ischaemic and reperfused myocardium. The isolated and reperfused rabbit hearts have been used as experimental models, and the protective effects of *N*-acetyl-cysteine have been determined in terms of mechanical function, whilst the occurrence of oxidative stress has been evaluated by measuring the tissue content of GSH and GSSG. *N*-Acetyl-cysteine is a sulphhydryl group donor which is transported in the cell where it is deacetylated, thus increasing the available thiol pool, including GSH [45]. Figure 5 shows that when *N*-acetyl-cysteine was added to the perfusate 60 min before ischaemia and continued during ischaemia and reperfusion, the rise in diastolic pressure during ischaemia and reperfusion was

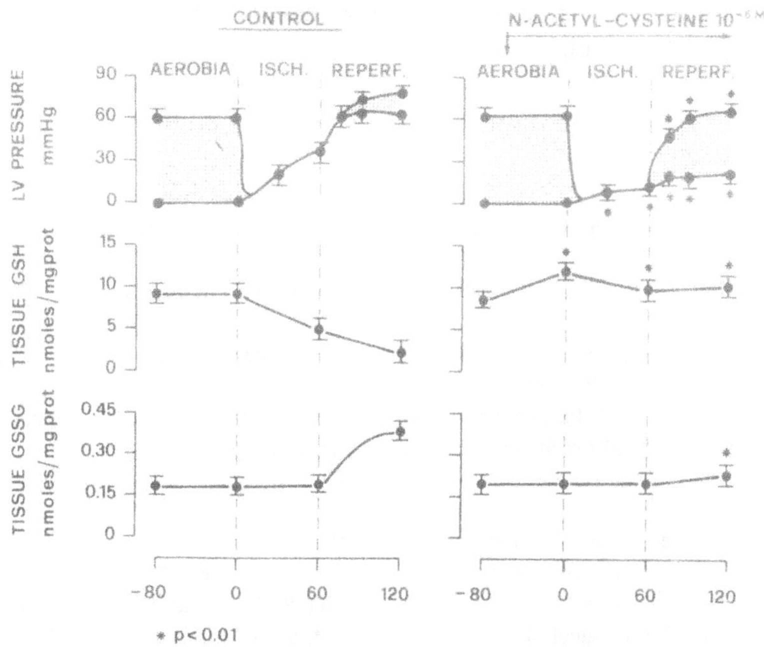

Fig. 6. Effect of *N*-acetyl-cysteine on mechanical function and tissue content of GSH and GSSG in isolated rabbit hearts perfused under ischaemic and reperfused condition. During aerobia and reperfusion the hearts were perfused at a mean coronary flow of 24 ± 0.9 ml/min. Ischaemia was started at time 0 by reducing coronary flow to 1 ml/min. Each point is the mean ± standard error of six experiments. *N*-Acetyl-cysteine was delivered to the hearts 60 min before ischaemia and through the ischaemic and reperfusion period. Significance (p) relates to the difference between control and the respective treated group

less ($p<0.01$) than that of control hearts, and that the percentage of recovery of developed pressure was increased. Figure 6 also shows that *N*-acetyl-cysteine, as expected, significantly increased tissue GSH values before the onset of ischaemia. In addition, at the end of ischaemia, tissue content of GSH in the hearts pretreated with *N*-acetyl-cysteine was significantly higher than that in the control. Pretreatment with *N*-acetyl-cysteine also had important effects on the changes in cellular redox state occurring on reperfusion: there was no further reduction of cellular GSH, and there was no increase of the tissue concentration of GSSG (Fig. 6).

The most likely explanation for this protective effect is that tissue GSH content was increased after aerobic perfusion by *N*-acetyl-cysteine. The ischaemia-induced decrease of GSH was therefore limited by pretreatment with *N*-acetyl-cysteine, and there was no accumulation of GSSG after reperfusion. This was concomitant with a better recovery of mechanical function, suggesting that maintenance of reduced thiol pool might represent an important development in cellular protection. This provides new insights into the physiological relevance of a fundamental regulatory mechanism constituted by oxidation-reduction of cellular thiol-disulphides.

References

1. Bors W, Saran M, Tait D (1984) Oxygen radicals in chemistry and biology. de Gruyter, Berlin
2. Halliwell B, Gutteridge JMC (1985) Free radicals in biology and medicine. Clarendon, Oxford
3. Johnson JE Jr, Walford R, Harman D, Miguel J (1986) Free radicals, aging, and degenerative diseases. Liss, New York
4. Rice-Evans C (1986) Free radicals, cell damage and disease. Richelieu, London
5. Sies H (1985) Oxidative stress. Academic, London
6. Taylor AE, Matalon S, Ward P (1986) Physiology of oxygen radicals. American Physiological Society, Bethesda
7. Halliwell B, Grootveld M (1987) The measurement of free radical reactions in humans: some thoughts for future experimentation. FEBS Lett 213:9 – 14
8. Edes I, Toszegi A, Csanady M, Bozoky B (1986) Myocardial lipid peroxidation in rats after chronic alcohol ingestion and the effects of different antioxidants. Cardiovasc Res 20:542 – 548
9. Dillard CJ, Downey JE, Tappel AL (1984) Effect of antioxidants on lipid peroxidation in iron-loaded rats. Lipids 19:127 – 133
10. Ferrari R, Ceconi C, Curello S, Guarnieri C, Caldarera CM, Albertini A, Visioli O (1985) Oxygen-mediated myocardial damage during ischaemia and reperfusion: role of the cellular defences against oxygen toxicity. J Mol Cell Cardiol 17:937 – 945
11. Ferrari R, Ceconi C, Curello S, Cargnoni A, Albertini A, Visioli O (1986) Oxygen utilization and toxicity at myocardial level. In: Benzi G, Packer L, Siliprandi N (eds) Biochemical aspects of physical exercice. Elsevier, Amsterdam, pp 145 – 156
12. Ferrari R, Ceconi C, Curello S, Cargnoni A, Medici D (1986) Oxygen free radicals and reperfusion injury: the effects of ischaemia and reperfusion on the cellular ability to neutralize oxygen toxicity. J Mol Cell Cardiol 18:67 – 69
13. Ferrari R, Ceconi C, Curello S, Cargoni A, Condorelli C, Raddino R (1985) Role of oxygen in myocardial ischaemic and reperfusion damage: effect of tocopherol. Acta Vitaminol Enzymol 7:61 – 70
14. Ferrari R, Ceconi C, Curello S, Cargnoni A, Albertini A, Visioli O (1987) Myocardial protection against oxygen free radicals. In: Benzi G (ed) Advances in myochemistry. Libbey, pp 263 – 277
15. Curello S, Ceconi C, Medici D, Ferrari R (1986) Oxidative stress during myocardial ischaemia and reperfusion: experimental and clinical evidences. J Appl Cardiol 1:311 – 327
16. Curello S, Ceconi C, Bigoli C, Ferrari R, Albertini A, Guarnieri C (1985) Change in the cardiac glutathione status after ischaemia and reperfusion. Experientia 41:42 – 43
17. Halliwell B, Gutteridge JMC (1985) The importance of free radicals and catalytic metal ions in human diseases. Mol Aspects Med 8:89 – 193
18. Halliwell B, Gutteridge JMC (1984) Lipid peroxidation, oxygen radicals, cell damage, and antioxidant therapy. Lancet I:1396 – 1397

19. Cross CL (1987) Oxygen radicals and human disease. Ann Intern Med 107:526 to 545
20. Freeman BA, Crapo MD (1975) Biology of disease. Free radicals and tissue injury. Lab Invest 47:412 – 426
21. Hochstein P, Jain SK (1981) Association of lipid peroxidase and polymerization of membrane proteins with erythrocyte aging. Fed Proc 40:183 – 188
22. Ferrari R, Cargnoni A, Ceconi C, Curello S, Albertini A, Visioli O (1987) Role of oxygen in the myocardial ischaemic and reperfusion damage: protective effects of vitamin E. In: Hayaishi O, Mino M (eds) Clinical and dietetic aspects of vitamin E. Elsevier, Amsterdam, pp 209 – 226
23. Turner JF, Boveris A (1980) Generation of superoxide anion by NADH dehydrogenase of bovine heart mitochondria. Biochem J 191:421 – 430
24. Ferrari R, Bongrani S, Cucchini F, Di Lisa F, Guarnieri C, Visioli O (1982) Effects of molecular oxygen and calcium on heart metabolism during reperfusion. In: Bertrand ME (ed) Coronary arterial spasm, pp 46 – 59
25. Braunwald E, Kloner RA (1985) Myocardial reperfusion: a double edged sword? J Clin Invest 76:1713 – 1719
26. McCord J (1985) Oxygen-derived free radicals in postischemic tissue injury. N Engl J Med 312:159 – 163
27. Kuehl FA, Humes JL, Torchiana ML (1979) Adv Inflammation Res I:419 – 430
28. Halliwell B, Gutteridge JMC (1984) Oxygen toxicity, oxygen radicals, transition metals and disease. Biochem J 219:1 – 14
29. Korthuis RJ, Granger DN, Townsley MI, Taylor AE (1982) The role of oxygen-derived free radicals in ischemia-induced increases skeletal muscle vascular permeability. Circ Res 57:599 – 611
30. Engler RL, Schmid-Schonbein GW, Pavelec RS (1983) Leukocyte capillary plugging in myocardial ischemia and reperfusion in the dog. Am J Pathol 111:98 – 111
31. Burton KP, McCord MJ, Ghai G (1984) Myocardial alterations due to free-radical generation. Am J Physiol 246:H776 – H783
32. Singal PK, Kapur N, Dhillon KS, Beanish RE, Dhalla NS (1982) Can J Physiol Pharmacol 60:1390 – 1397
33. Ferrari R, Ceconi C, Curello S, Cargnoni A, Agnoletti G, Boffa GM, Visioli O (1986) Intracellular effects of myocardial ischaemia and reperfusion: role of calcium and oxygen. Eur Heart J 7:3 – 12
34. Mullane KM, Read N, Salmon JA, Moncada S (1984) Role of leukocytes in acute myocardial infarction in anesthetized dogs: relationship to myocardial salvage by antiinflammatory drugs. J Pharmacol Exp Ther 228:510 – 515
35. Romson JL, Hook BG, Kunkel SL, Abrams GD, Schork MA, Lucchesi BR (1983) Reduction of the extent of ischemic myocardial injury by neutrophil depletion in the dog. Circulation 67:1016 – 1027
36. Werns SW, Shea MJ, Lucchesi BR (1986) Free radicals and myocardial injury: pharmacologic implication. Circulation 74:1 – 5
37. Werns SW, Shea MJ, Driscoll EM, Cohen C, Abrams GD, Pitt B, Lucchesi BR (1985) The independent effects of oxygen radical scavengers on canine infarct size: reduction by superoxide dismutase but not catalase. Circ Res 56:895 – 912
38. Chambers DE, Parks DA, Patterson G, Roy R, McCord JM, Yoschida S, Parmley LF, Downey JM (1985) Xanthine oxidase as a source of free radical damage in myocardial ischemia. J Mol Cell Cardiol 17:145 – 153

39. Werns SW, Shea MJ, Mitsos JE, Dysko RC, Fantone JC, Schok MA, Abrams GD, Pitt B, Lucchesi BR (1986) Reduction of the size of infarction by allopurinol in the ischemic-reperfused canine heart. Circulation 73:518 – 602
40. Reimer KA, Jennings RB (1985) Failure of the xanthine oxidase inhibitor allopurinol to limit infarct size after ischemia and reperfusion in dogs. Circulation 71:1069 – 1073
41. Ferrari R, Visioli O, Guarnieri C, Caldarera CM (1982) Vitamin E and the heart: possible role as antioxidants. Acta Vitaminol Enzymol 5:11 – 22
42. Guarnieri C, Ferrari R, Visioli O, Caldarera CM, Nayler WG (1978) Effect of tocopherol on hypoxic reperfused and reoxygenated rabbit. J Mol Cell Cardiol 10: 893 – 906
43. Mitsos SE, Askew TE, Fantone JC (1983) Protective effect of N2 mercaptopropionyl glycine against myocardial reperfusion injury after neutrophil depletion in the dog: evidence for the role of intracellular-derived free radicals. Circulation 73:1077 – 1086
44. Zhu WX, Bolli R, Myers ML, Hartley CJ, Roberts R (1985) Dimethyl-thiourea enhances recovery of post ischaemic myocardium (Abstract). Circulation 72 [III]:74
45. Maister A (1985) Methods for selective modification of glutathione metabolism and study of glutathione transport. In: Maister A (ed) Methods in enzymology. Academic, New York, pp 571 – 585
46. Curello S, Ceconi C, Cargnoni A, Cornacchiari A, Ferrari R, Albertini A (1987) Improved procedure for determining glutathione in plasma as an index of myocardial oxidative stress. Clin Chem 33/8:1448 – 1449

Calcium and the Stunned Myocardium*

J. K. Porterfield, H. Kusuoka, and E. Marban

Introduction

Reperfusion after myocardial ischemia of brief duration does not result in myocardial necrosis [24]. Nonetheless, the contractile function and metabolic properties of the previously ischemic tissue may exhibit a prolonged, but reversible, period of derangement after reperfusion [13, 22, 23]. This phenomenon of reversible myocardial contractile dysfunction following sublethal periods of ischemia has been termed myocardial "stunning" [9].

Reversible postischemic dysfunction has been observed clinically. Patients undergoing thrombolytic therapy for acute myocardial infarction demonstrate a delayed improvement in regional function after the restoration of perfusion [27, 44, 48]. Both an immediate and a delayed improvement in regional wall motion have been observed in ischemic segments revascularized surgically [53], presumably due to relief of myocardial ischemia. Chronic depression of ventricular performance due to recurrent ischemia has also been postulated as the mechanism underlying ischemic cardiomyopathy in patients without evidence of frank myocardial infarction [46].

The mechanism of stunning remains unclear. Early studies of regional ischemia demonstrated a close temporal correlation between contractile function and high-energy phosphate levels in reperfused myocardium [13, 14, 25]. This apparent relationship led to the suggestion that the contractile dysfunction of stunned myocardium results directly from inadequate energy stores. The suggestion was bolstered by experimental observations which suggested that the prolonged depression of ATP levels following ischemia and reperfusion may be due to loss of nucleotide precursors during reperfusion [51]. It was postulated that the pool of adenine nucleotide precursors must be replenished by either de novo synthesis or so-called "salvage" pathways. Reimer and his colleagues [42] noted that the time course of repletion of these nucleotide precursors roughly approximated the observed temporal course of functional recovery following reversible myocardial ischemic injury.

* Figures are reproduced from J Clin Invest 79:950–961 (1987) with permission of the American Society for Clinical Investigation.

Nevertheless, the pathogenetic role of ATP depletion has been thrown into doubt by the observation that β-adrenergic stimulation of postischemic stunned myocardium leads to improvement, or even complete reversal of the contractile dysfunction [4, 12, 15]. This apparent moment-to-moment reversibility of stunned myocardium argues against the concept that the decrease in ATP levels represents a critically limiting deficiency of energy stores.

While the ability of stunned myocardium to respond to inotropic stimulation argues indirectly against the concept that low ATP levels play a causative role in contractile dysfunction, other experiments in isolated Langendorff-perfused hearts have directly demonstrated a lack of correlation between functional recovery and intracellular ATP concentration [39, 52]. These studies suggest that the border between reversible and irreversible ischemic injury is not directly related to ATP levels, but to the ability of the hearts rapidly to resynthesize phosphocreatine [52] and to the accumulation of metabolic products of anaerobic glycolysis [39]. Experiments with low-calcium reperfusion or the administration of free radical scavengers [31, 41] have also demonstrated the lack of correlation between ATP levels and the recovery of function.

If the ATP depletion observed in stunned myocardium is not causally related to functional impairment, what other mechanisms could be responsible for post-ischemic dysfunction? The problem may lie in disruption of energy utilization rather than impairment of energy production [18]. The well-documented observation that creatine phosphate levels increase rapidly upon reperfusion following a brief ischemic insult supports this hypothesis since creatine phosphate can only be produced by phosphorylation of creatine by ATP [51, 52]. The concept of disrupted energy utilization in stunned hearts is supported by experimental studies which have found a decrease in the activity of both mitochondrial creatine kinase [5, 6] and myofibrillar creatine kinase [18] after a nonlethal period of ischemia followed by reperfusion. A close functional coupling of myofibrillar creatine kinase and actomyosin ATPase has been demonstrated and is thought to be critical for optimizing ATPase activity. Therefore, a decrease in activity of this creatine kinase could compromise ATP production at the myofibrils and thus alter myocyte function. This mechanistic explanation of myocardial stunning has been challenged, however, by other investigators who correctly point out that the aforementioned functional "reserve" of stunned myocardium, which can be reversed by β-adrenergic stimulation, implies that alterations in creatine kinase activity, either mitochondrial or myofibrillar, are not responsible for the contractile impairment [2].

Recent experimental work suggests that stunning represents a disturbance in excitation-contraction coupling. One recent study demonstrated depression of action potential parameters and reduced excitability in myocardial tissue salvaged after 15 min of ischemia [33], consistent with the hypothesis that myocardial stunning may be due to primary impairment in excitation. Studies focusing on sarcoplasmic reticulum (SR) function have demonstrated a defect in SR calcium transport after a 15-min period of ischemia [20, 21, 29]. This alteration in SR function is characterized by a significant depression and shift of the calcium sensitivity curve of Ca^{2+}-Mg^{2+} ATPase activity with a resultant higher concentration of calcium required to activate the enzyme.

The possible contribution of free radicals to reperfusion injury has attracted considerable attention. While the particular free radical species, as well as its site of generation, remains subject to speculation, several studies have demonstrated a reduction in infarct size by administration of so-called free radical scavengers [54, 55]. Recently, Ambrosio et al. [3] have demonstrated improved contractile recovery following a 30-min period of global normothermic ischemia by administering human recombinant superoxide dismutase at the time of reflow. In view of the demonstrated reduction in reperfusion-induced injury after prolonged ischemia, a number of investigators have recently implicated oxygen-derived free radicals in myocardial stunning. Myers and colleagues were able to demonstrate an improvement in contractile function following 15 min of regional ischemia in the dog by the administration of superoxide dismutase and catalase [37]. This attenuation of stunning has been confirmed by several other groups using a variety of free radical scavengers, and the improved functional recovery has been found not to correlate with improved high-energy phosphate content [8, 11, 41].

We undertook the current study to assess both the pathophysiology and the pathogenesis of myocardial stunning with particular regard to a possible etiologic role for cellular calcium overload. Calcium overload has been recognized as an important component of injury after prolonged episodes of ischemia followed by reperfusion [38], but its role in myocardial stunning had not been previously investigated.

Most studies of stunned myocardium have employed a regional model of ischemia, usually 15 min of coronary occlusion [22] or repetitive 5-min occlusions [40] in the dog, followed by reperfusion. In a regional model, the area of stunning can be observed for functional improvement over an extended time period (days to weeks). In addition, this regional model is presumed to simulate the effects of transient coronary occlusion in humans.

We chose instead to employ the globally ischemic isolated ferret heart perfused via a Langendorff apparatus because of the ability to render the heart homogeneously ischemic while simultaneously monitoring ventricular function and myocardial energy metabolism by phosphorus 31 nuclear magnetic resonance (NMR) spectroscopy [17]. Brief periods of ischemia (<20 min) induced by zero flow have been shown in this model to be associated with a reproducible impairment in contractile function without evidence of necrosis [2]. Ultrastructurally, we observed similar morphologic changes to those seen in regional stunning (primarily, loss of glycogen granules), as well as mild interstitial edema, likely due to prolonged crystalloid perfusion [45].

In the past, it has not been possible to characterize the pathophysiologic basis of stunned myocardium due to a lack of suitable methods in intact heart. A new approach has recently been described in our laboratory which enables the determination of maximal Ca^{2+}-activated force as reflected by isovolumic pressure in the isolated perfused ferret heart, using tetani elicited by rapid pacing after exposure to ryanodine [36]. This technique was previously employed to evaluate the mechanism of early contractile failure during hypoxia [30]. We applied this approach to determine whether myocardial Ca responsiveness and maximal Ca^{2+}-activated force are decreased in stunned myocardium produced by reperfusion after 15 min of global ischemia at 37 °C. Furthermore, we have utilized these measurements to assess the benefits of reperfusion with low-Ca solution and hence the role of cellular Ca overload in the pathogenesis of stunned myocardium.

Methods

The experimental preparation has been described previously [30, 36]. Hearts from young male ferrets (10–14 weeks of age) were rapidly excised following anesthesia with intraperitoneal sodium pentobarbital. After cannulation of the aorta, retrograde perfusion was instituted with standard Tyrode solution at 37 °C. Heart rate was maintained at 3 Hz by right ventricular pacing using a Grass S44 stimulator. A latex balloon tied to the end of a polyethylene tube was passed into the left ventricle through the mitral valve and connected to a Statham P23DB pressure transducer. The balloon was filled with aqueous solution to an end-diastolic pressure of 8–12 mmHg, then kept isovolumic throughout the experiment. Perfusion pressure was monitored at the cannulation point of the aorta. Left ventricular pressure and perfusion pressure were recorded with a direct-writing recorder, and following a 20- to 30-min stabilization period, the coronary flow rate, controlled by a peristaltic pump, was adjusted such that perfusion pressure equalled 90 mmHg. The flow rate was then kept constant throughout the experiment except during the ischemic period.

To induce myocardial stunning, hearts were subjected to 15 min of global ischemia at 37 °C after which they were reperfused until developed pressure (DP) recovered to a new steady state (20–30 min). Pacing was discontinued during ischemia and for the first 20 min of reperfusion, after which it was restored prior to any new experimental measurements.

The perfusate utilized was a bicarbonate- and phosphate-free HEPES-buffered Tyrode solution, which has the advantage that perfusate Ca levels can be varied over a wide range without inducing crystal precipitation. The pH of the solution was adjusted to 7.4, and the perfusate was bubbled continuously with 100% O_2.

The responsiveness of myocardium to Ca was determined by measuring DP during twitch contractions as a function of varying levels of $[Ca]_0$ (0.5, 1, 2, 5, and 7.5 m*M*). Maximal calcium-activated pressure (MCAP) was determined from the DP during tetani as $[Ca]_0$ was increased as previously described [36]. Briefly, hearts were exposed for 10–20 min to 3 μ*M* ryanodine, a plant-derived

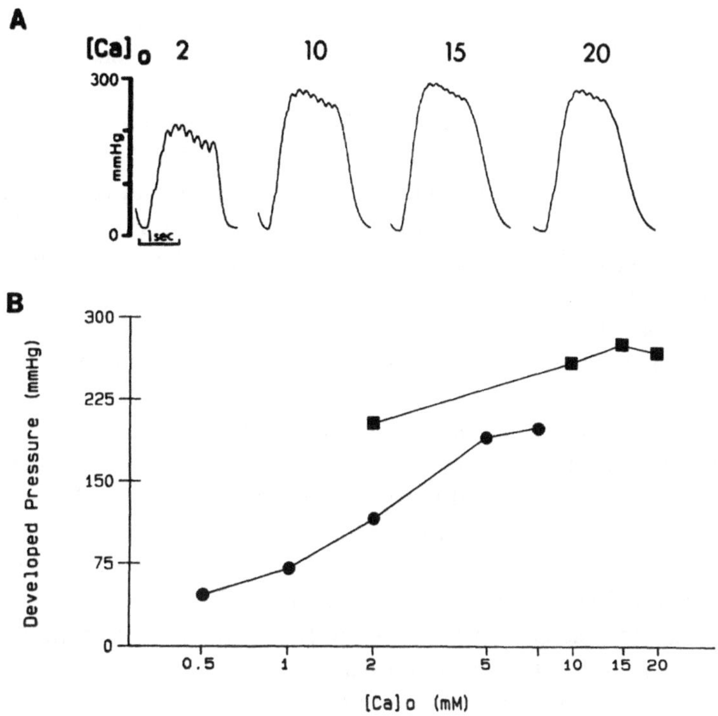

Fig. 1A,B. DP during tetani saturates with respect to $[Ca]_0$, yielding MCAP. **A** Recordings of tetani from typical experiment at 2, 10, 15, and 20 m*M* $[Ca]_0$. **B** DP during twitches (*solid circles*) and during tetani (*solid squares*), plotted as a function of $[Ca]_0$

alkaloid believed to inhibit the release of Ca from the SR [50]. Tetani were then elicited by high-frequency electrical stimulation (10–12 Hz) at two times the capture threshold.

MCAP was determined from the saturation of DP during tetani as $[Ca]_0$ was varied from 2 to 20 m*M*. The greatest value of DP achieved during each tetanus was measured, and saturation was inferred if the values at two or more distinct $[Ca]_0$ agreed within 5%. Figure 1 illustrates such an experiment. Figure 1A shows records of left ventricular pressure during tetani at $[Ca]_0$ from 2 to 20 m*M*. Tetanic pressure increased up to a $[Ca]_0$ of 10 m*M*, beyond which there was no further increase. DP during tetani is plotted in Fig. 1B, along with the DP during twitches measured in the same heart prior to ryanodine exposure. Each point represents the average of three or more consecutive records of DP during twitches or tetani at each $[Ca]_0$.

Ca_0 responsiveness, i.e., the relationship between $[Ca]_0$ and DP during twitches, is determined by both the Ca^{2+} transient and the myofilament properties, and thus alterations in Ca_0 responsiveness cannot be solely attributed to a change in the contractile apparatus unless Ca^{2+} transients remain unchanged. A major advantage of MCAP is that it directly reflects myofilament properties because $[Ca^{2+}]_i$ presumably reaches saturating levels, thus eliminating the potentially confounding effect of altered Ca^{2+} transients.

Phosphorus Nuclear Magnetic Resonance Measurements. The phosphorus 31 NMR methods have been described previously [17, 30]. Briefly, the preparation was lowered into a 25-mm diameter NMR tube and placed into the wide-bore superconducting magnet of a spectrometer (4.2 Tesla, 72.39 MHz for ^{31}P; model WH-180, Bruker Instruments, Inc., Billerica, Massachusetts). ^{31}P NMR spectra were obtained at a spectral width of 3 kHz using 45° pulses delivered at 2-s intervals. In NMR experiments, the balloon in the left ventricle was filled with a 15 m*M* solution of magnesium trimetaphosphate as a standard for quantification of high-energy phosphates.

The amount of inorganic phosphate (Pi), phosphocreatine (PCr), and ATP in the myocardium were obtained by planimetry of the areas under individual peaks using a digitizer (model 9810 A; Hewlett-Packard Co., Palo Alto, California). The tissue contents of Pi, PCr, and ATP in the myocardium were normalized by the peak for magnesium trimetaphosphate standard in the left ventricular balloon. The calculated amounts of Pi, PCr, and ATP were divided by heart weight to yield concentrations ([Pi], [PCr], and [ATP]) in units of micromole per gram wet weight. Intramyocardial pH was estimated from the chemical shift of the Pi peak measured relative to the resonance of PCr [17].

Experimental Design. Experiments were performed in a total of 27 hearts. Of these, 13 were subjected to stunning, 6 were nonischemic controls, and 8 were used to study the effects of reperfusion with low-$[Ca]_0$ solution. The experimental protocol is schematically illustrated in Fig. 2.

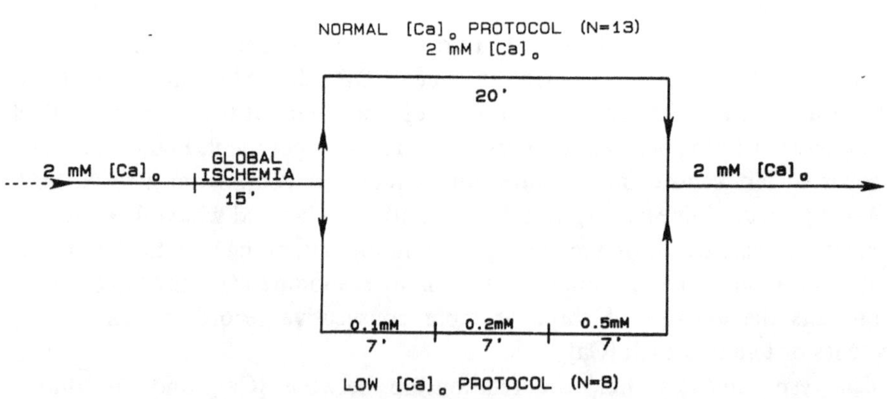

Fig. 2. Schematic illustration of experimental protocol, demonstrating initial control and ischemic periods followed by either standard ($[Ca_0]$ = 2 m*M*) or low-$[Ca]_0$ reperfusion. After reperfusion and a period of stabilization, functional recovery was assessed by measuring Ca_0 responsiveness and maximal Ca^{2+}-activated pressure (MCAP)

The design of the experiments in stunned myocardium is discussed first. During an initial control phase, i.e., prior to ischemia, Ca_0 responsiveness was measured. The heart was then subjected to 15 min of global ischemia. After 20 min of reperfusion with the standard solution ($[Ca_0] = 2$ m*M*), Ca_0 responsiveness was once again measured, this time in stunned myocardium. After the second assessment of Ca_0 responsiveness, ryanodine was added to the perfusate and MCAP was measured. In 5 of 13 hearts devoted to this protocol, myocardial high-energy phosphate compounds and pH were measured simultaneously with ^{31}P NMR.

In the nonischemic control group, the goal was to account for any time-dependent deterioration of function that might occur even in the absence of ischemia and reperfusion. After an initial control phase identical to that in the stunned group, hearts were perfused with the standard perfusate ($[Ca]_0 = 2$ m*M*) for 35 min (equivalent to the 15 min of global ischemia and 20 min of reperfusion in the stunned hearts). Ca_0 responsiveness was then determined for a second time, followed by measurements of MCAP after exposure to ryanodine.

In the third protocol, the initial control and ischemic periods were identical to those described for stunned hearts. The only difference was in the $[Ca]_0$ of the reperfusion solution. Hearts were reperfused stepwise with low-$[Ca]_0$ solutions, first 0.1 m*M* $[Ca]_0$, then 0.2 and 0.5 m*M* $[Ca]_0$, and finally with 2 m*M* $[Ca]_0$ solution, each for 7-min periods. After equilibration in 2 m*M* $[Ca]_0$ reperfusate, Ca_0 responsiveness was evaluated and tetanic pressure was measured as in the other two protocols. In three of eight hearts devoted to this protocol, metabolic changes in the myocardium were measured simultaneously using ^{31}P NMR.

Statistical Analysis. Data are presented as mean ± SEM. Statistical analysis was performed with paired or nonpaired *t* tests and the analysis of variance, including multivariate analysis of variance to compare Ca_0 responsiveness in the different experimental groups. Data from the initial control phase of all hearts ($n = 27$) was pooled to yield control data for statistical tests.

Results

Effect of Stunning on Ca_0 Responsiveness and MCAP. There was no time-dependent decrease in ventricular function in the nonischemic control hearts, confirming the stability of this preparation during the experimental period (Fig. 3A). In contrast, DP was decreased at all $[Ca]_0$ after ischemia and reperfusion (center panel, Fig. 3B). The right-hand panels show records of tetani at saturating levels of $[Ca]_0$ (MCAP) in control (Fig. 3A) and in stunned (Fig. 3B) hearts, demonstrating the depression of MCAP in stunned hearts when compared with the nonischemic control group.

Pooled data from control and stunned hearts for Ca_0 responsiveness and MCAP are shown in Fig. 4A and 4B, respectively. The force of contraction of

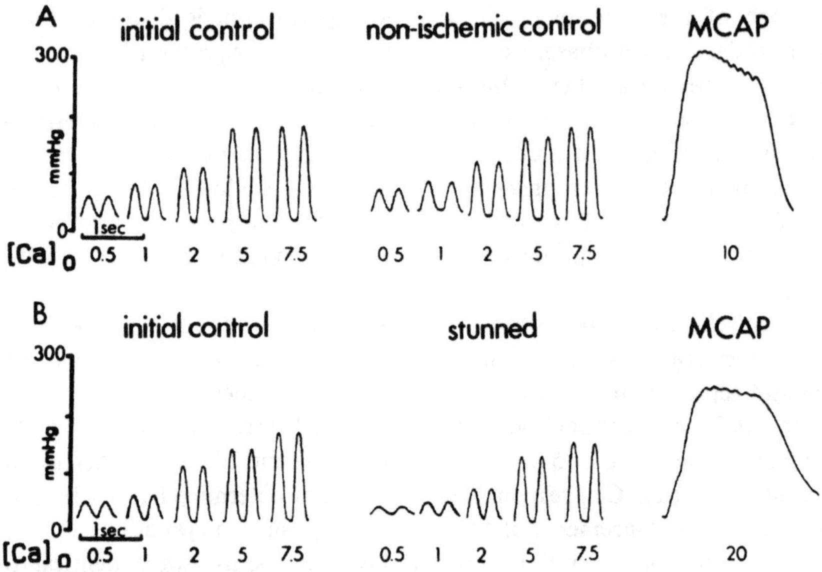

Fig. 3A,B. Ca_0 responsiveness and maximal Ca^{2+}-activated pressure (*MCAP*) in a nonischemic control and a stunned heart. Pressure recordings at various $[Ca]_0$ are shown during the initial control phase (equivalent in both groups), after a 35-min nonischemic period (**A**, nonischemic control), or after stunning (i.e., 20-min reperfusion after 15 min of global ischemia; **B**, stunned). The *right panels* show tetani at saturating $[Ca]_0$ (MCAP)

the twitch was significantly depressed at all $[Ca]_0$ after stunning ($p<0.001$). Likewise, tetanic pressure was depressed at all $[Ca]_0$ in the stunned hearts compared with the nonischemic control groups ($p<0.001$). The saturating pressure (i.e., MCAP) was different in the two groups: in stunned hearts, MCAP was significantly decreased compared with that in nonischemic controls (216 ± 10.2 mmHg versus 270 ± 15.3 mmHg, $p<0.05$).

Myocardial Metabolites as Potential Causes of a Change in Ca_0 Responsiveness. While it is well-known that both acidosis and increased levels of Pi can depress contractile function in skinned papillary muscles [16, 26], previous studies in regional models of stunned myocardium have shown that both [Pi] and pH_i rapidly return to normal levels. We reexamined this question in our preparation using ^{31}P NMR. Figure 5 shows typical ^{31}P NMR spectra obtained during the initial control phase (Fig. 5A), global ischemia (Fig. 5B), and after reperfusion (Fig. 5C) in the stunning protocol. During global ischemia, [Pi] increased markedly (from 1.33 µmol/g wet weight at control to 8.50 µmol/g wet weight), concomitant with the development of intracellular acidosis (from pH 7.06 to 6.26). [PCr] decreased from 7.33 µmol/g wet weight to an undetectably low level, and [ATP] decreased from 2.71 to 1.71 µmol/g wet weight. With reperfusion, [Pi], [PCr], and pH all quickly returned to control levels, but [ATP]

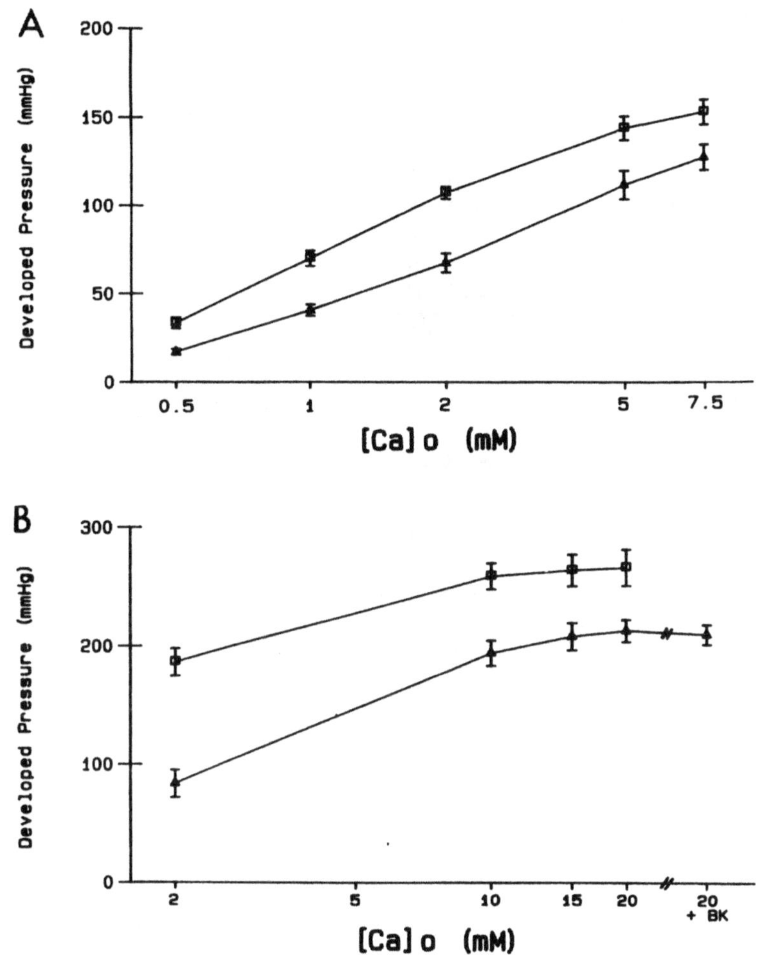

Fig. 4A,B. Characterization of altered contractility in stunned myocardium. **A** Ca_0 responsiveness during initial control period (*solid squares*) pooled from all experiments ($n = 27$) and after stunning (*solid triangles*) in 13 hearts. **B** DP during tetani measured in 6 nonischemic control hearts (*solid squares*) and in 13 stunned hearts (*solid triangles*). Note that saturation of tetanic pressure in stunned hearts was confirmed by adding Bay K 8644 (300 n*M*), a Ca-channel agonist, to 20 m*M* $[Ca]_0$ perfusate

remained depressed. Similar findings were obtained in all five stunned hearts examined with ^{31}P NMR. The persistent decline in ATP levels was consistent with the hypothesis that depletion of high-energy phosphates is causally related to the contractile depression in stunned myocardium, although other observations discussed below lead us to question this association.

Effects of Reperfusion with Low $[Ca]_0$ Solution on Stunning. Cellular Ca overload is known to be an important component of irreversible myocardial

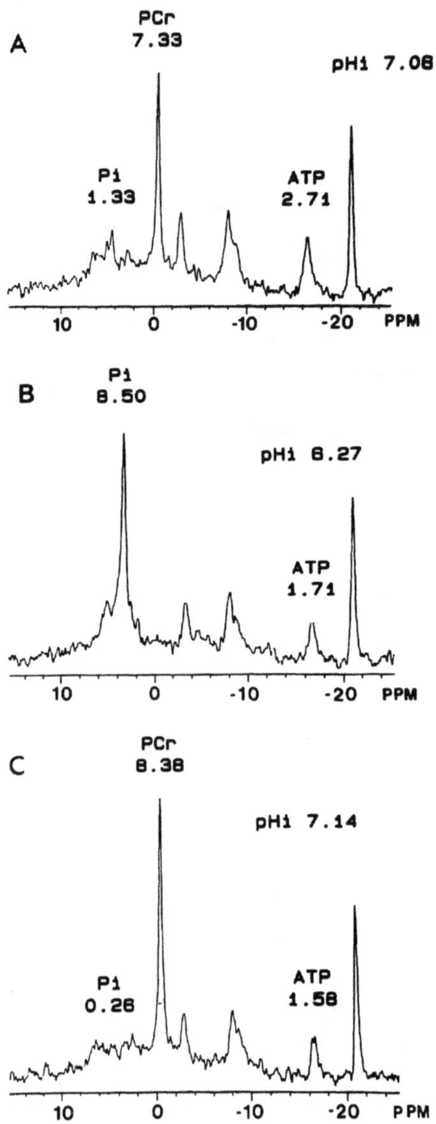

Fig. 5A – C. Phosphorus NMR spectra measured in stunning protocol (acquisition time of 5 min). **A** During initial control period. **B** During 10 – 15 min of global ischemia. **C** During 10 – 15 min of reperfusion. Note that PCr is undetectable during ischemic period

reperfusion injury [45]. Histologically, such injury is characterized by contraction band necrosis, mitochondrial calcium phosphate deposition, and the disruption of the intercalated disks by hypercontraction. Cellular Ca overload occurs if Ca influx pathways that are inhibited during ischemia are suddenly reactivated upon reperfusion. One specific hypothesis involves Na-Ca exchange [19, 43]. This pathway normally extrudes Ca from the cell at the expense of the transsarcolemmal Na gradient. During ischemia, inhibition of the Na-K ATPase results in accumulation of intracellular Na, while, simultaneously, Na-Ca exchange is inhibited by the intracellular acidosis. With reperfusion intracellular pH rapidly normalizes, reestablishing Na-Ca exchange. Because intracellular [Na] is still elevated, the Na gradient drives Ca into the cells. The resultant increase in $[Ca]_i$ can have a deleterious effect on cardiac performance both directly and indirectly, through activation of phospholipases or stimulation of free radical production. We hypothesized that stunning may share the same basic mechanism as irreversible reperfusion injury, with the major difference being one of degree of injury.

To test the hypothesis that stunning involves overload of intracellular Ca, we subjected hearts to the same ischemic protocol, but reperfused them with solutions containing lower $[Ca]_0$. If Ca influx occurring upon reperfusion causes stunning, then reduction of $[Ca]_0$ in the reperfusate will decrease stunning by decreasing the driving force for Ca influx. A prior study, employing a longer ischemic period, had shown a reduction in irreversible reperfusion injury with a similar experimental strategy [47].

Functional recovery, as assessed by measurement of Ca_0 responsiveness and MCAP, was significantly improved in hearts reperfused with low $[Ca]_0$ solution. Recovery of twitch responsiveness was significantly higher than in routinely stunned hearts ($p<0.05$) and statistically indistinguishable from nonischemic controls ($p>0.05$). Similarly, MCAP (257 ± 4.3 mmHg) was statistically indistinguishable from nonischemic controls ($p>0.05$) but significantly higher than in stunned hearts ($p<0.05$). While low-$[Ca]_0$ reperfused hearts did show mild evidence of stunning, i.e., end-diastolic pressure was significantly increased, the excellent preservation of Ca_0 responsiveness and MCAP shows that recovery of function is virtually complete after low-$[Ca]_0$ reperfusion. These experiments, documenting a protective effect of low-$[Ca]_0$ reperfusion, suggest a major pathogenetic role for cellular Ca overload in the stunning process.

Role of ATP Depletion in the Contractile Dysfunction of Stunned Myocardium. As previously mentioned, prolonged depletion of ATP was the only sustained metabolic abnormality in stunned myocardium. Does the beneficial effect of reperfusion with low $[Ca]_0$ result from a reduction of ATP depletion under these conditions? While pretreatment with Ca-channel blockers has been associated with improved functional recovery attributed to improved ATP levels [38], others have found the lower level of ATP in stunned myocardium to be an epiphenomenon rather than a causal factor in the stunning process [39]. In the low-Ca_0 reperfused hearts in which we measured intramyocardial metabolites with ^{31}P NMR, we found no statistical difference in [ATP] compared with hearts reperfused with standard solution. The absence of a unique correlation between [ATP] and MCAP is apparent in Fig. 6. Control hearts exhibit high [ATP] (2.81 ± 0.11 μmol wet weight) and high MCAP (270 ± 15.3 mmHg). Stunned myocardium shows low [ATP] (1.47 ± 0.15 μmol wet weight) and low MCAP (216 ± 10.2 mmHg). By themselves, these two observations are consistent with a cause-and-effect relationship between [ATP] and contractile function. However, the finding that low-$[Ca]_0$ reperfused hearts show reduced [ATP]

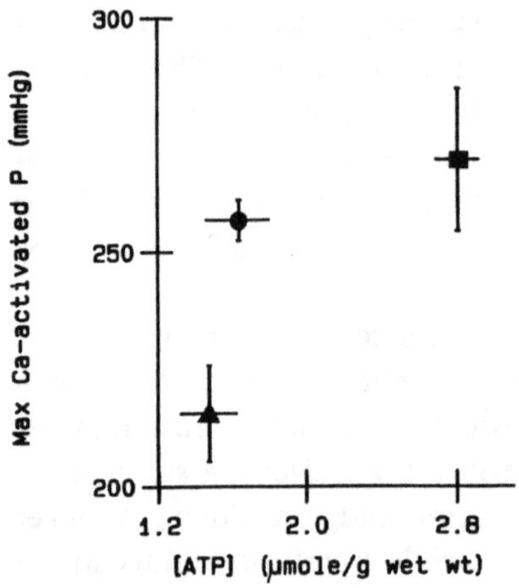

Fig. 6. Relationship between myocardial [ATP] and MCAP. Each point represents the mean ± SEM of [ATP] and MCAP in the initial control phase (*solid square*), after stunning (*solid triangle*), or following low-$[Ca]_0$ reperfusion (*solid circle*). The lack of correlation between [ATP] and MCAP is apparent

(1.63 ± 0.17 μmol wet weight), but near-baseline MCAP (257 ± 4.3 mmHg) suggests that there is no unique relationship between [ATP] and contractile function. Therefore, it is our belief that ATP depletion is not the cause of myocardial stunning.

Discussion

Pathophysiologic Basis of Stunned Myocardium. The abnormal contractile function of stunned myocardium is characterized by two distinctive features: (a) a decrease in MCAP and (b) diminished Ca_0 responsiveness. Figure 7 illustrates the potential pathophysiologic mechanisms involved in stunned myocardium based on our findings. Figure 7A depicts the relationship between intracellular calcium concentration ($[Ca^{2+}]_i$), as represented by a schematic aequorin signal, and twitch force in a normal heart. This relationship is defined by a sigmoid curve (illustrated above the arrow) as it might appear in this normal tissue. Figure 7B–D represents three ways, not mutually exclusive, in which the twitch can become depressed: (a) decrease in the amplitude of the Ca^{2+} transient (Fig. 7B) results in decreased force, even if the Ca^{2+}-force relation is unchanged. If however, myofilament Ca^{2+} sensitivity is decreased (as shown by the "shift-to-the-right" in the $[Ca^{2+}]_i$-force relation) without alteration in the Ca^{2+} transient (Fig. 7C), then at any given submaximal $[Ca^{2+}]$, less force is generated, although maximal force will remain the same. The third potential pathophysiologic mechanism is illustrated in Fig. 7D. Here, maximal force has been scaled down without alteration of the $[Ca^{2+}]_i$-force relation. Any one of these potential mechanisms, or perhaps a combination of two or more, could account for the diminished twitch force in stunned hearts.

Our experimental results can be usefully interpreted within this conceptual framework. Firstly, our finding that MCAP is depressed in stunned hearts

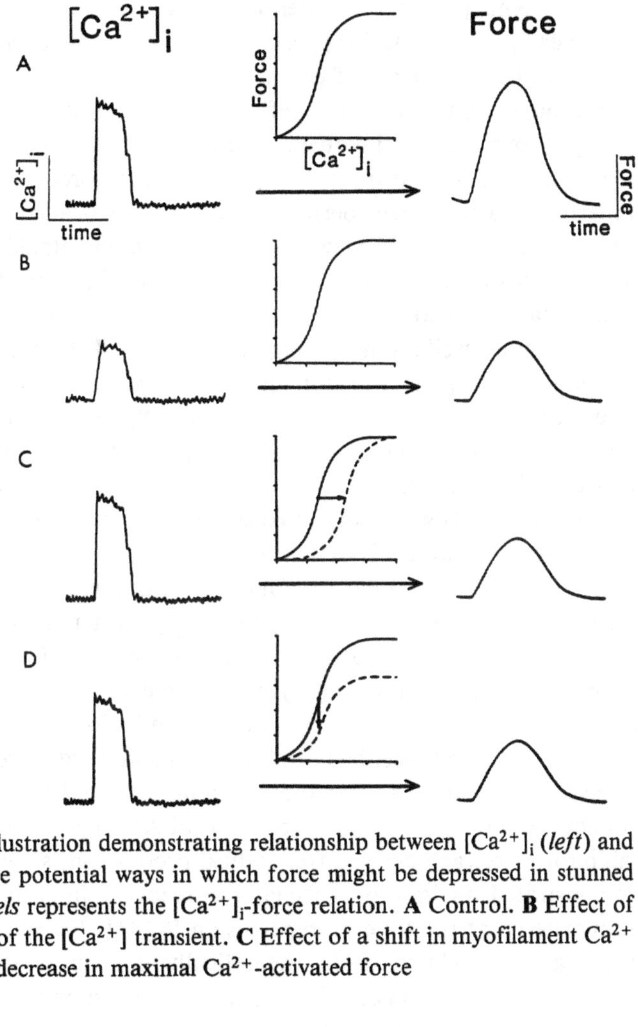

Fig. 7 A – D. Schematic illustration demonstrating relationship between $[Ca^{2+}]_i$ (*left*) and force (*right*) and the three potential ways in which force might be depressed in stunned myocardium. *Center panels* represents the $[Ca^{2+}]_i$-force relation. **A** Control. **B** Effect of decreasing the amplitude of the $[Ca^{2+}]$ transient. **C** Effect of a shift in myofilament Ca^{2+} sensitivity. **D** Effect of a decrease in maximal Ca^{2+}-activated force

demonstrates unequivocally that the hypothesis in Fig. 7D contributes to the contractile dysfunction. Our finding that Ca_0 responsiveness is decreased in stunned hearts could theoretically be due to an alteration in the Ca^{2+} transient, a shift in myofilament Ca^{2+} sensitivity, or a combination of these effects, as both potential mechanisms are subsumed within our measured Ca_0 responsiveness. Explicit determination of whether the primary change is in the Ca^{2+} transient or in myofilament Ca^{2+} sensitivity awaits reliable measurement of $[Ca^{2+}]_i$ in intact hearts [35].

Cellular Mechanism of Stunning. We have found that functional recovery following a brief period of ischemia is markedly improved by reperfusion with low-$[Ca]_0$ solutions. The fact that this intervention requires no pretreatment, which might potentially ameliorate the ischemic insult, makes this result particularly striking and suggests that the major determinant of stunning is not ischemia, but rather reperfusion.

Although the functional benefit observed with low-$[Ca]_0$ reperfusion suggests that Ca overload is involved in the pathogenesis of stunning, the precise mechanism of cellular injury is unclear. Calcium-related damage occurring with reperfusion after longer periods of ischemia, so-called "reperfusion injury," is easier to understand in view of the extensive histologic and metabolic damage [45]. The histologic changes observed in stunned myocardium are mild, however, and metabolic recovery is almost complete. Ca overload is characterized by asynchronous oscillations of intracellular $[Ca^{2+}]$ throughout cells [49, 56]. Such oscillations of $[Ca^{2+}]_i$ result in inhomogeneous contractile activation and attenuation of overall force production [28]. Nonetheless, it appears unlikely that $[Ca^{2+}]_i$ oscillations alone can be responsible for diminished force generation in stunned myocardium in view of the observation that Ca-overloaded myocardium responds with a paradoxical negative inotropic effect as $[Ca]_0$ is increased, whereas in stunned hearts, force increases as $[Ca]_0$ is increased [1].

It is possible that an increase in $[Ca^{2+}]_i$, occurring at the time of reperfusion, may indirectly lead to stunning by acting as a trigger for other intracellular events, such as the activation of phospholipases and/or the generation of free radicals. Several studies, employing different strategies, suggest that free radicals may play a role in stunning. A recent study from our institution, employing electron spin resonance, has demonstrated a marked increase in myocardial free-radical concentrations after only 10 min of global ischemia [57]. In addition, studies employing an oxygen-free radical scavenger, dimethylthiourea, and an inhibitor of oxygen-derived free radical production, superoxide dismutase, have demonstrated an improved functional recovery in stunned myocardium when administered at the time of reperfusion [8, 41]. Free-radical and phospholipid degradation products could theoretically contribute to myocardial stunning through their effect on cellular membranes including the sarcoplasmic reticulum [20, 21]. In this regard, one of the few electron-microscopic hallmarks of stunned myocardium is a moth-eaten appearance felt to represent edema of the SR [27].

Although the precise cellular mechanism underlying stunned myocardium remains to be elucidated, it is clear from our study that reperfusion-induced cellular calcium overload, either through direct or indirect actions, is a major contributing factor in the stunning process.

References

1. Allen DG, Eisner DA, Pirolo JS, Smith GL (1985) The relationship between intracellular calcium and contractions in calcium-overloaded ferret papillary muscle. J Physiol (Lond) 364:169–182

2. Ambrosio G, Jacobus WE, Bergman CA, Weisman HF, Becker LC (1987) Preserved high energy phosphate metabolic reserve in globally stunned hearts despite reduction of basal ATP content and contractility. J Mol Cell Cardiol 19:953–964
3. Ambrosio G, Weisfeldt ML, Jacobus WE, Flaherty JT (1987) Evidence for a reversible oxygen radical-mediated component of reperfusion injury: reduction by recombinant human superoxide dismutase administered at the time of reflow. Circulation 75: 282–291
4. Becker LC, Levine JH, DiPaula AF, Guarnieri T, Aversano TA (1986) Reversal of dysfunction in postischemic stunned myocardium by epinephrine and post-extrasystolic potentiation. J Am Coll Cardiol 7:580–589
5. Bittl JA, Ingwall JS (1985) Reaction rates of creatine kinase and ATP synthesis in the isolated rat heart. J Biol Chem 260:3512–3517
6. Bittl JA, Weisfeldt ML, Jacobus WE (1985) Creatine kinase of heart mitochondria. J Biol Chem 260:208–214
7. Bolli R, Zhu W, Myers ML, Hartley CJ, Roberts R (1985) Beta-adrenergic stimulation reverses postischemic myocardial dysfunction without producing functional deterioration. Am J Cardiol 56:964–968
8. Bolli R, Zhu W, Hartley CJ, Michael LH, Repine JE, Hess ML, Kukreja RC, Roberts R (1987) Attenuation of dysfunction in the postischemic "stunned" myocardium by dimethylthiourea. Circulation 76:458–468
9. Braunwald E, Kloner RA (1982) The stunned myocardium: prolonged, postischemic ventricular dysfunction. Circulation 66:1146–1149
10. Bush LR, Buja LM, Samowitz W, Rude RE, Wathen M, Tilton SD, Willerson JT (1983) Recovery of left ventricular segmental function after long-term reperfusion following temporary occlusion in conscious dogs. Circ Res 53:248–263
11. Charlat ML, O'Neill PG, Egan JM, Abernathy DR, Michael LH, Myers ML, Roberts R, Bolli R (1987) Evidence for a pathogenetic role of xanthine oxidase in the "stunned" myocardium. Am J Physiol 252:H566–H577
12. Ciuffo AA, Ouyang P, Becker LC, Levin L, Weisfeldt ML (1985) Reduction of sympathetic inotropic response after ischemia in dogs. J Clin Invest 75:1504–1509
13. DeBoer LMV, Ingwall JS, Kloner RA, Braunwald E (1980) Prolonged derangements of canine myocardial purine metabolism after a brief coronary artery occlusion not associated with anatomic evidence of necrosis. Proc Natl Acad Sci USA 77:5471–5475
14. Ellis SG, Henschke CI, Sandor T, Wynne J, Braunwald E, Kloner RA (1983) Time course of functional and biochemical recovery of myocardium salvaged by reperfusion. J Am Coll Cardiol 1:1047–1055
15. Ellis SG, Wynne J, Braunwald E, Henschke CI, Sandor T, Kloner RA (1984) Response of reperfusion-salvaged, stunned myocardium to inotropic stimulation. Am Heart J 107:13–19
16. Fabiato A, Fabiato F (1978) Effects of pH on the myofilaments and the sarcoplasmic reticulum of skinned cells from cardiac and skeletal muscles. J Physiol (Lond) 276:233–255
17. Flaherty JT, Weisfeldt ML, Bulkley BH, Gardner TJ, Gott VL, Jacobus WE (1982) Mechanism of ischemic myocardial cell damage assessed by phosphorus-31 nuclear magnetic resonance. Circulation 65:561–571
18. Greenfield RA, Swain JL (1987) Disruption of myofibrillar energy use: dual mechanisms that may contribute to post-ischemic dysfunction in stunned myocardium. Circ Res 60:283–289

19. Grinwald PM (1982) Calcium uptake during post-ischemic reperfusion in the isolated rat heart: influence of extracellular sodium. J Mol Cell Cardiol 14:354–365
20. Hess ML, Okabe E, Kantos HA (1981) Proton and free radical interaction with the calcium transport system of cardiac sarcoplasmic reticulum. J Mol Cell Cardiol 13:767–772
21. Hess ML, Manson NH (1984) Molecular oxygen: friend and foe. The role of the oxygen free radical system in the calcium paradox, the oxygen paradox and ischemia/reperfusion injury. J Mol Cell Cardiol 16:969–985
22. Heyndrickx GR, Millard RW, McRitchie RJ, Maroko PR, Vatner SF (1975) Regional myocardial function and electrophysiological alterations after brief coronary artery occlusion in conscious dogs. J Clin Invest 56:978–985
23. Heyndrickx GR, Baig H, Nellens P, Leusen I, Fishbein MC, Vatner SF (1978) Depression of regional blood flow and wall thickening after brief coronary occlusion. Am J Physiol 234:H653–H659
24. Jennings RB (1968) Early phase of myocardial ischemic injury and infarction. Am J Cardiol 24:753–765
25. Jennings RB, Hawkins HK, Lowe JE, Hill ML, Klotman S, Reimer KA (1978) Relation between high energy phosphate and lethal injury in myocardial ischemia in the dog. Am J Pathol 92:187–207
26. Kentish JC (1986) The effects of inorganic phosphate and creatine phosphate on force production in skinned muscles from rat ventricle. J Physiol (Lond) 370:585–604
27. Kloner RA, Ellis SG, Carlson NV, Braunwald E (1983) Coronary reperfusion for the treatment of acute myocardial infarction: postischemic ventricular dysfunction. Cardiology 70:233–246
28. Kort AA, Lakatta EG, Marban E, Stern MD, Weir WG (1985) Fluctuations in intracellular calcium concentration and their effect on tonic tension in canine cardiac Purkinje fibers. J Physiol (Lond) 367:291–308
29. Krause S, Hess ML (1984) Characterization of cardiac sarcoplasmic reticulum dysfunction during short-term, normothermic, global ischemia. Circ Res 55:176–184
30. Kusuoka H, Weisfeldt ML, Zweier JL, Jacobus WE, Marban E (1986) Mechanism of early contractile failure during hypoxia in intact ferret heart: evidence for modulation of maximal Ca^{2+}-activated force by inorganic phosphate. Circ Res 59:270–282
31. Kusuoka H, Porterfield JK, Weisman HF, Weisfeldt ML, Marban E (1987) Pathophysiology and pathogenesis of stunned myocardium. J Clin Invest 79:950–961
32. Lavallee M, Cox D, Patrick TA, Vatner SF (1983) Salvage of myocardial function by coronary artery reperfusion 1, 2, and 3 hours after occlusion in conscious dogs. Circ Res 53:235–247
33. Levine JH, Moore EN, Weisman HF, Kadish AH, Becker LC, Spear JF (1987) Depression of action potential characteristics and a decreased space constant are present in postischemic, reperfused myocardium. J Clin Invest 79:107–116
34. McCord JM (1985) Oxygen-derived free radicals in postischemic tissue injury. N Engl J Med 312:159–163
35. Marban E, Kitakaze M, Kusuoka H, Porterfield J, Yue DT, Chacko VP (1987) Intracellular free calcium concentration measured with ^{19}F NMR spectroscopy in intact ferret hearts. Proc Natl Acad Sci USA 84:6005–6009
36. Marban E, Kusuoka H, Yue DT, Weisfeldt ML, Weir WS (1986) Maximal Ca^{2+}-activated force elicited by tetanization of ferret papillary muscle and whole heart. Mechanism and characteristics of steady contractile activation in intact myocardium. Circ Res 59:262–269

37. Myers ML, Bolli R, Lekich R, Hartley CJ, Roberts R (1985) Enhancement of recovery of myocardial function by oxygen free-radical scavengers after reversible regional ischemia. Circulation 72:915–921
38. Nayler WG (1983) Calcium and cell death. Eur Heart J 4 [Suppl C]:33–41
39. Neely JR, Grotyohann LW (1984) Role of glycolytic products in damage to ischemic myocardium. Circ Res 55:816–824
40. Nicklas JM, Becker LC, Bulkley BH (1985) Effects of repeated brief coronary occlusion on regional left ventricular function and dimension in dogs. Am J Cardiol 56: 473–478
41. Przyklenk K, Kloner RA (1986) Superoxide dismutase plus catalase improve contractile function in the canine model of the "stunned myocardium". Circ Res 58:148–156
42. Reimer KA, Hill ML, Jennings RB (1981) Prolonged depletion of ATP and of the adenine nucleotide pool due to delayed resynthesis of adenine nucleotides following reversible myocardial ischemic injury in dogs. J Mol Cell Cardiol 13:229–234
43. Renlund DG, Gerstenblith G, Lakatta EG, Jacobus WE, Kallman CH, Weisfeldt ML (1984) Perfusate sodium during ischemia modifies post-ischemic functional and metabolic recovery in the rabbit heart. J Mol Cell Cardiol 16:795–801
44. Satler LF, Kent KM, Fox LM, Goldstein HA, Green CE, Rogers WJ, Pollas RS, Del Negro AA, Pearle DL, Rackley CE (1986) The assessment of contractile reserve after thrombolytic therapy for acute myocardial infarction. Am Heart J 111:821–825
45. Schaper J, Mulch J, Winkler B, Schaper W (1979) Ultrastructural, functional, and biochemical criteria for estimation of reversibility of ischemic injury: a study on the effects of global ischemia on the isolated dog heart. J Mol Cell Cardiol 11:521–541
46. Schuster EH, Bulkley BH (1980) Ischemic cardiomyopathy: a clinico-pathologic study of fourteen patients. Am Heart J 100:506–512
47. Shine KI, Douglas AM (1983) Low calcium reperfusion of ischemic myocardium. J Mol Cell Cardiol 15:251–260
48. Stack RS, Phillips HR III, Grierson DS, Bahar VS, Kong Y, Peter RH, Swain JL, Greenfield JC Jr (1983) Functional improvement of jeopardized myocardium following intracoronary streptokinase infusion in acute myocardial infarction. J Clin Invest 72:84–95
49. Stern MD, Kort AA, Bhatnagar GM, Lakatta EG (1983) Scattered-light intensity fluctuations in diastolic rat cardiac muscle caused by spontaneous Ca^{2+}-dependent cellular mechanical oscillations. J Gen Physiol 82:119–153
50. Sutko JL, Kenyon JL (1983) Ryanodine modification of cardiac muscle responses to potassium-free solutions: evidence for inhibition of sarcoplasmic reticulum calcium release. J Gen Physiol 82:385–404
51. Swain JL, Sabina RL, McHale PA, Greenfield JC Jr, Holmes EW (1982) Prolonged myocardial nucleotide depletion after brief ischemia in the open-chest dog. Am J Physiol 242:H818–H826
52. Taegtmeyer H, Roberts AFC, Raine AEG (1985) Energy metabolism in reperfused heart muscle: metabolic correlates to return of function. J Am Coll Cardiol 6:864–870
53. Topol EJ, Weiss JL, Guzman PA, Dorsey-Lima S, Blanck TJJ, Humphrey LS, Baumgartner WA, Flaherty JT, Reitz BA (1984) Immediate improvement of dysfunctional myocardial segments after coronary revascularization: detection by intraoperative transesophageal echocardiography. J Am Coll Cardiol 4:1123–1134
54. Werns SW, Shea MJ, Driscoll EM, Cohen C, Abrams GD, Pitt B, Lucchesi BR (1985)

The independent effects of oxygen radical scavengers on canine infarct size; reduction by superoxide dismutase but not catalase. Circ Res 56:895 – 898

55. Werns SW, Shea MJ, Mitsos SE, Dysko RC, Fantone JC, Schork MA, Abrams GD, Pitt B, Lucchesi BR (1986) Reduction of the size of infarction by allopurinol in the ischemic-reperfused canine heart. Circulation 73:518 – 524
56. Weir WG, Kort AA, Stern MD, Lakatta EG, Marban E (1983) Cellular calcium fluctuations in mammalian heart. Direct evidence from noise analysis of aequorin signals in Purkinje fibers. Proc Natl Acad Sci USA 80:7367 – 7371
57. Zweier JL, Flaherty JT, Weisfeldt ML (1987) Direct measurement of free radical generation following reperfusion of ischemic myocardium. Proc Natl Acad Sci USA 84:1404 – 1407

The No-Reflow Phenomenon

C.E. Ganote and R.S. Vander Heide

The no-reflow phenomenon following a severe ischemic episode was first described in the brain [1] and subsequently has been observed in other organs including the kidney [2] and the heart [3]. In the brain edema and increased intracranial pressure inside of the rigid skull have been shown to limit reflow. Likewise, the kidney is encapsulated in a fibrous sheath, and reflow may be limited by extrinsic compression. However, the heart has no constricting external capsule, and no-reflow must occur by mechanisms other than extrinsic compression of the organ.

No-reflow in the heart actually occurs under three quite different circumstances. The first can be labeled central no-reflow, and it occurs in the center of an infarct. The second type of no-reflow is limited flow due to granulocyte-mediated microvascular plugging at the margins of regional infarcts and may coexist with central no-reflow. Finally, no-reflow can occur following episodes of global ischemia leading to ischemic (adenosine triphosphate depletion) rigor contracture. This can occur in vivo as a result of ischemic cardiac arrest with subsequent reperfusion, which results in the "stone heart syndrome," or in vitro in isolated hearts made ischemic or perfused with anoxic buffer. Each of these three types of no-reflow appears to have a different pathogenesis and pathophysiologic significance.

Central Infarct No-Reflow in Regional Ischemia

The no-reflow phenomenon in regional ischemia was originally described in the open-chest dog model of temporary circumflex coronary artery ligation [4]. Sixty minutes of ischemia and reflow resulted in contraction-band necrosis of the posterior papillary muscle. The use of the albumin-bound fluorescent dye thioflavin S allowed visualization of blood flow patterns when fresh tissue was sectioned and examined under ultraviolet light. Whereas control myocardium showed uniform fluorescence following dye injection, an obvious perfusion deficit with an endocardial to epicardial gradient was observed in ischemic zones during coronary artery ligation. Uniform reflow was also observed in the infarct area following 60-min temporary coronary occlusions, but regional subendocardial zones of no-reflow were present if coronary ligations were extended to 90 min or longer.

These areas of no-reflow occurred within the infarct boundaries, and following periods of ischemia longer than 90–120 min infarcts were also associated with focal and sometimes extensive zones of hemorrhage [5]. In the no-reflow zones, myocardial cells usually do not show the contraction-banding characteristic of reperfusion infarctions, but rather show bland coagulation necrosis. Although the pathogenesis of this type of no-reflow is not fully established, it is believed due to ischemic microvascular damage with edema and blebbing of endothelial cell cytoplasm into vascular lumina [6]. Vascular compression from swelling of adjacent myocytes and thrombosis of vessels are also thought to play a role in vascular occlusion. The role of ischemic cellular swelling has been supported by experiments showing improvements in reflow upon infusion of hypertonic solutions as compared to isotonic reperfusions [7]. With longer periods of ischemia, microvascular damage becomes severe with ischemic necrosis of vessel walls. In this case, reperfusion results in a leakage of blood from damaged vessels into the interstitial spaces. The resultant hemorrhagic infarction is, however, not evidence of sustained reflow, and such areas do not contain blood flow markers such as radioactive microspheres or dyes injected at the time of reperfusion. Zones of hemorrhagic infarction always occur within the boundaries of regional infarctions and usually within no-reflow areas [8]. There is no convincing evidence to suggest that either no-reflow or hemorrhage causes either enlargement or extension of infarcts, or serious functional impairment of surrounding myocardium.

Granulocytic Capillary Plugging at Infarct Margins

Inflammation is essentially a vascular phenomenon that induces adherence of activated granulocytes to capillary and venule endothelium. Inflammation is an early component of myocardial cell death. Proteins released from dead myocytes can activate the complement system and elicit an inflammatory response. It has been shown that granulocytes can obstruct capillaries producing microscopic areas of no-reflow, as evidenced by colloidal carbon injections [9]. In species with significant collateral blood flow, for example, man and dogs, infarcts enlarge over a period of several hours so that there is opportunity for granulocyte infiltrates to develop in the low-flow zones of a developing infarct. Infiltrates can also occur in reperfused regions at borders of permanently ischemic infarcts which contain a mixture of viable and dead myocytes. It has been proposed that inflammation could lead to a perpetuating cycle of capillary obstruction and increasing ischemia which could extend infarctions beyond the area occupied by the cells dying from the original ischemic episode [10].

Evidence for this concept comes from several laboratories which have shown that (a) infarctions tend to be smaller in granulocyte-depleted animals than in control animals; (b) collateral flow to regions of ischemia is greater in granulocyte-depleted animals than in control animals [11]; and (c) agents that inhibit leucocyte-mediated lipoperoxidation reduce infarct size in animal models, particularly in those which induce critical stenosis in the artery supplying the infarct area [12].

Although it is uncertain what extent the role that capillary obstruction and microscopic zones of no-reflow at infarct borders plays in determining ultimate infarct size in man, it has become clear that this mechanism of injury is an important component of some experimental infarct models.

Endocardial No-Reflow in Global Ischemia

Hearts subjected to global ischemia can produce high-energy phosphates for a time utilizing anaerobic glycolysis and nucleotide phosphate exchange. Eventually, however, adenosine triphosphate becomes exhausted, and hearts undergo rigor contracture. Early rigor contracture is reversible, and if blood flow is restored, myocytes, following a period of recovery, can resume normal function. In globally ischemic hearts, however, contracture causes sustained elevation of intramural pressures, particularly in the subendocardium. Subendocardial blood flow is compromised during systole during the normal cardiac cycle, and a heart in ischemic or anoxic contracture is physiologically similar to a heart in perpetual systole, leading to impaired subendocardial reflow.

The role of ischemic contracture in causing endocardial no-reflow is demonstrated by two lines of evidence. First, the extent of no-reflow correlates with the magnitude of developed contracture force. Hearts which undergo rigor contracture under conditions of low extracellular calcium ion concentration develop weaker contractures than control hearts and have correspondingly smaller subendocardial zones of no reflow. Secondly, if left ventricular cavities of hearts are maintained at a diastolic volume by an inflated intraventricular balloon during development of rigor, the ventricle becomes stiff and maintains the distended configuration upon deflation of the balloon. The deflation of the balloon reduces the intramural tension of the endocardium and allows reperfusion of the endocardium [14]. If the cells are reversibly injured, reperfusion causes relaxation of the myocardium and recovery of endocardial flow is maintained. If, however, the ischemic insult is severe enough to cause irreversible myocyte injury, then reperfusion induces a secondary contracture of cells with contraction-band necrosis. This reperfusion-induced contracture of irreversibly injured cells causes a reduction in ventricular volume and redevelopment of subendocardial no-reflow.

Contracture-induced subendocardial no-reflow is probably not a clinically important component of regional infarctions because ischemic cells are stretched during systole as a manifestation of dyskinesis, resulting in the so-called wavy fibers, and intramural contracture forces are not present. In experimental ischemic models, using isolated perfused hearts, subendocardial no-reflow may seriously impede functional recovery of otherwise reversibly injured hearts. The mechanisms of contracture and secondary no-reflow also may contribute to the pathophysiology of the "stone heart syndrome" [15] in man.

Summary. The no-reflow phenomenon is not a single entity but can be divided into three types, each with a different pathogenic mechanism and pathophysiologic significance. The central no-reflow in regional infarcts appears to result from severe ischemic damage to blood vessels and occurs following onset of irreversible myocardial injury. Capillary plugging by granulocytes in areas of low flow at infarct margins results from inflammation and could contribute to restricted reflow or could be a factor in infarct extension. The subendocardial no-reflow following global ischemia is related to contracture and sustained intramural pressures. This type of no-reflow may contribute to subendocardial infarctions during global ischemia and is a factor to be considered in perfused heart models of experimental ischemia.

References

1. Chaing J, Kowada M, Ames A, Wright RL, Majno G (1968) Cerebral ischemia, III. Vascular changes. Am J Pathol 52:455–476
2. Summers WK, Jamison RL (1971) The no-reflow phenomenon in renal ischemia. Lab Invest 25:635–643
3. Kloner RA, Ganote CE, Jennings RB, Reimer KA (1975) Demonstration of the "no-reflow" phenomenon in the dog heart after temporary ischemia. In: Roy PE, Rona C (eds) Recent advances in studies on cardiac structure and metabolism, vol 10. University Park Press, Baltimore, pp 463–473
4. Kloner RA, Ganote CE, Jennings RB (1974) The "no-reflow" phenomenon after temporary coronary occlusion in the dog. J Clin Invest 54:1496–1508
5. Braunwald E, Kloner RA (1985) Myocardial reperfusion: a double-edged sword? J Clin Invest 76:1713–1719
6. Jennings RB, Kloner RA, Ganote CE, Reimer KA (1982) Changes in capillary fine structure and function in acute myocardial ischemic injury. In: Tillmanns H, Kübler W, Zebe H (eds) Microcirculation of the heart. Springer, Berlin Heidelberg New York, pp 87–97
7. Willerson JT, Powell WJ Jr, Gruiney TE, Start JJ, Sanders A, Leaf A (1972) Improvement in myocardial function and coronary blood flow in ischemic myocardium after mannitol. J Clin Invest 51:2989–2998
8. Reimer KA, Jennings RB (1979) The "wave front phenomenon" of myocardial cell death. II. Transmural progression of necrosis within the framework of ischemic bed size (myocardium at risk) and collateral flow. Lab Invest 40:633–644
9. Engler RL, Schmid-Schönbein GW, Pavelec RS (1983) Leucocyte capillary plugging in myocardial ischemia and reperfusion in the dog. Am J Pathol 111:98–111
10. McCord J (1987) Oxygen-derived radicals: a link between reperfusion injury and inflammation. Fed Proc 46:2402–2406
11. Engler R (1987) Consequences of activation and adenosine-mediated inhibition of leucocytes during myocardial ischemia. Fed Proc 46:2407–2412

12. Simpson PJ, Mickelson JK, Lucchesi BR (1987) Free radical scavengers in myocardial ischemia. Fed Proc 46:2413–2421
13. Humphrey SM, Gavin JB, Herdson PB (1980) The relationship of ischemic contracture to vascular reperfusion in the isolated rat heart. J Mol Cell Cardiol 12:1397–1406
14. Humphrey SM, Thomson RW, Gavin JB (1982) The effect of an isovolumic left ventricle on the coronary vascular competence during reflow after global ischemia in the rat heart. Circ Res 49:784–791
15. Cooley DA, Reul GJ, Wukasch DA (1972) Ischemic contracture of the heart: "stone heart". Am J Cardiol 29:575–577

Microcirculation in Myocardial Ischemia and Reperfusion

H. Tillmanns, H. Leinberger, F.-J. Neumann, M. Steinhausen, N. Parekh, R. Zimmermann, R. Dussel, and W. Kübler

Introduction

The microcirculatory consequences of severe or extended myocardial ischemia are quite well documented [1, 3, 4, 6, 7]. In contrast, however, relatively little is known about the consequences of mild or transient ischemia, terminated well within cardiac resuscitation time. According to Kloner and Braunwald [6, 7], ischemic damage arises first in the myocyte, and this is followed by microvascular injury. This claim is based on morphologic data and does not consider disturbances of microvascular function.

A study was designed in our laboratory to investigate brief myocardial ischemia of the rat and cat heart, as induced by 10- to 20-min occlusion of the left anterior descending coronary artery, and subsequent reperfusion. We sought to determine whether there are functional microcirculatory disturbances occurring before the onset of detectable morphologic alterations of both the myocyte and the microvasculature.

Materials and Methods

The in vivo microscopic studies were performed by means of epi-illumination [12] or transillumination [13] of the left ventricular myocardium of the rat and cat heart. Motion pictures were recorded by a highly sensitive television-camera tape system or by means of high-speed cinematography. Additionally, fluorescence microscopic methods – intravenous injection of fluorescent dextrans and latex particles – were applied to improve contrast of the microvascular system and to measure blood flow velocity. Following intravenous bolus injection of fluorescein isothiocyanate (FITC) labeled high-molecular dextran, larger cardiac vessels could be readily distinguished at lower magnifications. Venules could easily be differentiated from arterioles because of the direction of flow at areas of bifurcation. At higher magnifications, the proximity and diameters of capillaries and the direction of blood flow could be visualized. Intraluminal pressures in the microvascular bed were obtained by micropuncture of arterioles and venules of the beating left ventricular myocardium [16]. Pressures were continuously recorded by a resistance servo mechanism nulling system according to Wiederhielm [18]. Diameters of small vessels were measured by digital video subtraction angiography [10].

Results and Discussion

In considering ischemia-induced changes in the hemodynamics of the microcirculation, we have been particularly interested in determining whether the reduction in coronary blood flow arising from a coronary artery stenosis [2, 5] is a consequence of a decrease in blood flow velocity in individual capillaries or a decrease in the number of capillaries being perfused. As expected, poststenotic myocardial areas exhibited dilatation of smaller coronary arterioles (A_3 and A_4, with diameters of less than 30 μm). In contrast, capillary and venular diameters did not change significantly. Despite arteriolar dilatation, the decline in perfusion pressure resulted in a marked reduction of mean blood flow velocity in capillaries and venules of both the cat and rat heart [17]. Furthermore, the drop of perfusion pressure in poststenotic arterioles could be shown to cause an increase in the distances between plasma-perfused capillaries, as visualized by fluorescein-labeled high-molecular dextran [17]. This increase of functional intercapillary distances in ischemic myocardium results in deterioration of regional myocardial oxygen supply, since, according to the Krogh model [8], a rise of diffusion distances leads to a decline of oxygen supply to the third power.

Ten minutes after coronary artery ligation (in the rat) or severe artery narrowing (in the cat), the red cell content of plasma-perfused capillaries decreased [14, 17]. Thus, while under physiological conditions approximately 78% of plasma-perfused capillaries contain red cells, in myocardial areas supplied by a stenosed vessel the ratio of capillaries filled with red cells to those containing plasma alone was markedly diminished [15]. In addition, temporary myocardial ischemia was occasionally found to provoke red cell aggregation in terminal arterioles and capillaries, thereby exaggerating the severity of regional myocardial malperfusion.

During reperfusion after 10- to 15-min occlusion of the left anterior descending coronary artery, functional intercapillary distances in the myocardial region supplied by the previously occluded vessel returned to normal values. During reperfusion, a rise of red cell content of plasma-perfused capillaries was recognized in each experiment compared to the values obtained in the course of myocardial ischemia. In 9 of 14 animals, however, the preischemic control values were not reached, which establishes a functional no-reflow phenomenon. This is mainly due to the augmented appearance of red cell aggregates and leukocytes, which already after 15 min of ischemia and especially during postischemic reperfusion often were observed in slow-flow capillaries of the ischemic zone [15]. Due to their lower deformability compared to red cells, during ischemia and reperfusion leukocytes tended to plug capillary branches. Under these circumstances we noted that capillaries downstream were still filled with fluorescent dextran,

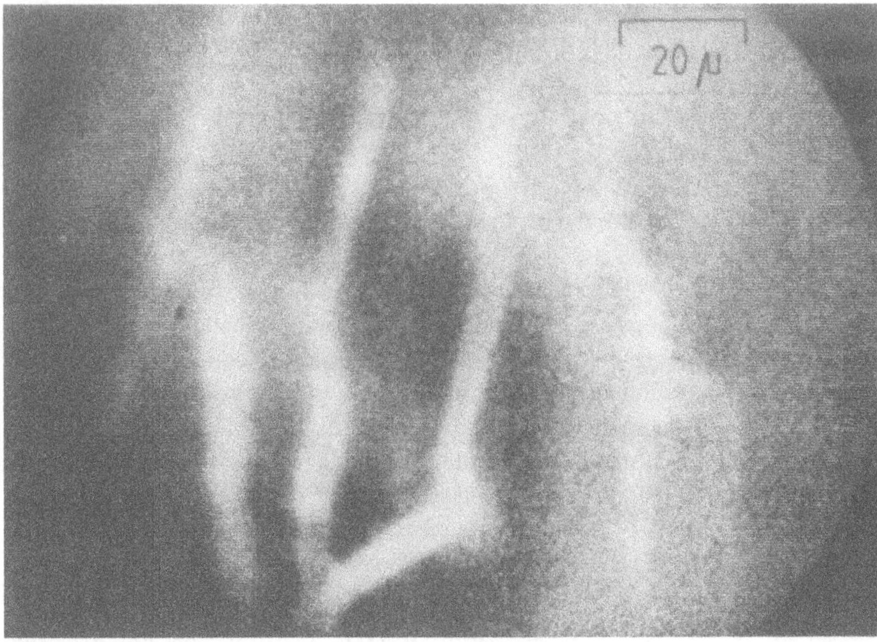

Fig. 1. In vivo fluorescence microphotograph of the rat heart obtained 10 min after ligation of the left anterior descending coronary artery. As can be seen, already after this short time there is an increase of permeability of capillaries and postcapillary venules, as indicated by extravascular clouds of fluorescent dextran

i.e., they were still experiencing plasma flow; red cells, however, were not detectable since they could not pass the leukocytes that were trapped at the capillary branch. Thus, leukocyte plugging, in addition to diminished red cell deformability, may be an important contributer to regional malperfusion in the ischemic and especially in the reperfused myocardium.

In addition to the hemodynamic and rheological changes induced by ischemia, impairment of microvascular function may arise as a consequence of changes in capillary permeability. After 10 min of myocardial ischemia and reperfusion, a rise of postcapillary venular and capillary permeability was indicated by extravascular clouds of fluorescent dextran [15] (Fig. 1). This increase of microvascular permeability was quantified using iodine-125 labeled albumin. In these experiments we noted that after 10 and 20 min of coronary artery ligation, myocardial extravascular albumin activity rose to 199% and 372%, respectively, of the value observed in control tissue. Prolongation of the ischemic period to 40 min did not result in any further increase of iodine-125 accumulation [14]. Varying the reperfusion period between 5 and 30 min revealed peak albumin activity at 10 min. Thereafter, the activity gradually decreased, indicating a washout of extravascular albumin. The data indicate that the rise of permeability to albumin is reversible during the first 30 min of reperfusion. The increase of microvascular permeability in the ischemic and reperfused myocardium was not influenced by indomethacin (10 μg/kg i.v.) and the thromboxane A_2 synthetase inhibitor dazoxyben (30 μg/kg i.v.).

Myocardial platelet accumulation after prolonged ischemia is claimed to be an important pathogenic factor contributing to disturbances of microvascular flow [9, 11]. After brief myocardial ischemia for 10 min, peripheral areas of ischemic myocardial regions showed accumulation of platelets. After varying periods of reperfusion, chromium-51 platelet activity in the previously ischemic myocardium rose significantly, with a maximum reached after 10 min of reperfusion. In contrast to indomethacin, which proved to be ineffective, the thromboxane A_2 synthetase inhibitor dazoxyben provoked a marked reduction of chromium-51 platelet activity in the ischemic (and reperfused) myocardium.

The aforementioned data indicate that after brief periods (10 – 20 min) of myocardial ischemia major changes occur in the flow characteristics of red cells and leukocytes, and that platelet trapping and major changes of capillary and especially postcapillary venular permeability can also occur. Therefore, microcirculatory disturbances occurring before the onset of detectable structural changes of the microvasculature may well be the primary cause of myocardial cell death.

The clinical significance of these experimental findings during postischemic reperfusion was investigated in patients with single-vessel coronary artery disease (left anterior descending coronary artery, ⩾75% stenosis) and without transmural myocardial infarction who underwent coronary angioplasty (PTCA). Noninvasive radionuclide studies were performed in 16 patients with single-vessel coronary artery disease before and 1 week after successful PTCA of the left anterior descending coronary artery (residual stenosis ⩽25%). Twelve patients were reinvestigated 6 months later. Thallium-201 serial scintigraphy was taken as reference for perfusion imaging, and tracer uptake (LAO 30° projection) was assessed by relating the tracer uptake in the diseased territory supplied by the left anterior descending coronary artery, to the tracer uptake in the nondiseased left circumflex territory within the respective scintigram using an operator-independent computer algorithm. Before PTCA, in myocardial areas with exercise-induced ischemia – as indicated by an initially decreased thallium-201 uptake and subsequent redistribution within 3 h – regional ^{13}N glutamate uptake was increased, either relatively compared to the same region in the poststress thallium-201 scintigram, or even absolutely compared to nonischemic segments within the respective scintigram, as was reported in a previous study from our laboratory [19].

Mean thallium-201 uptake (poststress images) was significantly increased 1 week after successful PTCA (78 ± 8% versus 72 ± 7%; $p>0.001$) and stayed fairly constant during the next 6 months. ^{13}N glutamate uptake was likewise increased 1 week after PTCA (103 ± 11% versus 94 ± 12%; $p<0.01$). After 6 months, however, ^{13}N glutamate uptake was diminished to the pre-PTCA level (94 ± 12%). Thus, repeated studies of poststenotic ^{13}N glutamate extraction reveal a delayed metabolic recovery of human myocardium despite successful coronary angioplasty. This phenomenon might be explained by disturbances of the myocardial microcirculation which disappeared within 6 months after successful coronary angioplasty.

References

1. Armiger LC, Gavin JB (1975) Changes in the microvasculature of ischemic and infarcted myocardium. Lab Invest 33:51–56
2. Gould KL, Lipscomb K, Hamilton GW (1974) Physiologic basis for assessing critical coronary stenosis. Instantaneous flow response and regional distribution during coronary hyperemia as measures of coronary flow reserve. Am J Cardiol 33:87
3. Jennings RB, Kloner RA, Ganote CE, Hawkins HK, Reimer KA (1982) Changes in capillary fine structure and function in acute myocardial ischemic injury. In: Tillmanns H, Kübler W, Zebe H (eds) Microcirculation of the heart, theoretical and clinical problems. Springer, Berlin Heidelberg New York, pp 87–96
4. Jennings RB, Sommers H, Smyth GA, Flack HA, Linn H (1960) Myocardial necrosis induced by temporary occlusion of a coronary artery in the dog. Arch Pathol 70: 68–78
5. Klocke FJ (1976) Coronary blood flow in man. Prog Cardiovasc Dis 19:117–166
6. Kloner RA, Braunwald E (1980) Observations on experimental myocardial ischemia. Cardiovasc Res 14:371–395
7. Kloner RA, Ganote CE, Jennings RB, Reimer KA (1974) The "no-reflow" phenomenon after temporary coronary occlusion in the dog. J Clin Invest 54: 1496–1508
8. Krogh A (1919) The number and distribution of capillaries in muscles with calculations of the oxygen pressure head necessary for supplying the tissue. J Physiol (Lond) 52:409
9. Leinberger H, Suehiro GT, McNamara JJ (1979) Myocardial platelet trapping after coronary ligation in primates. J Surg Res 27:3–40
10. Möller P, Tillmanns H, Steinhausen M, Dart AM, Parekh N, Kübler W (1983) Digital video subtraction imaging of myocardial microvasculature during hypoxia and reactive hyperemia. Circulation 68 [Suppl III]:82
11. Moschos CB, Lahiri K, Lyons M, Weisse AB, Oldewurtel HA, Regan TJ (1973) Relation of microcirculatory thrombosis to thrombus in the proximal coronary artery: effect of aspirin, dipyridamole and thrombolysis. Am Heart J 86:61–68
12. Steinhausen M, Tillmanns H, Thederan H (1978) Microcirculation of the epimyocardial layer of the heart. I. A method for in vivo observation of the microcirculation of superficial ventricular myocardium of the heart and capillary flow pattern under normal and hypoxic conditions. Pflügers Arch 378:9–14
13. Tillmanns H, Ikeda S, Hansen H, Sarma JSM, Fauvel JM, Bing RJ (1974) Microcirculation in the ventricle of the dog and turtle. Circ Res 34:561–569
14. Tillmanns H, Kübler W (1984) What happens in the microcirculation? In: Hearse DJ, Yellon DM (eds) Therapeutic approaches to myocardial infarct size limitation. Raven, New York, pp 107–124
15. Tillmanns H, Leinberger H, Neumann FJ, Steinhausen M, Parekh N, Zimmermann R (1984) Early microcirculatory changes during brief ischemia – primary events in ischemic myocardial injury? Circulation 70 [Suppl II]:88

16. Tillmanns H, Steinhausen M, Leinberger H, Thederan H, Kübler W (1981) Pressure measurements in the terminal vascular bed of the epimyocardium of rats and cats. Circ Res 49:1202 – 1211
17. Tillmanns H, Steinhausen M, Leinberger H, Thederan H, Kübler W (1981) Hemodynamics of the coronary microcirculation during myocardial ischemia. Circulation 64 [Suppl IV]:40
18. Wiederhielm CA, Woodbury JW, Kirk ES, Rushmer RF (1964) Pulsatile pressures in the microcirculation of frog's mesentery. Am J Physiol 207:173 – 176
19. Zimmermann R, Tillmanns H, Knapp WH, Helus F, Georgi P, Rauch B, Neumann FJ, Girgensohn S, Maier-Borst W, Kübler W (1988) Regional myocardial N-13 glutamate uptake in patients with coronary artery disease: inverse post-stress relation to thallium-201 uptake in ischemia. J Am Coll Cardiol 11:549 – 556

Reperfusion Injury*

K. A. Reimer and R. B. Jennings

It is our intention to discuss briefly some of the possible consequences of reperfusing myocytes which have been ischemic. (For a more detailed discussion of this subject, the reader is referred to [1 – 3].) At the outset, one must understand that ischemic myocardium is heterogenous. Thus, different myocytes even within the same ischemic region may be affected quite differently by reperfusion. The principal determinants of the myocardial response to reperfusion are (a) the duration of ischemia and (b) the severity of ischemia. By severity of ischemia we refer here to the degree to which collateral blood flow is inadequate to provide for the metabolic demands of the myocardium.

Back in the 1950s, Dr. Jennings began to study the pathophysiology of myocardial ischemia and reperfusion and defined cell injury – in very simple, biologic terms – as being reversible if reperfusion prevent cellular necrosis and as being irreversible if cells undergo necrosis despite reperfusion. In an experimental model in which the circumflex artery is occluded in open-chest anesthetized dogs, if the artery is never reperfused, a substantial part of the ischemic region undergoes infarction. In contrast, if the circumflex artery is occluded for 15 min or less and is then reperfused, the entire ischemic region is reversibly injured; reperfusion prevents necrosis. If ischemia persists for 40 min, the subendocardial zone becomes irreversibly injured; a subendocardial infarct develops despite reperfusion. Nevertheless, there is still a large amount of reversibly injured myocardium in the mid- and subepicardial zones which can be salvaged by reperfusion. As the ischemic episode is prolonged, the transmural extent of irreversible injury increases; reperfusion salvages fewer myocytes, and infarcts are correspondingly larger.

For any given duration of occlusion, there is substantial variation in myocardial infarct size; variation in infarct size is related to variation in the severity of ischemia. In other words, there is a substantial range of infarct sizes, related to a substantial range of collateral blood flows. Large infarcts occur when there is little flow, small infarcts occur when there is substantial collateral flow.

A few characteristics of reversibly injured myocardium following reperfusion include the following: viability is retained (by the definition given above); ultrastructure is rapidly restored (within minutes); adenine nucleotides are slowly

* Supported in part by NIH grants HL27416 and HL23138.

restored (perhaps requiring several days); and contractile function is slowly restored (this may also require several days, i.e., the myocardium is "stunned").

The characteristic ultrastructural features of reversible injury include the following: there is mild peripheral aggregation of nuclear chromatin; myofibrils are in a relaxed state; the sarcoplasm is moderately swollen, as are many of the mitochondria; and there is loss of particulate glycogen from the sarcoplasm. By 20 min of reperfusion following 15 min or less of ischemia, these changes disappear; these reperfused myocytes are virtually indistinguishable from the control nonischemic myocytes except for an occasional degenerate mitochondrion.

Metabolic recovery takes considerably longer. After 15 min of severe ischemia and no reperfusion, 50% – 60% of the tissue ATP has been utilized, and nearly half of the adenine nucleotide content has been lost by degradation to purine nucleosides and bases. After reperfusion, AMP and ADP are rapidly rephosphorylated to ATP, but adenine nucleotide resynthesis is very slow. Minimal repletion occurs during the first 24 h, and repletion is not quite complete even 4 days after a single 15-min coronary occlusion.

Two ultrastructural characteristics of irreversibly injured myocardium are the development of amorphous matrix densities in swollen mitochondria and overt damage to the sarcolemma. The sarcolemma is composed of the trilaminar unit membrane, i.e., the plasmalemma, with its overlying basal lamina. In irreversibly injured myocytes, the basal lamina is structurally intact, but the plasmalemma is missing in some areas. These features distinguish irreversibly from reversibly injured myocytes and are detectable before reperfusion. If such cells are reperfused, they undergo an accelerated form of necrosis which we call contraction band necrosis. Some of the early features of this type of necrosis include: more severe sarcolemmal disruption; severe cell swelling, often with formation of edematous blebs beneath the sarcolemma; washout of soluble intracellular catabolites and enzymes such as creatine kinase; disruption of myofibrils resulting in the formation of myofibrillar contraction bands; and mitochondrial calcification. Damage to the microvasculature also may occur during ischemia and may lead to intramyocardial hemorrhage during reperfusion.

On the basis of this brief review of the biology of reperfusion, we will now consider the concept of "reperfusion injury." This term is now in widespread use; unfortunately, however, it seems to mean different things to different people. Buckberg et al. have provided a good general definition of the term; to them, reperfusion injury refers to "those metabolic, functional and structural consequences of restoring coronary flow, that can be avoided or reversed by modification of the conditions of reperfusion." These investigators have studied reperfusion primarily in a surgical setting of global myocardial ischemia during cardiopulmonary bypass, followed by reperfusion. Their general definition seems applicable to regional myocardial ischemia as well. However, in actual practice reperfusion injury often takes on a more specific definition, depending on the experimental or clinical setting:

1. In the surgical setting, and with certain experimental models, reperfusion injury is defined as postischemic contractile dysfunction or postischemic metabolic abnormalities, if caused by reperfusion.
2. In some cases, reperfusion injury has been used to refer to failed reperfusion, the no-reflow-phenomenon, or reduced reperfusion due to microvascular compression or obstruction.
3. In other circumstances reperfusion injury is used to refer to the accelerated necrosis or contraction band necrosis, described above.
4. In the case of myocardial infarction, and the goal of limiting myocardial infarct size by reperfusion, with or without adjuvant pharmacologic therapy, reperfusion injury refers specifically to the death of myocytes which were viable at the end of a period of ischemia, but were killed by some deleterious aspect of reperfusion per se.
5. Finally, reperfusion injury may refer to weakening of the infarct or the scar by some deleterious effect of reperfusion, such as myocardial hemorrhage, that could occur independently of any effect of reperfusion on myocardial infarct size.

Evidence favoring the existence of reperfusion injury according to any one of these definitions is not evidence for the existence of reperfusion injury according to the other definitions. We want to consider now reperfusion injury specifically from the point of view of the fourth of these definitions.

There is a general hypothesis that some myocytes which undergo necrosis do so because of ischemic injury per se, while others die because of some deleterious effect of reperfusion, superimposed on the preceding ischemic injury. A currently popular specific hypothesis is that some ischemic cells are killed by free radicals produced during reperfusion. Although there are a number of possible sources of free radicals in postischemic myocardium, the two that have received the most attention have been (a) the xanthine-oxidase reaction, in which free radicals are produced by the oxidation of hypoxanthine to xanthine and (b) neutrophils which accumulate in the injured myocardium. Production of oxygen-centered free radicals by the xanthine-oxidase reaction is plausible inasmuch as a substrate for xanthine oxidase, hypoxanthine, and its immediate precursor inosine accumulate rapidly in ischemic myocardium. The neutrophil hypothesis also is plausible because neutrophils accumulate rapidly in myocardium during reperfusion following either 40 or 90 min of ischemia. In recent results from our laboratory, neutrophils were isolated and labeled with indium 111 and then reinjected into the same dogs at the end of either a 12-, 40-, or 90-min episode of ischemia. Tissue neutrophil content was then quantitated at the end of 1 h of reperfusion. Neutrophils accumulated in the previously ischemic region during this 1st h of reperfusion. Accumulation was most pronounced in the inner (subendocardial) and midmyocardial zones of greatest anticipated necrosis.

However, we have been unable to find any protective effect of administering superoxide dismutase (SOD) in the same animal model, using a 40-min period of ischemia and quantitating infarct size histologically after 4 days of reperfusion. The circumflex vascular bed, i.e., the area at risk of infarction was the same average size in both groups. Infarct size, as a percentage of the size of the LV and of the AAR, also was the similar in both groups.

Because infarct size is so variable among dogs, it is essential to evaluate infarct size with respect to the amount of collateral blood flow in the same animal. As mentioned earlier, there is an inverse relationship between infarct size and collateral blood flow, i.e., low flow causes large infarcts, and high flow causes small infarcts. If SOD had been protective, infarct size should have been smaller than predicted for any given amount of collateral blood flow. However, this was not the case; the relationship was similar for SOD-treated and for control animals. We have also found no protective effect in this model of the xanthine-oxidase inhibitors allopurinol and oxypurinol. Thus, to date we have been unable to detect reperfusion injury caused by superoxide radicals in an experimental model characterized by 40 min of ischemia and 4 days of reperfusion.

Summary. Reperfusion certainly does limit myocardial infarct size if it is initiated sufficiently early. Reperfusion permits the rapid ultrastructural recovery and the slower metabolic and functional recovery of reversibly injured myocytes. Modified conditions of reperfusion may be beneficial in that they can accelerate functional recovery. Reperfusion also accelerates the disintegration of irreversibly injured myocytes. Reperfusion may kill some myocytes, which are still potentially salvagable prior to the onset of reperfusion. Dr. Lucchesi has presented evidence suggesting that this does in fact occur. However, to date we have not been able to find similar protective effects of free radical scavengers in our experimental models. Reperfusion may alter infarct or scar strength independent of any effect on myocardial infarct size. The latter statement is an hypothesis that has considerable clinical importance but to date there is little experimental evidence, either for or against it.

References

1. Reimer KA, Jennings RB (1986) Myocardial ischemia, hypoxia, and infarction. In: Fozzard HA, Haber E, Jennings RB, Katz AM, Morgan HE (eds) The heart and cardiovascular system. Raven Press, New York, pp 1133–1201
2. Reimer KA, Ideker RE (1987) Myocardial ischemia and infarction: anatomic and biochemical substrates for ischemic cell death and ventricular arrhythmias. Hum Pathol 18:462–475
3. Uraizee A, Reimer KA, Murry CE, Jennings RB (1987) Failure of superoxide dismutase to limit myocardial infarct size in a 40 minutes ischemia/four days reperfusion model in dogs. Circulation 75:1237–1248

Discussion: Session I – Pathophysiology of Salvage of Ischemic Myocardium by Reperfusion

Chairman: R.B. Jennings

Dr. Jennings: I would like to ask Dr. Tillmanns a question: What is the explanation for the increased glutamate uptake and/or delayed clearance of glutamate from reversibly injured myocardium?

Dr. Tillmanns: The increased glutamate uptake was confirmed by studies of Heinrich Taegtmeyer on the hypoxic myocardium. He also used ischemic heart muscle and under experimental conditions confirmed the following hypothesis: under hypoxic or ischemic conditions, lactate accumulates by reduction of pyruvate (impaired oxidative metabolism). Glutamate as an amino nitrogen donor can reduce lactate accumulation by formation of alanine from pyruvate. On the other hand, energy metabolism of heart muscle is improved by glutamate as an amino nitrogen donor for the transaminase reaction from α-ketoglutamate to aspartate. These are the beneficial effects of glutamate on high-energy phosphate metabolism in ischemic heart muscle. Experimental data by Mudge and coworkers (1976) led in the same direction; these authors demonstrated alanine release from the coronary sinus during acute myocardial ischemia.

With regard to the delayed recovery of glutamate extraction following successful PTCA, these are two possibilities of explanation: (a) Changes of vessel diameter after PTCA; here I would like to mention data obtained by Patrick Serruys and his group. (b) Disturbances of the myocardial microcirculation despite the absence of coronary artery stenosis following successful PTCA. In our study, only patients with diameter narrowing below 25% were included.

Dr. Jennings: Thank you very much. That would be very significant because it would allow you to identify that you successfully reperfused living myocardium. Next question:

Dr. Olsson: I would like to ask Dr. Jennings three short questions, the first one concerns the electron-microscopic and histological changes in the myocardium following coronary artery occlusion. Are the changes an all-or-none phenomenon, or are there different time periods within the given areas? The second question is: it is well-known from experimental models and also from studies on man that there is a well recognized time sequence of cell injury; given the explanation that Dr. Reimer has presented so beautifully, I do not think that the factors he mentioned can be the sole explanation: what in your opinion, Dr. Jennings, is the difference between the experimental model and man when reperfusion starts after 3 or 4 h following total occlusion of the coronary vessel? And the last question is: do catecholamines ever play a role in ischemic damage at all?

Dr. Jennings: For various reasons, these three questions are difficult to answer. The difficulty with the first is the fact that we have only studied severely ischemic myocardium. Within the severely ischemic myocardium, virtually all the myocytes show the same changes at about the same time. When cell death first begins to appear 18 – 20 min after the onset of ischemia, very few myocytes are dead. The number of myocytes dying increases exponentially until 90% or more of them in the zone of severe ischemia are dead some 60 min after the onset. The mechanism of cell death throughout this zone almost certainly is identical from myocyte to myocyte. It is clear that myocytes in the zone of moderate ischemia eventually die, and that they die more slowly than the severely ischemic myocytes. We assume that the same changes occur in both severely and moderately ischemic tissue but have little data to support this conclusion. The reason for the assumption is the fact that there is no reliable way to identify moderately ischemic tissue with certainty at the time it is sampled for analysis. Nevertheless, regardless of whether moderately ischemic myocytes die by the same mechanism, they die on a slower time scale. In summary, we think that cell death is an "all-or-none" phenomenon in the sense that the myocyte is dead when the sarcolemma is disrupted. Cell death, however, occurs as a function of the severity of the ischemia. Severity, however, is a variable which changes transmurally in most dogs as well as in many human hearts. Therefore, all ischemic myocytes do not die simultaneously. In fact, mildly ischemic myocytes often survive.

As to the effects of reperfusion 3 – 4 h after the onset of ischemia, the changes seen are those described by Dr. Reimer. I believe that the same pattern probably exists in man.

The role of catecholamines in ischemic injury remains difficult to ascertain. I vascillate between believing that they are involved and believing that they are not. At the present time, my enthusiasm is rising relative to the role of catecholamines. Again, I have no solid data on this point.

Dr. Ganten: I would like to draw your attention to one system which has not been discussed, and which might actually bear on the question of Dr. Olssen, and that is the renin-angiotensin system. There is very good evidence now that renin is not just a circulating hormone, but that the renin gene and the angiotensinogen gene are expressed in the heart. Renin mRNA and angiotensin mRNA are present in myocardial tissue. There is also angiotensin in the heart itself at relatively high concentrations. We have performed studies with converting enzyme inhibitors and have seen that in the isolated Langendorff heart preparation, where the circulating angiotensin is completely excluded, converting enzyme inhibitors have a beneficial effect on the reperfusion arrythmia and also on reperfusion metabolic changes, namely energy-rich phosphates are increasing, lactate is decreasing, and glycogen is increasing in converting enzyme inhibitor treated animals as opposed to untreated controls. We therefore suggest that in addition to the mechanisms being discussed this morning, an interference with local angiotensin in the heart and possibly other peptide systems such as kinins, which of course are also affected by converting enzyme inhibitors, might have to be considered.

Dr. Jennings: Do you think those are localized primarily in the myocytes or in the nerves in the heart?

Dr. Ganten: I think there are both possibilities. There is indication that angiotensin acts via stimulation of neuronal activity, but of course there is also a direct action of angiotensin on the microcirculation. In vivo the possibility of an activation of circulating angiotensin in contact with the endothelium and/or paracrine activation of angiotensin within the heart has to be considered.

Dr. Verstraete: I would like to address three brief questions to Dr. B.R. Lucchesi. Why is that in using polyethylene glycol, SOD would adhere more readily if not selectively to the endothelium cells? My second question is whether SOD protects tissue against both the xanthine oxidase and neutrophil-generated oxygen? My last query concerns the rationale of monoclonal antibodies directed against receptors on MO1. You nicely indicated that ibuprofen prevents the development of the receptor. Is it not more logical to prevent the formation of MO1 receptors than to let them develop and then impede their function?

Dr. Lucchesi: First let me answer the last question. The advantage of using the MO1 antibody over ibuprofen is that ibuprofen is being claimed – and I'm not quite sure whether this is correct – to interfere with the healing process, and the MO1 antibody should not do this, because neutrophil function is restored relatively quickly.

Now to the second question: as far as I know, human SOD has not been used in man. Dr. Pitt has some answer to that quickly.

Dr. Pitt: The pilot studies examining the safety of superoxide dismutase in patients have been completed. A multicenter trial of superoxide dismutase in patients with acute infarction is ready to begin involving the TAMI and Johns Hopkins University groups.

Dr. Lucchesi: To answer the first question, it has been shown that polyethylene glycol causes cell fusions because of its ability to adhere to cell surfaces, and it is used in a lot of fusion-type experiments for this very purpose. When you congregate it to protein such as glutathione peroxidase, it facilitates not only the adherence to the cell surface, but also the incorporation into the cell – if you give it intravascularly. I'm not saying that it is not incorporated into myocytes; we don't have data on that. There are data, however, to show that it is incorporated into the endothelial cell.

Summary of Session I

R. B. Jennings

This session was arranged to provide the audience with the background required to understand some of the phenomena which occur in ischemic myocardium. It is clear that, although much is known of the molecular mechanisms involved in ischemia and reperfusion, much remains to be learned. Moreover, new phenomena, such as stunning, preconditioning, and reperfusion injury, now need molecular or pathophysiologic explanations. New therapies, including free radical scavenger therapy, have come onto the scene as controversial contributions to our understanding of the pathogenesis of either ischemic or reperfusion injury.

Biology of Regional Ischemia. The sequential changes in myocardial metabolism, structure, and function occurring in a zone of acute regional ischemia have been established in the dog heart using severely ischemic subendocardial left ventricular tissue. Within seconds of the onset of severely depressed or absent coronary arterial flow, aerobic metabolism ceases and anaerobic glycolysis becomes the source of virtually all new high-energy phosphates (HEP) available in the tissue. A net of 3 μmol HEP are captured as 1 μmol glucose from glycogen is converted into 2 μmol lactate. This amount, plus that available from the preexisting pool of CP and ATP is inadequate to meet the demand of the tissue for HEP. ATP is depleted and adenine nucleotides are degraded to nucleosides and bases. The metabolic changes occurring in the ischemic myocytes leads to the production of many new intracellular particles, which are termed the osmolar load. The myocytes become edematous as a consequence of the osmolar load and declining levels of ATP.

In this system, lethal injury is characterized by an ATP of <2 μmol/g dry, cessation of anaerobic glycolysis, rupture of the sarcolemma, high lactate, H^+, and AMP, etc., and low glycogen. The critical event, i.e., the lethal event, is considered to be membrane disruption. Reversibly injured cells exhibit similar but less marked changes. The ATP is >5 μmol/g dry. Anaerobic glycolysis persists, but at a depressed rate. The sarcolemma is intact. The net level of H^+, phosphate, AMP, lactate, etc. is lower than in irreversibly injured tissue, while glycogen and ATP levels are higher.

Reversibly injured myocytes exhibit mild changes in structure consistent with cell edema and ongoing anaerobic glycolysis. Reperfusion quickly restores the ultrastructure towards normal. Mild cell edema persists for hours. The stunning phenomenon, i.e., depressed contractile efficiency, persists for days; also, the adenine nucleotide pool requires days before resynthesis is complete.

Dr. Tillmanns showed that myocardium reversibly injured by a brief episode of ischemia in man may exhibit a metabolic change which allows the presence of living damaged reperfused myocytes to be recognized. These myocytes accumulated ^{13}N glutamate. A metabolic marker of this type may be very valuable in assessing the effects of successful thrombolysis.

Early in the phase of lethal injury, reperfusion of the tissue is usually successful, i.e., all vessels are reperfused with arterial blood. This results in the prompt development of the histologic pattern of contraction-band necrosis. The cells become very edematous and accumulate Na^+, Ca^{2+}, Cl^-, and H_2O while losing K^+, Mg^{2+}, and phosphate. The mitochondria of such cells accumulate much calcium phosphate in the form of hydroxyapatite.

If the period of ischemia is extended, some vascular death occurs in the center of the zone of severe ischemia. Such tissue cannot be reperfused; it exhibits the no-reflow phenomenon. Dr. Ganote also showed that cell edema and rigor contracture contribute to no-reflow.

It seems likely that the accumulation of leukocytes in the zone of severe ischemia contributes to perfusion defects including the no-reflow phenomenon. Dr. Reimer has shown that when such tissue is reperfused with arterial blood, leukocyte infiltration increases in proportion to the duration of the injury. This increase is probably because the number of lethally injured myocytes present is increasing as the period of ischemia is extended from 60 – 90 min. Much remains to be learned about the potential role leukocytes play in so-called reperfusion injury. Reimer showed data which indicated that there are fewer leukocytes in reperfused reversibly injured tissue than in control tissue. The role leukocytes play in causing persistent ischemia by capillary obstruction or by causing direct vascular injury is discussed further under reperfusion injury.

Consequences of Reperfusion: Concept of Reperfusion Injury. The effects of reperfusion were described in a number of experimental models. Although reperfusion clearly salvages living reversibly injured ischemic myocytes, it also may damage some myocytes which would potentially be salvageable if the conditions of reperfusion had been altered. This theoretical effect of reperfusion is termed reperfusion injury.

Reperfusion injury is not a well-defined process. It has been studied in a variety of dissimilar experimental models employing different end points, including cell death defined by histology or enzymatic techniques (TTC), oxidative loads, and contractile defects. In order to avoid confusion, aspects of each of the three types of reperfusion injury will be summarized separately below.

Reperfusion Injury as Defined by Cell Death. Data presented by Reimer and Jennings clearly establishes that reperfusion with arterial blood salvages living ischemic myocytes. On the other hand, other authors have presented data which suggest that there are myocytes in the reperfused tissue which are killed by the reperfusion procedure. If this phenomenon exists, it represents a form of reperfusion injury which might be prevented if its pathogenesis were known. Successful treatment would result in an increase in the number of myocytes salvaged by reperfusion over the number which is salvaged in untreated hearts.

In analyzing this question in experimental studies of transient ischemia in the dog heart, Reimer emphasized that one must control for the major variables which affect infarct size, namely, the volume of collateral flow and the amount of myocardium at risk, if an accurate answer is to be obtained to the question of whether additional cell death occurred as a consequence of the reperfusion procedure. Up to the present time, most studies of this problem in in vivo ischemia have not controlled for both of these variables. Accordingly, it was his opinion that the phenomenon of reperfusion injury remains unproved at this point in time.

On the other hand, Lucchesi summarized a series of studies of reperfusion injury in the open-chest anesthetized dog which strongly suggest that free radical generation may cause the death of myocytes which were alive, although badly damaged by ischemia, at the time of reperfusion. He emphasized that free radical generation from activated leukocytes attracted to the ischemic tissue during the reperfusion procedure, might be the cause of some cell death in this system. The evidence included reduction in infarct size by: (a) administration of superoxide dismutase prior to the time of reperfusion, (b) induction of neutropenia, (c) pretreatment with ibuprofen to prevent activation of leukocytes, and (d) treatment with antibody to leukocyte-adherence receptor. Each of these procedures reduced the amount of damage from leukocyte-derived free radicals. It seems clear that vascular damage or obstruction induced by leukocytes could induce local ischemia in the reperfused tissue and thereby kill potentially salvageable myocytes.

The studies of Lucchesi's group were done in a model of ischemia in which a critical stenosis was placed on the vessel distal to the planned occlusion site. This stenosis was of sufficient magnitude to prevent the reactive hyperemia which occurs immediately after reflow in vascular beds in which no stenosis is present. Since arterial collateral flow was not controlled in the reperfusion injury studies of this group, these data remain to be confirmed in appropriately controlled analyses of infarct size. However, the mass of data suggests that reperfusion injury is a significant feature of reperfusion when it is performed after 90 min of ischemia in the open-chest anesthetized dog.

Reperfusion Injury as Defined by Oxidative Loads. Ferrari presented data on intracellular free radical generation in the isolated heart subjected to episodes of ischemia of various duration followed by reperfusion. Most of the free radicals generated in the system originate from mitochondrial respiration. He believes that free radical production increases in mitochondria that have been damaged by ischemia and measures the stress of intracellular free radicals by studying shifts in the glutathione peroxidase system. Changes in the proportion of reduced (GSH) and oxidized glutathione (GSSG) occurred as a function of the duration of ischemia. The longer the ischemia, the greater the proportion of GSSG. In addition, mitochondrial superoxidase dismutase activity was reduced by 50% in mitochondria damaged by ischemia and subjected to reperfusion.

An alternate approach to the evaluation of the role of intracellular free radical production on cell injury was made by preloading the myocyte with *N*-acetylcysteine to provide SH groups in support of GSH production. Ferrari reported marked improvement in function and energy production in hearts pretreated with this SH compound and subjected to reperfusion.

Reperfusion Injury Defined by Contractile Defects. The term reperfusion injury was developed by Buckberg to describe the deleterious effects of the reperfusate on the capacity of a totally ischemic arrested heart to resume function when it was reperfused with arterial blood. Buckberg clearly showed that left ventricular function of such hearts could be improved by specific alterations in the composition of the perfusate, including making it hypertonic, transiently lowering its content of ionized Ca^{2+}, and providing substrates designed to support metabolism in a heart emerging from the ischemic state.

Stunning Phenomenon. Braunwald and Kloner coined the term "stunning" to describe the fact that living myocardium damaged by ischemia and successfully salvaged by reperfusion, i.e., reversibly injured myocardium contracts less efficiently than it did prior to the episode of ischemia. By definition, the stunned myocardium, contains no necrotic tissue, has been successfully reperfused in the sense that no residual ischemia is present in the tissue, and eventually fully recovers contractile function.

The contractile machinery seems to be intact in the stunned myocardium in the sense that contractile function can be restored transiently by catecholamine stimulation or by intra-arterial Ca^{2+} infusion. Also, energy production and utilization appears to be uninvolved even though the adenine nucleotide pool is depleted in the stunned myocardium.

Marban reported on studies of the mechanism of stunning in the isolated perfused heart. His results suggest that it may be caused by a transient Ca^{2+} overload occurring during the episode of ischemia.

Session II
Thrombolysis in Acute Myocardial Infarction

Chairman: M. Verstraete

Thrombolysis in Acute Myocardial Infarction

M. Verstraete

There is by now a consensus that thrombolytic treatment in the first hours after the acute symptoms of myocardial infarction is reducing short-term and 1-year mortality. The evidence is based mainly on the Italian GISSI trial, the results of the ISIS-2 study and data pooled from other, smaller trials with intracoronary and intravenous streptokinase. The reduction in mortality is 15% – 20% in patients treated with thrombolytic drugs within the first 5 h. During this period not only is coronary reperfusion more readily and rapidly achieved (the fresher the thrombus, the faster the lysis), but there is also the critical time for reperfusion to salvage of myocardium ("time is muscle"). For the patient having continuing ischemia (as shown by continuing ischemic pain or by electrocardiographic changes), benefit may extend beyond this time. Efforts to reduce the time delay from the onset of symptoms to the institution of thrombolytic therapy, such as giving these agents in the patient's home or in the coronary ambulance, are likely to have a major impact on survival.

To offer the benefit of effective thrombolytic treatment to a greater proportion of patients as soon as possible after myocardial infarction, short and simple therapeutic schemes must be developed. Logistical considerations favour the intravenous route as the safest for thrombolytic drugs.

Management of residual stenosis in the affected artery remains an unresolved issue. Recent studies have cast some doubts on the usefulness of immediate angioplasty after thrombolysis, and the pharmacological prevention of rethrombosis is less than ideal.

Many questions still remain to be answered concerning which thrombolytic drugs should be used. What is the role of adjunctive therapy, such as β-blockers, α-blockers or free radical scavengers?

Streptokinase in Acute Myocardial Infarction – Benefits and Risks

H. Schmutzler

Thirty years ago in 1958 the first experience with intravenous administration of fibrinolytic agents in 22 patients with acute myocardial infarction was reported by Fletcher and coworkers in the United States [6]. The next step was intermittent diastolic administration of fibrinolysin through a catheter in Valsalva's sinus in 1960, reported by Boucek and Murphy [1]. In the period between 1960 and 1966 uncontrolled and controlled studies were reported, involving intravenous administration of streptokinase with initial dose of 250×10^3 U followed by maintenance doses of 100×10^3 U/h for periods of 12–24 h in patients with acute myocardial infarction. As a result, successful treatment by thrombolysis or fibrinolysis was suspected but not proven in individual cases. Although all investigators recognized the necessity of coronary angiography, prevailing opinion at that time held that angiography in the setting of acute infarction was associated with unacceptably high risk. Randomized and controlled multicenter studies with large groups of patients were initiated to allow statistical analysis of mortality in this situation.

It was soon demonstrated that patients treated within 12 h had better results than those treated up to 24 h after the onset of chest pain. The authors reported significantly better survival in the treatment group when therapy was instituted within a few hours after the onset of infarction. This was already verified by the first Swiss-German streptokinase study in 1966 [18].

In 1976 the Russian cardiologist Chazev was the first to provide angiographic evidence of reperfusion in 16 patients treated with intracoronary administration of 5×10^3 U fibrinolysin [3]. The breakthrough in thrombolytic treatment came with Rentrop in 1978 [10], after it was demonstrated by DeWood that coronary angiography in acute myocardial infarction is not associated with additional risk but provides the advantages of an exact diagnosis and the possibility of confirming therapeutic effect [5].

Intracoronary administration of streptokinase is associated with a higher recanalization rate than intravenous administration, but the logistical requirements are so great that the application of this method is necessarily limited, while short-term lysis by intravenous administration of $500-1500 \times 10^3$ U streptokinase has proven its broad applicability in the clinical setting. Patel and Kloner [9] have recently performed a pooled analysis of ten randomized studies published since 1981, seven with intracoronary and three with intravenous

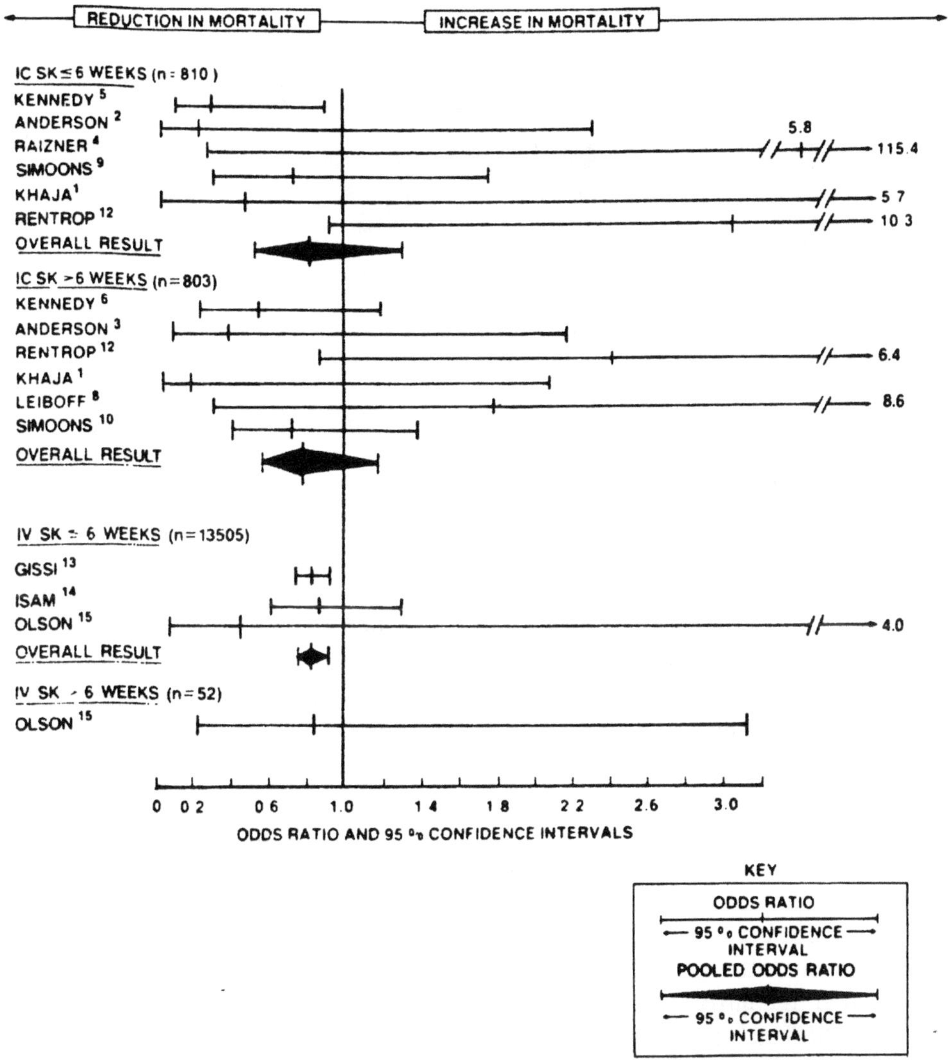

Fig. 1. Pooled analysis of 10 randomized studies ($n = 14335$). To increase comparability among the trials, analysed trials with a clearly defined endpoint of mortality were separated into 2 groups: one with follow-up of 6 weeks or less, and another with more than 6 weeks follow-up. Assessment of mortality was done by calculating pooled odds ratio and 95% confidence interval (by the Mantel-Haenszel methods). When the pooled odds ratio is less than 1.0 the reduction in risk of death is significant

administration of thrombolytic agents, to review survival rates. The studies comprise a total of 14335 patients and are the basis for an evaluation of benefits and risks (Fig. 1). All studies of intravenous and intracoronary streptokinase administration within 3–4 h of the onset of chest pain have demonstrated a significant reduction in hospital mortality (up to 6%) [7, 13]. Failure to demon-

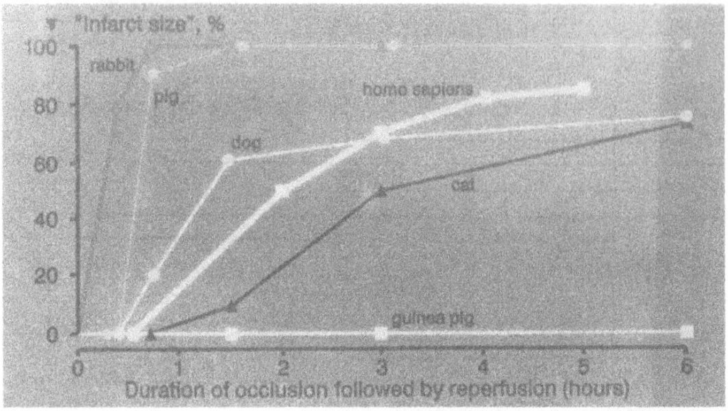

Fig. 2. Duration of occlusion followed by reperfusion in coronary arteries (Schaper W, Eur. Heart J 4 (Suppl D): 73 (1983), Hugenholtz P.G., Texas Heart Institute J 13: 433 (1986)

strate therapeutic effect was associated with too late administration of the thrombolytic agent after the zone of infarction had attained its full extent. The relation between time and extent of myocardial infarction in different species and the relative position of humans here was demonstrated first by Schaper (Fig. 2).

The most important factor in successful treatment is thus early initiation of therapy. When treatment is started early, the recanalization rate is higher, and this provides the possibility of limiting the extent of infarction. The shorter the period of occlusion, the greater is the chance of salvaging ischemic tissue. In other words, limitation of infarction is associated with limited loss of function and with reduced mortality [2, 7, 19]. The GISSI study has demonstrated the relationship between the start of treatment and therapeutic effect most impressively with significantly lower mortality in the streptokinase-treated group compared to controls (only) in the first few hours (Table 1) [21].

It is difficult to demonstrate limitation of functional loss in patients with successful reperfusion. The global ejection fraction is an unsuitable parameter due to the compensatory hyperkinesia found in the noninfarcted region. Thus, analysis of regional wall motion is more useful for estimation of myocardial salvage, but evaluation for functional recovery is affected by timing of the diagnostic procedure and sensitivity of the method for detecting regional abnormalities. In addition, coronary anatomy also determines outcome, so that infarct location, collateral circulation, and the degree of coronary obstruction require consideration [15]. As concerns differences in the possible benefit from recanalization in myocardial infarction at different locations I would argue the recanalization of an occluded vessel is potentially beneficial if ischemic tissue can be preserved from necrosis. On the other hand, significant reductions in infarct size are achieved better in patients with large areas of myocardial involvement than in those with smaller areas of infarction. Moreover, an untreated small

Table 1. Short-term mortality (21 days) in streptokinase-treated and control groups following acute myocardial infarction

Duration of occlusion (h)	Streptokinase	Control	p
	10.7 628/5860	13.0 758/5852	0,0002
<1	8.2% 52/635	15.4% 99/642	0,0001
<3	9.2% 278/3016	12.0% 369/3078	0,0005
>3–6	11,7% 217/1849	14,1% 254/1800	0,03
>6–9	12.6% 87/693	14,1% 93/659	n.s.
>9–12	15,8% 46/292	13.6% 41/302	n.s.

Streptokinase dose: 1.5×10^6 U/100 ml, per hour intravenously. Treatment in control group was determined by attending physician. The category "<1 h" is also included in the category "<3 h." $n = 11712$. (From [21])

inferior infarction may result in practically no loss of function. It may be worth defining which subgroups of patients are more likely to benefit from this therapy. The decision whether to treat or not is facilitated by knowledge of the coronary anatomy.

There remains a question as to whether the short-term reduction in mortality with streptokinase therapy would result in a long-term improvement in survival. Long-term success depends initially on early recanalization, but maintenance of blood flow and prevention of reocclusion and reinfarction are decisive [11, 17]. Reocclusion rates of 10% – 15% within the first few days following recanalization are usual despite administration of anticoagulants. This rate seems to be related to the degree of residual vessel stenosis. The long-term effect of an effective thrombolytic treatment – whether with streptokinase or other agents – depends mainly on the follow-up procedure, which has as its goal the maintenance of restored coronary blood flow by PTCA and/or adjuvant drug to support the healing process of the endothelium to prevent reocclusion or to diminish recurrence of narrowing (Table 2) [4, 8, 12, 23].

As concerns the risk of hemorrhage associated with streptokinase therapy, one can refer to the GISSI study [21], which reflects previous experience with a 10% – 15% incidence of minor bleeding and hematomas and 1% – 2% of major bleeding complications (0% – 8% gastrointestinal hemorrhage and 0.3% intracranial hemorrhage) (Table 3). Immunologic and allergic complications and pyrogen reactions are virtually never encountered and do not exceed 1%.

All thrombolytic agents are associated with hemorrhagic complications when administered in effective doses. This also includes so-called clot-specific agents

Table 2. Studies of short- and long-term effects on mortality of streptokinase (SK) treatment in acute myocardial infarction

Study	Early mortality (30 days)					Late mortality (1 year)		
	Duration of Occlusion (h)	Procedur	SK treatment	Control	p	SK treatment	Control	p
KENNEDY USA, 1985	<12	i.c.	3.7	11,2	0,02	8.2	14,7	0,10 n.s.
SCHMUTZLER Berlin, 1986	< 3	i.v./i.c.	4,9	12.3	<0.05	12,3	16,2	n.s.
SIMOONS NL, 1985	< 4	i.v./i.c.	6.0	12.0	0.03	9.0	16,9	<0.05
V. ESSEN Aachen, 1985	< 8	i.c. + PTCA + Bypass	7,8 3,1 2.6	14,0	<0.05 <0,01	21,2 9.3 6.4	20,0	n.s. <0.01

Table 3. Adverse reactions (AR) to streptokinase treatment (SK) GISSI trial

	AR leading to withdrawal of SK infusion		AR attributed to SK after completion of infusion	
	n	%	*n*	%
Minor bleeds	30	0.5	188	3.2
Major bleeds	0	-	19	0.3
Allergic reactions	99	1.6	42	0.7
Anaphylactic shock	7	0.1	0	-
Hypotension	96	1.6	82	1.4
Shivering and fever	21	0.4	41	0.7
Ventricular arrhythmias	0	-	70	1.2
Stroke	0	-	10	0.2

$n = 5860$
(From [21])

since heparin must be administered concurrently, however, whether this theoretically based demand is essential or not has yet to be established. In view of the development of newer thrombolytic agents one of the unsolved and interesting questions is whether a hemostatic defect is a disadvantage. The agents which produce the greatest effect on hemostasis are those with less clot selectivity and with long half-lives. Simultaneous therapy is not required, and one can frequently wait until recovery begins (at approximately 4 h) before administering heparin.

The longer the half-life, the longer thrombolytic activity persists; this implies longer duration of thrombolytic treatment and more complete dissolution of the coronary thrombus, which is an important consideration in the prevention of reocclusion. Other possible contributions to effective fibrinolysis are a reduction in plasma viscosity, which may improve flow in the microcirculation where plasma skimming may be important, and a possible improvement in collateral flow to the marginal zone of ischemia [16].

Table 4. Advantages and disadvantages of various thrombolytic agents in acute evolving myocardial infarction

Agent	Advantages	Disadvantages
Streptokinase	Effective Least expensive Proved value	Severe hemostatic defect Antigenic Occasional allergic reaction Hypotensive when given too rapidly Least clot selective
Urokinase	Effective Modest clot selectivity Nonantigenic Bolus injection	Moderately severe hemostatic defect Expensive
APSAC	Effective Rapid injection Prolonged action	Severe hemostatic defect Antigenic Occasional allergic reaction Moderately expensive
rt-PA	Effective Activatory nonantigenic Highly clot selective	Moderate hemostatic defect Simultaneous heparin Rx required Short half-life—prolongs Rx Antigens? Probably very expensive
r-Prourokinase	Effective Activatory nonantigenic Highly clot selective	Mild hemostatic defect usual Simultaneous heparin Rx required Very short half-life—prolonged Rx Antigens? Probably very expensive

APSAC, Anisoylated plasminogen-streptokinase activator complex; rt-PA, recombinant tissue-plasminogen activator.

To ascertain the current position of streptokinase in the field of thrombolytic agents we should take into consideration the qualities of the main agents under study (Table 4). Each of these has potential advantages and disadvantages. The advantages of streptokinase therapy outweigh the risks, and streptokinase – properly administered – has maintained its place in the therapeutic armamentarium even after the advent of newer fibrinolytic agents. We consider the combination of intravenous and intracoronary administration with the additional advantages of coronary angiography status to be the ideal treatment regimen, since this provides a recanalization rate of 80% – 90% with the possibility of immediate evaluation of therapeutic result and of the necessity for follow-up treatment [11, 12, 13, 17]. Should logistical considerations preclude this therapeutic strategy, one can still recommend intravenous treatment with streptokinase or acylated [20]. With streptokinase, however, one must bear in mind that – concerning APSAC – in spite of the fast application by rapid injection, the time of onset of effective lysis is prolonged. The main advantages of early treatment may thus be lost. The potential for using prourokinase seems to be limited because it is slow to initial lysis. In combination with urokinase it acts much faster. Clinical experience provides little superiority of tissue-plasminogen activator because it includes selectivity and moderate hemostatic effect [14, 22, 24, 6]. However, an ideal thrombolytic agent, according to Verstraete [25], should be "highly effective, nontoxic, nonimmunogenic, non-antigenic, fibrin-specific, and also able to distinguish the fibrin in a thrombus from that in a hemostatic plug, convenient to administer, probably given in a bolus intravenously (or possibly even intramusculary or subcutaneously) without the need for laboratory monitoring and priced acceptably."

References

1. Boucek RJ, Murphy WP (1960) Segmental perfusion of the coronary arteries with fibrinolysin in man following a myocardial infarction. Am J Cardiol 6:525
2. Braunwald E (1983) Thrombolytic therapy in patients with acute myocardial infarction. Summary and comments. Circulation 68 [Suppl 1]:67 – 69
3. Chazov EJ, Matveeva LS, Mazaev AV, Ruda MY (1975) Intracoronary administration of fibrolysin in myocardial infarction. Therapy-Archiv Kardiolog. Fragen 48:7
4. Erbel R, Pop T, Heinrichs KJ, von Olshausen K, Schuster CJ, Rupprecht HJ, Steuernagel C, Meyer J (1986) Percutaneous transluminal coronary angioplasty after thrombolytic therapy: a prospective controlled randomized trial. J Am Coll Cardiol 8 [3]:485 – 495
5. DeWood MA, Spores J, Notske R et al. (1980) Prevalence of total coronary occlusion during the early hours of transluminal myocardial infarction. N Engl J Med 303:897 – 902
6. Fletcher AP, Alkjaersig N, Smyrniotis FE, Sherry S (1958) The treatment of patients suffering from early myocardial infarction by massive and prolonged streptokinase therapy. Tr Assoc Am Physicians 71:287
7. Hugenholtz PG (1987) Acute coronary artery obstruction in myocardial infarction: overview of thrombolytic therapy. J Am Coll Cardiol 9 [6]:1375 – 1384
8. Miller HI, Almagor J, Keren G, Chernilas J, Roth A, Eschar Y, Shapira I, Shagorodsky B, Berenfeld D, Laniado S (1987) Early intervention in acute myocardial infarction: significance for myocardial salvage of immediate intravenous streptokinase therapy followed by coronary angioplasty. J Am Coll Cardiol 9 [3]:608 – 614
9. Patel B, Kloner RA (1987) Analysis of reported randomized trials of streptokinase therapy for acute myocardial infarction in the 1980s. Am J Cardiol 59:501 – 504
10. Rentrop P, De Vivie ER, Karsch KR, et al. (1978) Acute coronary occlusion with impending infarction as an angiographic complication relieved by a guide wire recanalization. Clin Cardiol 1:101 – 107
11. Rutsch W, Jatzkewitz A, Schartl M, Eichstädt H, Schmutzler H (1985) One-year

follow-up after thrombolytic therapy in acute myocardial infarction. Eur Heart J 6:187–192

12. Rutsch W, Schartl M, Schmutzler H (1986) Percutaneous transluminal angioplasty in acute myocardial infarction with and without prior systemic fibrinolytic therapy. In: Höfling B (ed) Current problems in PTCA. Steinkopff, Darmstadt
13. Rutsch W, Schmutzler H (1986) Intracoronary thrombolysis: organizational prerequisites, technique, and results. Cardiovasc Intervent Radiol 9:245–252
14. Rutsch W, Schartl M, Schmutzler H (1987) Die Europäischen rt-PA-Studien beim akuten Myokardinfarkt. In: De Bono DP, Bronchier ML, Hugenholtz P, Kübler W, Verstraete M (eds) Thrombolytische Therapie des akuten Herzinfarktes. Springer, Berlin Heidelberg New York, p 75
15. Sheehan FH (1987) Determinants of improved left ventricular function after thrombolytic therapy in acute myocardial infarction. J Am Coll Cardiol 9 [4]:937 to 944
16. Sherry S (1987) Recombinant tissue plasminogen activator (rt-PA): Is it the thrombolytic agent of choice for an evolving acute myocardial infarction? Am J Cardiol 59:984–989
17. Schmutzler H, Rutsch W, Schartl M, Eichstädt H, Jatzkewitz A (1986) Langzeitergebnisse nach Therapie mit Streptokinase bei Myokardinfarkt. Herz 11 [1]:1–8
18. Schmutzler R, Heckner F, Körtge P, van Deloo J, Pezold FA, Poliwoda H, Praetorius TF, Zekorn D (1966) Zur thrombolytischen Therapie des frischen Herzinfarktes. (I. deutsch-schweizerische Studie) Dtsch Med Wochenschr 91:581
19. The TIMI Study Group (1985) Special report. The thrombolysis in myocardial infarction (TIMI) trial. N Engl J Med:932–936
20. Timmis AD, Griffin B, Crick JCP, Sowton E (1987) Anisoylated plasminogen streptokinase activator complex in acute myocardial infarction: a placebo-controlled arteriographic coronary recanalization study. J Am Coll Cardiol 10 [1]:205–210
21. Tognoni F, Rovelli F et al. for GISSI (Gruppo Italiano per lo Studio della streptochinasi nell'infarcto myocardio) (1986) Effectiveness of intravenous thrombolytic therapy in acute myocardial infarction. Lancet I:397–402
22. Topol EJ, Morris DC, Smalling RW, Schumacher RR, Taylor CR, Nishikawa A, Liberman HA, Collen D, Tufte ME, Grossbard EB, O'Neill WW (1987) A multicenter, randomized, placebo-controlled trial of a new form of intravenous recombinant tissue-plasminogen activator (activase) in acute myocardial infarction. J Am Coll Cardiol 9:1205–1213
23. Topol EJ, Califf RM, George BS, Kereiakes DJ, Abbottsmith CW, Candela RJ, Lee KL, Pitt B, Stack RS, O'Neill WW (1987) A randomized trial of immediate versus delayed elective angioplasty after intravenous tissue plasminogen activator in acute myocardial infarction. N Engl J Med 10 [317]:581–588
24. Verstraete M, Bernard R, Bory M, et al. (1985) Randomised trial of intravenous recombinant tissue-type plasminogen activator versus intravenous streptokinase in acute myocardial infarction. Lancet I:842–847
25. Verstraete M, Arnold AER, Brower RW, Collen D, de Bono DP, de Zwaan C, Erbel R, Hillis WS, Lennane RJ, Lubsen J, Mathey D, Reid DS, Rutsch W, Schartl M, Schofer J, Serruys PW, Simoons ML, Uebis R, Vahanian A, Verheugt FA, von Essen R (1987) Acute coronary thrombolysis with recombinant human tissue-type plasminogen activator: initial patency and influence of maintained infusion on reocclusion rate. Am J Cardiol 60:231–237

Results from ISAM and GISSI

R. Schröder

The Intravenous Streptokinase in Acute Myocardial Infarction Trial (ISAM) was a double-blind placebo-controlled study. The recruitment period was from March 1982 to March 1985. Within 6 h after the onset of symptoms of myocardial infarction (MI), 1741 patients (aged up to 75 years) were randomly assigned either to a 1-h intravenous infusion of 1.5×10^6 U streptokinase (STK) or to placebo [1]. The Gruppo Italiano per lo Studio Della Streptochinasi Nell'Infarto Miocardico (GISSI) was an open controlled trial. A total of 11806 patients (without age limit) within 12 h of the onset of MI symptoms were randomly assigned either to a 1-h intravenous infusion of 1.5×10^6 U STK or to conventional treatment [2].

In the ISAM trial, limitation of infarct size was confirmed by three independent parameters:

1. Significantly smaller integrated area under the serum CK-MB and CK-enzyme activity curves.
2. Reduced loss of R wave potentials and less development of new Q waves. There was an increasing difference between STK and placebo groups up to 7 months after MI.
3. Higher global and regional ejection fraction in angiograms performed 3–4 weeks after MI.

The differences between the STK group and the placebo group were highly significant overall and for those treated within 3 h after symptom onset. In patients treated within 3–6 h after onset of MI there was only a trend to a lower infarct size in the STK group.

In-Hospital Mortality. In patients treated within 3 h of symptom onset in ISAM, there was a difference of 20% in favor of STK. In those treated 3–6 h after symptom onset, the difference was 11%. The differences between the two treatment groups were not statistically significant. The in-hospital mortality in the placebo group was lower than expected – only 7.1%.

In the GISSI study, the difference in those treated within 3 h after symptom onset was 23% and in those treated between 3–6 h 17% in favor of STK. The difference in the early-treated patients was highly significant, in those treated at 3–6 h marginally significant ($p = 0.03$). A difference of 47% in favor of STK was observed in the 1277 patients treated within 1 h from symptom onset.

The in-hospital mortality in the control group in GISSI (13%) was higher than in ISAM. This might in part be explained by the fact that in GISSI more older patients were included who had a very high mortality rate (33.1% in 623 placebo patients older than 75 years of age). For younger patients the differences in mortality between the two studies were not so striking: in ISAM patients ⩽69 years of age 5.1% for STK and 6.6% for placebo, and in GISSI in patients ⩽65 years of age for STK 5.7% and 7.7% for placebo.

What is the reduction in mortality due to? Most probably, the limitation of infarct size is responsible for the reduction of mortality. This suggestion is supported by the fact that the differences in mortality are caused almost exclusively by a lower incidence of death from cardiac failure in the STK group. In both studies, more than 50% of the in-hospital deaths were due to pump failure. In ISAM, the corresponding figure was 2.9% in the STK group and 4.0% in the placebo group. In GISSI, cardiac failure was the cause of death in 5.6% of STK and 6.7% of control patients.

Serious Side-Effects. Bleedings occurred in ISAM in 5.9% of patients given STK versus 1.5% in those given placebo. In GISSI, serious bleedings occurred in 0.3% of STK patients. What we are most concerned about are cerebral bleedings. Cerebral hemorrhage was the cause of death in 2 of 859 (0.23%) in ISAM, and in GISSI in 5 of 5860 (0.09%) patients treated with STK. In the placebo and control groups, none of the patients had cerebral hemorrhage.

Long-Term Mortality. It has been apparent in all postinfarction studies that the degree of left ventricular dysfunction at hospital discharge has a considerable influence on long-term mortality in patients with acute MI. Since the limitation of infarct size had been demonstrated for STK-treated patients, an increasingly favorable long-term outcome as compared with non-treated patients could have been anticipated. However, in both studies after hospital discharge the mortality rates in the two respective treatment groups were similar (i.e., benefit obtained in hospital was in general maintained during long-term follow-up – but without further improvement in STK-treated patients). At an average follow-up time of 31 months, in ISAM the proportion of patients who died was 17.6% in the STK group and 18.6% in the placebo group [3]. In GISSI, the 1-year mortality rate was 19% in the STK group and 21.2% in the control group [4]. The mortality after hospital discharge at an average follow-up time of 31 months in those treated within 3 h from symptom onset in ISAM was 10.4% for those given STK versus 11.8% for those given placebo. In those in whom treatment was started 3–6 h after onset of symptoms, the corresponding figures were 14.1% versus 12.3%. In GISSI, the 1-year mortality after hospital discharge in those treated within 3 h was 7.4% in STK-treated patients versus 7.1% control patients. In those in whom treatment was started 3–6 h after the onset of symptoms, the corresponding figures were 8.8% versus 9.5%. A trend to a more favorable outcome after hospital discharge, however, was noted in those treated within 1 h of the onset of symptoms (5.7% versus 8.1% given placebo).

Reinfarction. In ISAM, the 7-month probability of reinfarction in patients assigned to STK (7.2%) was significantly higher than that in those assigned to placebo (4.5%). The 6-month nonfatal reinfarction rate in GISSI was 7.5% in STK and 4.4% in placebo patients. Thus, like in other thrombolysis trials, the reinfarction rates were significantly higher in those treated as compared with those without thrombolytic therapy.

Potential Clinical Instability in Streptokinase-Treated Patients. Although there is a favorable long-term outcome for many patients, others have an increased risk of dying. Death from reinfarction is only the tip of the iceberg. The main ischemic event leading to death after hospital discharge from acute MI is sudden death. Subgroup mortality analysis of data from the ISAM trial showed that an increased risk of dying after hospital discharge cumulated in patients with anterior MI who had earliest reperfusion according to the CK-MB peaking $\leqslant 9$ h after start of treatment [5]. Duration of ischemia is the major determinant of infarct size. Logically, the earliest reperfusion of an infarct-related coronary artery should provide the greatest potential for salvage of ischemic but nonnecrotic fractions of at-risk myocardium. Without additional mechanical revascularization, such as percutaneous transluminal coronary angioplasty (PTCA) in patients with proximal obstructions involving 1 or 3 arteries and bypass surgery in those with more extensive lesions, after hospital discharge STK-treated patients apparently are in an unstable situation, with greater vulnerability to recurrent fatal infarction and sudden death.

Conclusion. In addition to ISAM and GISSI, preliminary data from the Second International Study of Infarct Survival (ISIS-2) were disclosed in February 1987 [6]. Among the nearly 4000 patients randomized within 4 h after symptom onset either to 1.5×10^6 U STK intravenously or to placebo, mortality was significantly reduced in STK-treated patients (from about 12% among placebo patients to about 8% among those given STK). Thus, there is proof beyond reasonable doubt that intravenous STK administered within the first 4–6 h of acute myocardial infarction is effective in reducing in-hospital mortality. During long-term follow-up this beneficial effect of mortality is in general maintained. However, an increasingly favorable outcome for STK-treated patients is lacking. After successful thrombolytic therapy in acute MI, patients are potentially unstable, with greater vulnerability to recurrent MI and sudden death [3, 5]. In certain patients reperfusion has only "bought time." Apparently, in all suitable patients additional mechanical revascularisation is required. However, prospective studies are needed to ascertain the true impact of such "definitive" treatment.

General Recommendations. Intravenous thrombolysis within the first 4–6 h after onset of acute MI is recommended for all patients with clinical symptoms of acute MI and significant persistent ST-segment elevation. As a personal statement, based on nonrandomized follow-up studies I would add: (a) angiography within the first 5 – 10 days and (b) PTCA (or CABG) in all suitable patients regardless of actual symptoms.

References

1. The ISAM Study Group (1986) A prospective trial of intravenous streptokinase in acute myocardial infarction (ISAM). Mortality, morbidity, and infarct size at 21 days. N Engl J Med 314:1465 – 1471
2. Gruppo Italiano per lo Studio della Streptochinasi nell'Infarto Miocardico (GISSI) (1986) Effectiveness of intravenous thrombolytic treatment in acute myocardial infarction. Lancet I:397 – 401
3. Schröder R, Neuhaus KL, Leizorovicz A, Linderer T, Tebbe U, for the ISAM Study Group (1987) A prospective placebo-controlled double-blind multicenter trial of intravenous streptokinase in acute myocardial infarction (ISAM): long-term mortality and morbidity. JACC 9:197 – 203
4. Gruppo Italiano per lo Studio della Streptochinasi nell'Infarto Miocardico (GISSI) (1987) In-hospital results and one-year follow-up of GISSI trial. G Ital Cardiol 17 [1]:20 – 29
5. Schröder R, Neuhaus KL, Linderer T, Leizorovicz A, Wegscheider K, Tebbe U, for the ISAM Study Group (1987) Risk of death from recurrent ischemic events after intravenous streptokinase in acute myocardial infarction: results from the ISAM-study. Circulation 76 [II]:44 – 51
6. ISIS Steering Committee (1987) Intravenous streptokinase given within 0 – 4 hours of onset of myocardial infarction reduced mortality in ISIS-2. Lancet I:502

Prehospital Thrombolysis in Acute Myocardial Infarction: The Jerusalem Experience*

M.S. Gotsman, A.T. Weiss, D. Sapoznikov, D. Applebaum, S. Rosenheck, C. Lotan, and S. Welber

Acute myocardial infarction is usually a consequence of thrombotic occlusion of a coronary artery [1–4]. Myocardial necrosis starts 20 min after abrupt occlusion of the coronary artery and spreads as a wave front from endocardium to epicardium. Irreversible damage is complete after 6 h, but most of the necrosis has occurred within 1 h [5, 6]. Thrombolytic therapy can reopen 40%–90% of obstructed arteries [7–9]. If thrombolytic therapy is to be successful and salvage myocardium, it must be applied early and quickly, often within the 1st h after the onset of chest pain [10–13].

We have shown that myocardial infarction size increases progressively from the initial time of pain onset until streptokinase administration, and that a delay of 2 h is the watershed point between myocardial survival and important necrosis. Two-thirds of patients treated within 2 h have small infarcts whereas all patients treated after 2 hours have large ones (Fig. 1) [11, 13, 14]. We have also shown that infarct size is related to the total duration of pain – from pain onset until pain is relieved suddenly or decreases in intensity. This period corresponds to the total duration of ischemia – the delay until the thrombolytic drug is administered and then a further delay while the chemical reaction initiates clot lysis and reperfusion occurs in the coronary artery. The crucial time interval for myocardial salvage appears to be 3.5 h (Fig. 2). And, finally, we have demonstrated regarding residual stenosis in the infarct-related coronary artery that patients with less than 75% residual stenosis have small infarcts whereas patients with more than 75% stenosis have larger infarcts. This applies only to patients in whom therapy is started within 2 h of pain onset. Patients who receive delayed treatment (over than 2 h) have irreversible myocardial necrosis, and adequate reperfusion has little influence on infarct size (Fig. 3).

This paper describes a strategy of prehospital thrombolysis to demonstrate how the time interval until the onset of treatment can be reduced, and how this salvages myocardium. It examines short-term mortality, the incidence of complications, and the amount of myocardial salvage in a consecutive group of 200 patients and the long-term prognosis in the first 88 patients followed for a period of 18 months.

---

* Financial support was received from the Rita and Max Altura Memorial Fund, Los Angeles, California, USA.

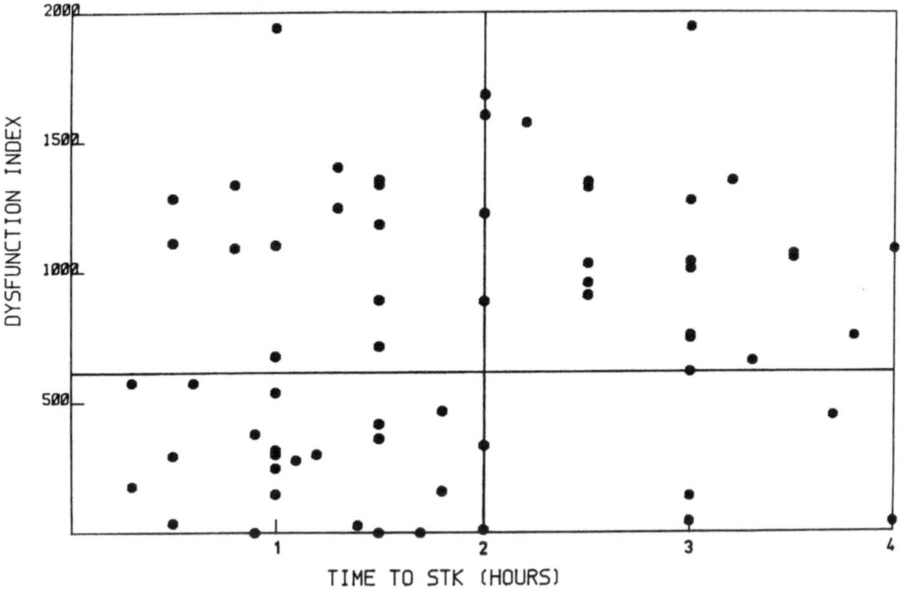

Fig. 1. Comparison of time from initial pain onset until streptokinase administration and dysfunction index. Myocardial infarction increases with the delay until treatment, and a delay of 2 h is the watershed point between myocardial survival and important necrosis. Two-thirds of patients treated within 2 h have small infarcts, whereas all the patients treated after 2 h have large ones

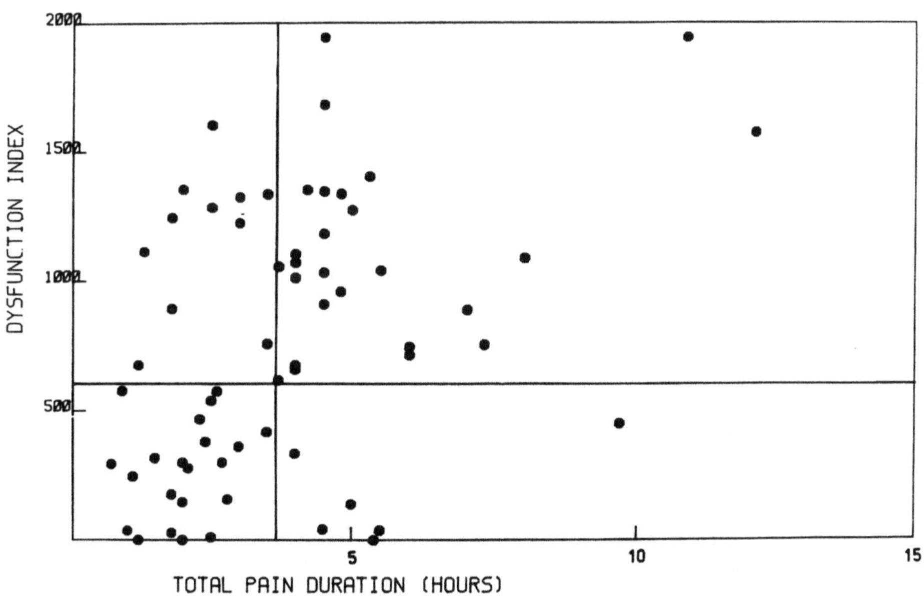

Fig. 2. Relationship between infarct size (dysfunction index) and the total duration of pain, from pain onset until pain is relieved suddenly or decreases in intensity. Infarct size is related to the total duration of pain, and 3.5 h appears to be the crucial time interval for myocardial salvage

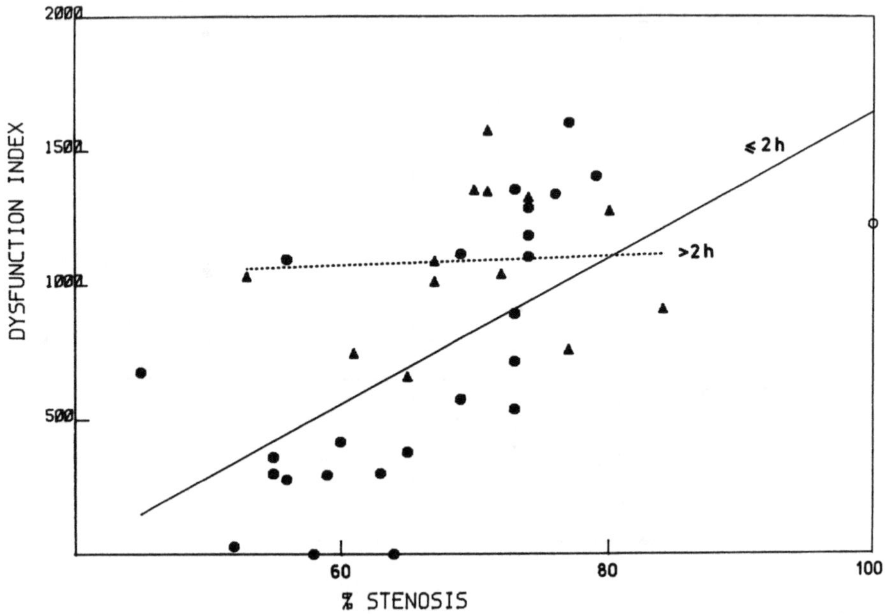

Fig. 3. Relationship between infarct size and residual stenosis in the infarct related coronary artery. Residual stenosis is an important determinant of myocardial reperfusion and residual infarct size. Patients treated in less than 2 h are shown as *solid circles,* and those treated after 2 h as *solid triangles.* The *solid regression line* shows that there is a linear relationship between infarct size and residual stenosis in patients treated in less than 2 h. The *dotted line* is the regression line of patients treated after 2 h and shows that these patients had developed their infarct, and that there was no relationship to residual stenosis

Physician-Operated Mobile Intensive Care Unit

A physician-operated mobile intensive care unit (MICU) was first established in 1972, and the city population is aware of the importance of the ambulance in acute myocardial infarction, sudden collapse, motor vehicle accidents, and mass casualties. The MICU ambulance is equipped with facilities for diagnosis, resuscitation, and management. This includes a 12-lead single-channel electrocardiogram, a portable monitor-defibrillator-external pacemaker and all drugs for management and resuscitation. A trained emergency physician experienced in cardiovascular diagnosis supervises two paramedical assistants and an ambulance driver who is also trained in resuscitation. A 24-h physician cover is available, and the physicians work in two shifts. The city is small and compact and has excellent arterial highways. Although the roads are congested with heavy traffic, particularly at rush hour, the ambulance has a fast response time. The mean arrival time after ambulance call is 6 min, and once the unit has arrived at the patient's home, it can diagnose myocardial infarction, set up intensive coronary care, monitor and treat all arrhythmias, and administer thrombolytic drugs (Fig. 1). The unit was established to serve as a mobile diagnostic-therapeutic care unit to treat patients in the street or at home and as a monitored transport system. Its value in resuscitation and immediate care has been established [15].

Patient Selection and Method of Prehospital Administration of Thrombolytic Drug Therapy

Consecutive patients were included in the study if they had:

1. Ischemic chest pain of less than 4-h duration.
2. ST segment elevation of >2 mm in at least two leads.
3. No response to sublingual vasodilators.

Patients were excluded if they were older than 75 years, had hypertension (>180/100 mm Hg) and a bleeding tendency, a peptic ulcer, or a previous cerebrovascular accident.

One-quarter of the patients received treatment at home, and three-fourths were treated routinely in the emergency room. The ambulance (MICU) is activated by a patient- or family-initiated call to the central ambulance station. The physician takes the clinical history, makes a careful physical examination, and then records a routine 12-lead ECG. If the patient has classical anginal chest pain, with or without acute ischemia on the ECG, he is given sublingual isorbide dinitrate (5 ml) to assess the response of the chest pain, and the ECG is repeated after a further 10–15 min, to exclude coronary artery spasm. The presence of classical ST segment elevation with persistent chest pain is an indication of early acute myocardial infarction. Diagnosis and triage are made at home or the site of the event. ECG monitoring to detect arrhythmias is started, and appropriate treatment given. Two intravenous lines are placed: one for infusion and a second for blood withdrawal. The patient receives 500 mg intravenous hydrocortisone to prevent allergic reactions and then intravenous streptokinase, 750×10^3 U in initial bolus of 250×10^3 U followed by a slow infusion over 30 min to prevent hypotensive reactions. Coronary care is started in the patient's home or at his place of work, and the patient is then transferred leisurely to the intensive care unit which had been warned by radio of patient arrival. In hospital, the emergency room is by-passed and the patient admitted directly to the coronary care unit. Treatment then includes standard routine coronary care and intravenous heparin (approximately 300 mg per day), titrated to maintain the partial thromboplastin time (PTT) at twice normal value.

Left ventricular function and coronary artery angiography are performed on day 6. The maximum percentage diameter stenosis of the infarct related coronary artery in any view is used for analysis.

Left ventricular function and size of the infarct in the left ventricle are assessed from:

1. The ECG using the QRS score of Selvester et al. [16].
2. Left ventricular ejection fraction measured from the contrast ventriculogram in the right anterior oblique position.
3. Left ventricular infarct-related regional ejection fraction [17, 18].
4. Left ventricular dysfunction index to determine the size and extent of the poorly contractile segment of the left ventricle [19].

Results

A total of 200 consecutive patients were treated. Their mean age was 57 ± 11 years; 172 were men and 28 were women. The mean time delay to streptokinase administration was 1.3 ± 0.5 h. Streptokinase was administered to 143 patients in less than 2 h and to 57 in 2–4 h. Of the 200 patients, 48 received streptokinase at home and 152 in hospital. Patients who received streptokinase at home did so 1.1 ± 0.6 h after pain onset and those in hospital 2.0 ± 0.9 h. For 163 patients it was the first infarct, and for 106 patients the infarct was anterior.

On average, patients waited 33 ± 18 min from the onset of pain to MICU (ambulance) call. The MICU response time was 5 ± 3 min. The attending physician took 25 min to make the diagnosis, exclude contraindications, place the intravenous lines, and administer streptokinase. The total delay to streptokinase administration was 63 min (Fig. 4).

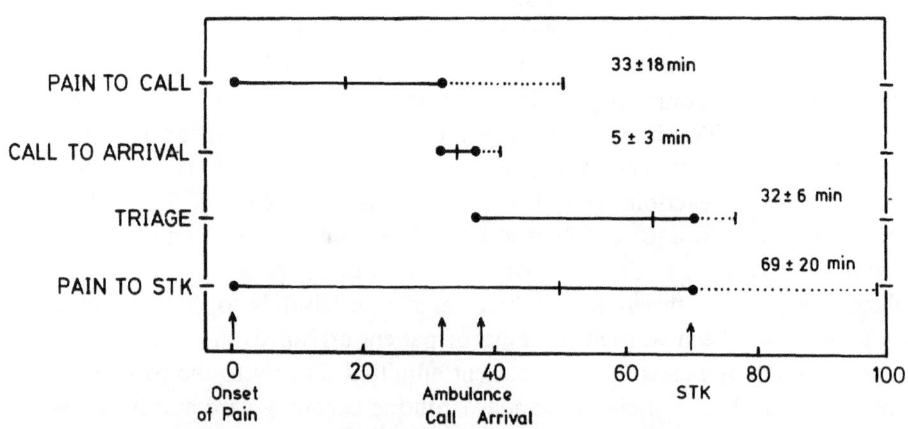

Fig. 4. Delay times for the administration of streptokinase using out-of-hospital treatment and a medical intensive care unit (MICU). Times in minutes are shown on *horizontal axis*. The time delay from pain onset to MICU alert is 33 ± 18 min. MICU travel time to the patient is 5 ± 3 min. The physician requires 25 ± 10 min to take a history, perform a physical examination and 12-lead ECG, administer vasodilators, repeat the ECG, set up two intravenous lines, and administer the thrombolytic drug. The total delay time is 63 ± 19 min. (Reprinted with permission from *Chest*)

Six patients died in hospital. Two had intracerebral hemorrhage; two others had early cardiogenic shock, and it is uncertain whether the thrombolytic therapy was effective. Two died later of cardiogenic shock from recurrent infarction. There were six late deaths during the first 18 months of follow-up: three died of reocclusion of the artery after satisfactory reperfusion or in relation to mechanical interventions (PTCA or CABG).

Hemorrhage occurred in 19 patients. Major hemorrhage occurred in four: intracerebral in two, major gastrointestinal in one, and severe neck swelling from an intravenous line placed in the internal jugular vein in one. Hemorrhage was minor in 15. None of these patients was treated in the prehospital phase. Arrhythmias were also common. Ventricular fibrillation occurred in 17, usually before streptokinase was administered and most commonly with a large infarction. Ventricular tachycardia occurred in 48 patients and was usually a reperfusion arrhythmia. Complete heart block occurred in six patients and usually cleared after streptokinase administration.

Of the 200 patients, 186 had an angiogram on day 6, and in 14 the patients either died or refused angiography. The patency rate of the infarct-related coronary artery in these patients was 85%. Of the 62 patients who underwent an early PTCA at the time of the first angiogram, 38 had a routine second angiogram (after 4 months), and in 21 of these a delayed PTCA was performed.

Myocardial Salvage

Table 1 compares the patients treated before and after admission to hospital. There was no difference in the age, sex, infarct number, infarct site, and infarct-related coronary artery patency rate or CPK values between the two groups. When patients with a first anterior infarct were compared, infarct size was much smaller if the patient was treated at home. The differences are summarized in Table 2. Approximately one-fourth of the infarct was prevented and myocardium salvaged if the patient was treated in hospital, and about one-half if the patient was treated at home. Nonetheless, all the patients had an important infarct. The comparison of ECG score, ejection fraction, regional ejection fraction, and dysfunction index are shown graphically in Fig. 5, which compares infarct size in patients treated at home, those treated in hospital and those with an established anterior myocardial infarct.

The 18-month follow-up in the first 88 patients studied showed that they had important residual symptoms. Ten patients had severe residual angina pectoris (grade 3 or 4) and nine were short of breath (grade 3 or 4). Twenty-two had been hospitalized a second time; this was for angina pectoris (11 cases), recurrent infarction (2), congestive cardiac failure (5), and arrhythmia (4). Forty-three required a mechanical intervention: 10 had coronary artery bypass grafting (CABG), 13 underwent an early PTCA, and 20 a delayed PTCA. The residual symptoms of angina pectoris or shortness of breath were related to the severity of

Table 1. Comparison of Home and Hospital Streptokinase Treatment

	Home	Hospital
Number of patients	48	152
Age	57 ± 10	56 ± 11
Men	40	121
Number of first anterior infarcts	21	84
Number of first inferior infarcts	27	68
Patent IRCA	37	117
Time to STK (h)	1.1 ± 0.6	2.0 ± 0.9**
Total pain duration (h)	3.0 ± 1.8	3.7 ± 2.1*
QRS Score	5.0 ± 3.5	6.7 ± 4.5*
LVEF	61 ± 12	56 ± 14*
IRREF	49 ± 24	47 ± 22
DI	506 ± 524	713 ± 528*
CPKr	1503 ± 1246	1676 ± 1267

STK, Streptokinase; IRCA, Infarct-related coronary artery; LVEF, left ventricular ejection fraction; IRREF, Infarct-related regional ejection fraction; DI, Dysfunction index; CPKr, Cumulative CPK release; QRS, score EKG scoring (Selvester et al. [16]).

* $p<0.05$.

** $p<0.001$.

Table 2. Comparison of Home and Hospital Treatment with Streptokinase (First Anterior Infarct with Patent Artery) Compared to Patients with a Classical Anterior Infarction

	Home	Hospital	Classical anterior infarction
Number of patients	17	48	16
Age (years)	58 ± 8	58 ± 12	48 ± 8
Men	16	39	14
Number of first anterior infarcts	17	48	
Patent IRCA	17	48	
Time to STK (h)	1.2 ± 0.6	2.1 ± 1.0*	
Total pain duration (h)	3.2 ± 2.4	4.0 ± 2.2	
QRS score	5.4 ± 3.4	8.5 ± 4.7*	13 ± 12.7
LVEF	60 ± 12	53 ± 14	46 ± 12
IRREF	55 ± 24	45 ± 21	36 ± 23
DI	602 ± 600	812 ± 509	1285 ± 572
CPKr	1612 ± 1740	1829 ± 1270	

IRCA, Infarct-related coronary artery; STK, Streptokinase; QRS score, EKG scoring (Selvester et al. [16]); LVEF, Left ventricular ejection fraction; IRREF, Infarct-related regional ejection fraction; DI, Dysfunction index.

* $p<0.05$.

** $p<0.001$.

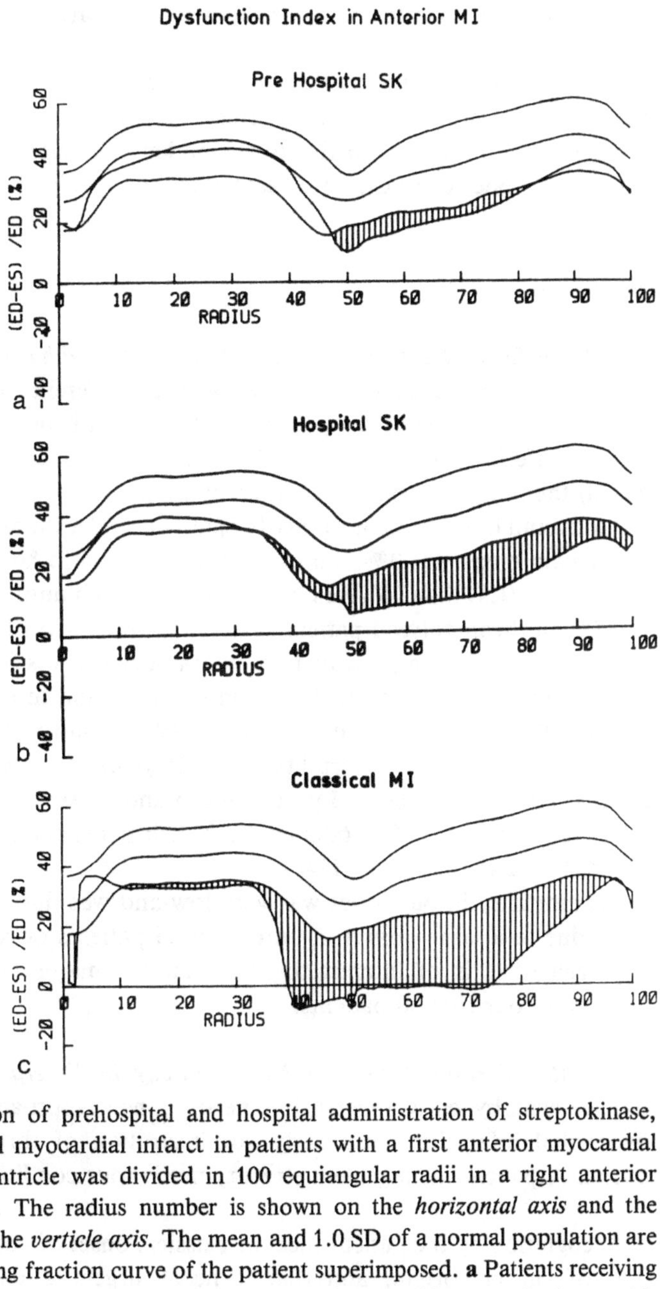

Fig. 5a–c. Comparison of prehospital and hospital administration of streptokinase, compared to a classical myocardial infarct in patients with a first anterior myocardial infarction. The left ventricle was divided in 100 equiangular radii in a right anterior oblique cineangiogram. The radius number is shown on the *horizontal axis* and the shortening fraction on the *verticle axis*. The mean and 1.0 SD of a normal population are shown and the shortening fraction curve of the patient superimposed. **a** Patients receiving prehospital streptokinase. **b** Patients receiving hospital streptokinase. **c** Patients with classical anterior myocardial infarction. *Hatched area* shows infarct size. Infarct size was very small in patients treated at home and moderate in patients treated in hospital

the residual stenosis in the infarct-related coronary artery or the underlying myocardial dysfunction.

In a nonselected group of 30 patients studied twice, the proportion stenosis in the patent infarct-related coronary artery increased from 68% ± 17% at 6 days to 76% ± 17% at 4 months. In five of the patients the artery had obstructed completely; only one reocclusion was associated with a significant clinical episode.

Discussion

Early Reperfusion Reduces In-Hospital Mortality and has Few Complications. It is difficult to compare mortality rates between different studies since the results depend on (a) the age of the patients, (b) the site of the infarcts (anterior compared to inferior and lateral infarctions), (c) the number of previous infarctions and (d) the time to thrombolytic therapy [15].

Our overall in-hospital mortality for patients under the age of 75 treated within 4 h of pain onset was 3%. This corresponds to an in-hospital mortality in the ISAM study (less than 75 years old and less than 6 h until thrombolytic therapy) of 6.3% in thrombolyzed patients and 7.1% in controls [20, 21]. In the GISSI study, the mortality in patients treated in under 1 h was 8.1% in streptokinase-treated patients compared to 15.3% in controls; and in patients treated in less than 3 h, 9.3% in treated patients and 11.9% in controls [22, 23]. Age was also very important since the mortality under 65 years was 5.6% in treated patients and 7.3% in controls; 66 – 75 years, 16.8% and 17.3%; and over 75 years, 29% and 32%, respectively. Schröder et al., in their patients treated in the prehospital period, had a 4% mortality [24].

The mortality in our series was very low and was due mainly to cardiogenic shock due to a large infarct in unreperfused patients or to major intracerebral hemorrhage. It is of interest to note that the major hemorrhagic problems occurred in our first 50 patients.

Prehospital Thrombolysis is a New Strategy in Emergency Coronary Care. Management by early reperfusion needs a new approach to handling acute myocardial infarction since early administration of thrombolytic therapy is crucial. A patient management strategy needs four conditions.

1. Recognition by the patient that the classical onset of abrupt severe chest pain is of cardiac origin, and that it needs urgent attention, diagnosis, and treatment.
2. A therapeutic team who can perform early thrombolytic therapy [11, 14, 15, 24, 25, 26].
3. Simple clinical and ECG methods to diagnose the earliest stages of myocardial infarction.
4. The availability of cheap, safe, and rapidly acting thrombolytic drugs.

The ENIM study conducted in France between November 1985 and 1986 showed that the mean delay between the onset of symptoms and hospitalization was 9 h 53 min. This consisted of a patient delay of 4 h 44 min and a physician and transfer delay of 5 h 9 min. They examined a series of 1105 patients to determine who might be a potential candidate for thrombolytic therapy. Of these, 414 patients were aged under 65 years without a contraindication to thrombolytic therapy, 205 were hospitalized within 6 h, and only 170 were hospitalized within 6 h in a CCU or ICU. This means that only 15.4% of the patients were eligible for thrombolytic therapy.

Medical Education – The Patient or Bystander Must Alert the MICU. The general population needs mass reeducation about the significance of chest pain and its relationship to acute myocardial infarction, since the nature of their awareness and reaction will determine their response [15].

In about 60% of patients, the chest pain has a sudden and abrupt onset and builds in a crescendo, with excruciating discomfort, sweating, nausea, and vomiting. Usually the patient, his family, or fellow workers recognize the impending myocardial infarction, apply first aid measures and call for medical assistance. In other patients, pain occurs in waves: appears, disappears, and then reappears – corresponding to plaque rupture, thrombus formation with partial occlusion of the vessel, and then reperfusion by mechanical dissolution of the clot by the flowing blood or spontaneous fibrinolysis. After several waves the vessel closes completely and severe established pain follows. The patient's threshold and response to pain varies, and this determines his subsequent behavior. Patients with a low pain threshold or anxious relatives call the medical team early. Stoic patients, or those who deny their illness, often wait for hours before calling for medical aid. Patient response time is so variable that, if this delay is to be decreased, there is the need for intensive education of the local population: about the nature and pathogenesis of myocardial infarction, its clinical presentation, and the potential for myocardial salvage if early thrombolytic therapy is administered. Education can be undertaken in schools and through training classes but the press and television are much more effective.

Physician Reeducation. Physician reaction depends on the stage at which the patient calls for medical care. It is related to the nature of the chest pain and the initial ECG. The latter may be normal or temporarily abnormal and return to normal and only in the later stages ST segment elevation becomes apparent.

The Physician-Operated Mobile Intensive Care Unit. Many cities have intensive care ambulances which respond rapidly to patient alert calls. They aim to provide immediate first aid for victims of acute myocardial infarction, diagnose and manage out-of-hospital arrhythmias, and supply urgent transport with ECG monitoring to the nearest hospital with a coronary care unit.

We elected to provide physician care in 1972, initially by an intern rotating through our coronary care unit and later by a dedicated trained physician. The response to ambulance alert is rapid, and the delay to treatment delivery is remarkably shortened. The initial response is made by a trained medical team with facilities for resuscitation, monitoring, diagnosis of myocardial infarction, and the administration of intravenous thrombolytic therapy. Similar facilities have been provided in Paris, Creteil, Antwerp, and Berlin [24, 25, 26].

Herve et al. in Creteil have shown that the ambulance can save 35 min in the administration of thrombolytic therapy [26]. Their average time from pain onset until SAMU (MICU) call was 54 min; MICU arrival time was 13 min; triage, diagnosis, and treatment at home needed 54 min; and ICU transfer time a further 31 min. The time delay from pain onset to the injection of the thrombolytic drug was 120 min. In a control group of patients treated in hospital, an extra 35 min was needed in the emergency room for the physician to respond, make an ECG, and give treatment [26].

Villemante et al. in Paris, showed that in-home thrombolysis could be given within 135 min [25]. This consisted of a 77-min delay until ambulance call, 9-min until the ambulance arrived, and a further 49-min delay for diagnosis and treatment at home. Patients treated in the ICU also waited 77 min to call the ambulance, ambulance arrival time was 9 min, physician delay in diagnosis was 43 min at home, transport time was 17 min, and a further 63 min was lost in the emergency room. The time interval for ICU management with thrombolytic therapy was 198 min. At-home thrombolysis saved 74 min. The Berlin Group showed a time saving of 46 min [24].

Nonphysician-operated ambulances have a short response time, but lack of a physician presence and medicolegal ethical problems – as to whether a paramedic can make a diagnosis and administer treatment – introduces potential difficulties. Numerous computer-aided ECG or telephone transmission systems have been described and are under trial.

Early response in the emergency room is the simpliest solution, but unfortunately experience has shown that few emergency room physicians attend to the patients with sufficient alacrity and speed. They cannot provide the undivided attention given by the physician in the MICU who treats a single patient and does not have the distraction of a busy emergency room. Moreover, the emergency room physician is a generalist who must call an on-duty internal medicine or cardiology resident to make the initial diagnosis and give treatment. Nonetheless, where physician-operated MICUs are not available, a crash emergency room alarm system is essential. The attending nurse and orderly should recognize impending myocardial infarction and call the physician immediately; the physician should give the patient his immediate attention and then administer intravenous streptokinase or another thrombolytic drug if he fulfills the criteria for early myocardial infarction.

Prehospital Thrombolysis is Cost-Effective. Vermeer et al. have shown how intravenously administered thrombolysis reduces mortality, shortens hospital stay, and improves quality of life after discharge from hospital [27]. They have calculated the cost of intravenous thrombolysis, intravenous thrombolysis followed by intracoronary treatment, and immediate and late PTCA for each patient survival. There is little doubt that the saving can be applied to other cities and conurbations. The annual cost of a single MICU in Jerusalem is approximately U.S. $ 1 million. The MICU responds to 15 calls per day and treats, in addition to arrhythmias and acute myocardial infarction, mass accidents, trauma, and other sudden cardiac and metabolic emergencies. The cost is approximately $ 50 per call. In Jersualem the ambulance sees the majority of patients with acute myocardial infarction, so that no additional expense is entailed in patient management. An additional $ 100 needs to be added for drug therapy, so that the cost is $ 150 per call.

Adjuvant Therapy also Reduces Myocardial Infarct Size. This study has not focused on adjuvant therapy in acute myocardial infarction: management of arrhythmias; drug therapy to control pain, blood pressure, and heart rate; and reperfusion injury. These adjuvant measures are important in individual patients and complement early thrombolytic therapy.

Long-Term Management of the Offending Atheromatous Plaque. Early thrombolytic therapy dissolves all or part of the thrombus overlying a ruptured atheromatous plaque but all the original initiating factors remain and rethrombosis is a continuous threat [29 – 33]. Earlier thrombolysis preserves myocardium, and reocclusion can thus potentially cause further massive infarction of the area salvaged. If adequate vessel reopening has been achieved, rapid blood flow and anticoagulation preserve vessel patency until endothelial continuity is restored, but where severe residual stenosis remains, mechanical dilatation with PTCA or bypass grafting should be undertaken to prevent reocclusion and further infarction or to ameliorate subsequent angina pectoris [28 – 36].

Conclusions

Prehospital thrombolytic therapy can, in the average patient, save 40 min between pain onset and the delivery of thrombolytic therapy. This apparently short period of time is crucial to save myocardium and reduce mortality. Prehospital therapy is simple and safe.

References

1. DeWood MA, Spores J, Notske R, Mouser LT, Borroughs R, Golden MS, Lang Ht (1980) Prevalence of total coronary occlusion during the early hours of transmural myocardial infarction. N Engl J Med 303:897 – 902
2. Woolf N (1982) Pathology of atherosclerosis. Butterworth, London
3. Davies MJU, Fulton WFM, Robertson WB (1979) The relation of coronary thrombosis to ischemic myocardial necrosis. J Pathol 127:99 – 110
4. Falk E (1983) Plaque rupture with severe pre-existing stenosis precipitating coronary thrombosis. Br Heart J 50:127 – 134
5. Jennings RB, Reimer KA (1981) Lethal myocardial ischemic injury. Am J Pathol 102:241 – 255
6. Reimer KA, Jennings RB (1979) The "wave front phenomenon" of myocardial ischemic cell death. II. Transmural progression of necrosis within the framework of ischemic bed size (myocardium at risk) and collateral flow. Lab Invest 40:633 – 644
7. Rentrop KP, Feit F, Blanke H, Stecy P, Schneider R, Rey M, Horowitz S, Goldman M, Karsch K, Meilman H, Cohen M, Siegel S, Sanger J, Slater J, Gorlin R, Fox A, Fagerstrom R, Calhoun WF (1984) Effects of intracoronary streptokinase and intracoronary nitroglycerine infusion on coronary angiographic patterns and mortality in patients with acute myocardial infarction. N Engl J Med 311:1457 – 1463
8. Yusuf S, Collins R, Peto R, Furberg C, Stamper MJ, Gaddhaber ST, Henmekens CH (1985) Intravenous and intracoronary fibrinolytic therapy in acute myocardial infarction: overview of results on mortality, re-infarction and side-effects from 33 randomized controlled trials. Eur Heart J 6:556 – 585
9. The TIMI Study Group (1985) The thrombolysis in myocardial infarction (TIMI) trial – phase I findings. N Engl J Med 312:932 – 936
10. Mathey DG, Sheehan FH, Schofer J, Dodge HT (1985) Time from onset of symptoms to thrombolytic therapy: a major determinant of myocardial salvage in patients with acute transmural infarction. J Am Coll Cardiol 6:518
11. Koren G, Weiss AT, Hasin Y, Applebaum D, Welber S, Rozenman Y, Lotan C, Mosseri M, Sapoznikov D, Luria MH, Gotsman MS (1985) Prevention of myocardial damage by very early treatment with intravenous streptokinase. N Engl J Med 313:1384 – 1389
12. Simoons ML, Serruys PW, van den Braud M, Res J, Verheugt FWA, Hanno Krauss X, Remme WJ, Bar F, DeZwaan Ch, van den Larse A, Vermeer F, Lubsen J (1986) Early thrombolysis in acute myocardial infarction: limitations of infarct size and improved survival. J Am Coll Cardiol 7:717 – 728
13. Fine DG, Weiss AT, Sapoznikov D, Welber S, Applebaum D, Lotan C, Hasin Y, Ben-David Y, Koren G, Gotsman MS (1986) Importance of early initiation of intravenous streptokinase therapy for acute myocardial infarction. Am J Cardiol 58:411 – 417
14. Weiss AT, Fine DG, Applebaum D, Welber S, Sapoznikov D, Lotan C, Mosseri M, Hasin Y, Gotsman MS (1987) Prehospital coronary thrombolysis: a new strategy in acute myocardial infarction. Chest 92:124 – 128
15. Gotsman MS, Weiss AT (1986) Immediate reperfusion in acute myocardial infarction. Bibl Cardiol 40:30 – 51
16. Hindman NB, Schocken DD, Windman M, Anderson WD, White RD, Leggett S, Ideker RE, Hinchara T, Selvester RH, Wagner GS (1985) Evaluation of a QRS scoring system for estimating myocardial infarct size. V. Specificity and method of application of the complete system. Am J Cardiol 55:1485 – 1490

17. Sapoznikov D, Halon DA, Lewis BA, Gotsman MS (1981) Regional ejection fraction of the normal left ventricle. Isr J Med Sci 17:1027 – 1034
18. Sapoznikov D, Halon DA, Lewis BS, Weiss AT, Gotsman MS (1983) Frame by frame analysis of the left ventricular function: quantitative assessment of regional and temporal function. Cardiology 70:61 – 72
19. Sapoznikov D, Welber S, Lotan C, Mosseri M, Shimoni Y, Gotsman MS: Quantitation of variations in regional left ventricular function in isolated disease of the left anterior descending coronary artery. Cardiology (in Press)
20. ISAM Study Group (1986) A prospective trial of intravenous streptokinase in acute myocardial infarction. N Engl J Med 314:1465 – 1471
21. Schröder R, Neuhaus KL, Linderer T, Leizorovicz A, Wegscheider K, Tebbe U, for the ISAM Study Group (1987) Risk of death from recurrent ischemic events after intravenous streptokinase in acute myocardial infarction: results from the intravenous streptokinase in myocardial infarction (ISAM) study. Circulation 76 [Suppl II]:44
22. The GISSI Study Group (1986) Effectiveness of intravenous thrombolytic treatment in acute myocardial infarction. Lancet I:397 – 401
23. Bippus PH, Haux R, Schröder R (1987) Prehospital intravenous streptokinase in evolving myocardial infarction: a randomised study about feasibility, safety, and time-gain. Eur Heart J 8 [Suppl 2]:103
24. Schröder R, Voringer M, Linderer T, Blamino G, Bruggermann T, Leitner ER (1985) Follow up after coronary arterial reperfusion with intravenous streptokinase in relation to residual myocardial infarct artery narrowing. Am J Cardiol 55:313 – 317
25. Villemante D, Barriot P, Bodenan P, Brunet F, Lafay Ph, Noto R, Monsallier JF (1987) At home thrombolysis and myocardial infarction: a real saving of time. Eur Heart J 8 [Suppl 2]:103
26. Herve C, Gaillard M, Desfemmes C (1984) Emergency medical care in France. Acta Anaesthesiol Belg 35 [Suppl]:137 – 144
27. Vermeer F, Simoons ML, de Zwaan C, van Es GA, Verheugt Freek WA, van der Laarse A, van Hoogenhuyze DCA, Azar AJ, van Dalen FJ, Lubsen J, Hugenholtz PG (1987) Cost benefit analysis of early thrombolytic therapy with intracoronary streptokinase. In: Vermeer F (ed) Thrombolysis in acute myocardial infarction. Van Gorcum, Assen
28. Serruys PW, Suryapranata H, Simoons ML, Vermeer F, van Den Brand M, DeFeyter PJ, van Domburg R, van Der Laarse A, Bar F, Verheugt FWA, Res J, Remme WJ, De Zwaan C, Hugenholtz PG (1987) Intracoronary thrombolysis in patients with acute myocardial infarction: the Netherlands randomized trial and current status. Circulation 76 [Suppl II]:63
29. Kennedy JW, Ritchie JL, Davis KB, Fritz JK (1983) Western Washington randomized trial of intracoronary streptokinase in acute myocardial infarction. N Engl J Med 308:1477 – 1482
30. Gold HK, Leinbach RC, Garabedian HD, Tsunheiro-Yasuda Sin, Johns JA, Grossbard EB, Palacios I, Collen D (1986) Acute coronary reocclusion after thrombolysis with recombinant human tissue-type plasminogen activator: prevention by a maintenance infusion. Circulation 23:347 – 352
31. Sheehan FH, Mathey DG, Schofer J, Dodge HT, Bolson EL (1985) Factors that determine recovery of left ventricular function after thrombolysis in patients with acute myocardial infarction. Circulation 71:1120 – 1121
32. Gash AK, Spann JF, Sherry S, Belber AD, Carabello BA, McDonough MT, Mann RH, McCann WD, Gault JH, Gantzler RD, Kent RL (1986) Factors influencing

reocclusion after coronary thrombolysis for acute myocardial infarction. Am J Cardiol 57:175 – 177

33. Sheehan FH, Mathey DG, Schofer J, Krebber HJ, Dodge HT (1983) Effect of interventions in salvaging left ventricular function in acute myocardial infarction: a study of intracoronary streptokinase. Am J Cardiol 52:431 – 438
34. Serruys PW, Wign SW, van der Brand M (1983) Is transluminal coronary angioplasty mandatory after successful thrombolysis? Quantitative coronary angiographic study. Br Heart J 50:257
35. Hartzler GO, Rutherford BD, McConahay DR, Johnson WL, McCallister BD, Gura GM, Conn RC, Crockett JE (1983) Percutaneous transluminal coronary angioplasty with and without thrombolytic therapy for treatment of acute myocardial infarction. Am Heart J 106:965 – 973
36. DeWood MA, Crna JS, Notske RN, Lang HT, Shields JP, Simpson CS, Rudy LW, Grunwald R (1979) Medical and surgical management of myocardial infarction. Am J Cardiol 44:1356 – 1364

Extracorporal Plasma Therapy in the Treatment of Severe Hyper-β-lipoproteinemia: The HELP System

D. Seidel

A large and convincing body of evidence links coronary risk with elevated plasma levels of both low-density lipoprotein (LDL) cholesterol and fibrinogen. Cholesterol in atherosclerotic lesions originates mainly from cholesterol circulating in the blood bound to LDL. Most forms of hyper-β-lipoproteinemia result from a defect in extraction of LDL from plasma by the liver, and the LDL receptor is now being recognized as the crucial element in the control of cholesterol homeostasis [1]. Elevated levels of fibrinogen, a common phenomenon in hypercholesterolemia increases the viscosity of the blood and thereby further alters perfusion of tissues in severe atherosclerotic disease. Furthermore, fibrinogen and its degradation products can both influence prostaglandin metabolism by inhibiting PGI_2 synthesis by endothelial and vascular smooth muscle cells, thereby facilitating platelet aggregation, and can also cause injury to endothelial cells.

Treatment of familial hypercholesterolemia by diet and drug therapy alone is often ineffective. Encouraging results have, however, been obtained in the treatment of this disorder and atherosclerosis by plasma exchange. Conventional plasma exchange requires replacement of some plasma proteins, which may bring problems due to the introduction of foreign protein and the transmission of infectious diseases.

We have now developed a procedure for the continuous elimination of LDL and fibrinogen from plasma based on their precipitation at low pH in the presence of heparin. The mechanism of the technique is based on an increase of the +/− charge of the LDL particles at low pH, allowing them to form a network with fibrinogen [2, 3].

This procedure has been named heparin-induced extracorporal LDL precipitation (HELP). Its major characteristic steps are as follows (Fig. 1). In a continuous flow system, plasma is obtained by filtration of whole blood through a 0.2-μm plasmareparator. This is then mixed continuously with a 0.2 *M* acetate buffer (pH 4.85) containing 100 iU/ml of heparin. Precipitation occurs at a final pH of 5.12 in a precipitation chamber, after which the suspension is circulated through a polycarbonate membrane filter to retain the precipitated material. The LDL-and fibrinogen-free filtrate is then passed to a heparin adsorber to remove excess heparin. This ion exchange resin is capable of completely binding heparin at pH 5.12 while plasma proteins are not retained at this pH. Finally, the buffer

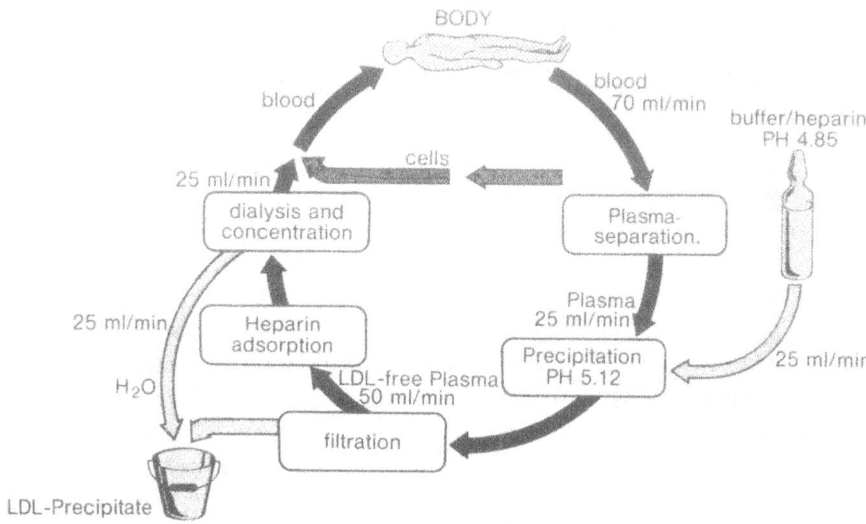

Fig. 1. Flow sheet of the HELP procedure

plasma mixture is subject to a bicarbonate dialysis filtration to restore physiological pH and to remove acetate and water before the LDL- and fibrinogen-free plasma is mixed with the blood cells and returned to the patient. The various parts used for a treatment (tubings, filter, etc.) are all disposable and intended for single use, which makes it easy and reliable to work with and guarantees a standard quality for each treatment independent of the clinic performing the treatment. Safety is assured by two microprocessors in parallel operating (Fig. 2). We clear 10 – 15 g LDL cholesterol and fibrinogen in one treatment, which turns the filter yellow. We treat 3 l plasma in 1.5 – 2 h.

At present, five patients with familial hypercholesterolemia (among them is one homozygous child) have been treated by HELP for more than 1.5 years. More than 60 patients are now under treatment in 12 different centers. At present we oversee approximately 900 single treatments. The frequency of treatments has averaged one every 8 days. Average pretreatment LDL cholesterol levels have been reduced by approximately 50% compared with the values prior the therapy. The mean LDL cholesterol concentration to which the vascular wall is exposed are, of course, lower (approximately 40%) since the posttreatment values are as low as 22% compared with the values prior to the start of the HELP therapy. The data for fibrinogen are very similar to the LDL data (Fig. 3). Plasma high-density lipoprotein (HDL) concentrations are unaffected by the HELP procedure; in some case an increase of approximately 10% – 22% may take place.

Despite the long-term treatment pretreatment values of plasminogen C-4 and C-3 complement – also heparin-binding proteins – have remained stable, indicating that treatment does not lead to deficiency in these proteins. In the case

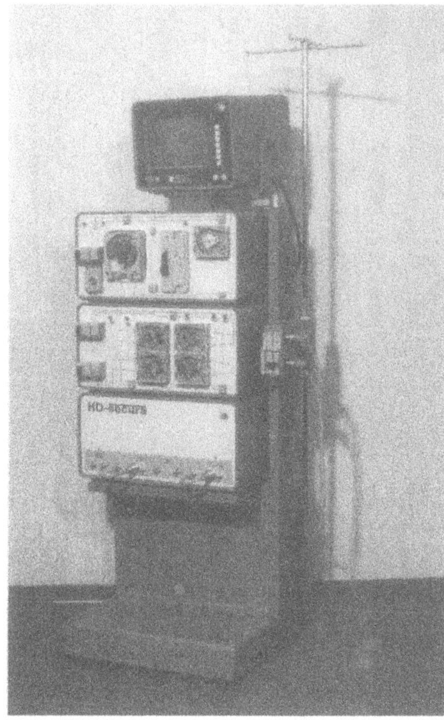

Fig. 2. Microprocessor used in carrying out the HELP procedure

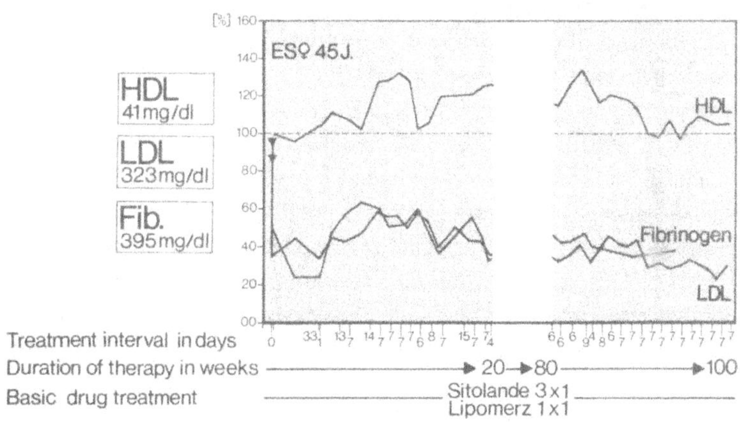

Fig. 3. Course of mean LDL, HDL, and fibrinogen levels during HELP therapy. Values expressed as percentage of pretreatment levels

of proteins that do not bind to heparin at low pH, plasma concentrations at the end of the HELP therapy were generally in the range of 80% – 90% of initial values. Samples taken 24 h after the end of the treatment showed that these proteins have retained their original level. Substitution of any kind, including vitamins, has not been necessary in 2 years of experience.

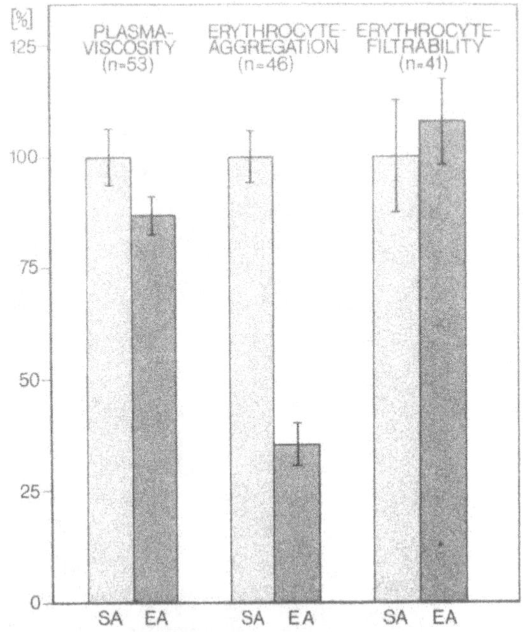

Fig. 4. Effect of HELP treatment on various hemorheological parameters. Values before each treatment are set at 100%. *SA*, Start of apheresis; *EA*, end of apheresis

The HELP treatment also significantly improves plasma viscosity, erythrocyte aggregation and erythrocyte filtration, indicating a positive change in membrane fluidity, a result which is of great clinical importance in subjects suffering from atherosclerosis. The improvement in these parameters by each treatment is also significant under the course of the HELP therapy (Fig. 4).

Special attention has been focused on the effect of HELP on homeostasis. All posttreatment controls were typical for extracorporal procedures. Plasma heparin levels at the end of the treatment averaged 0.17 iU/ml. No bleeding complications have been observed. Plasma electrolyte, hormones, vitamins, enzymes, immunoglobulin concentrations, and hematological parameters were virtually unchanged at the end of each treatment and after more than 100 weeks of treatment.

Overall treatment tolerance has been very good. No patient dropped out, and no major complications have been observed after approximately 900 treatments. No coronary infarction or other events have occurred after the start of the therapy. No alterations in pulse rate or blood pressure were observed either under the therapy or soon thereafter.

All subjective and some objective clinical signs of coronary heart disease (angina attacks, regression of xanthomata, etc.) have improved impressively under the HELP therapy.

It remains to be established whether such a drastic lowering of LDL and fibrinogen can lead to a regression of atherosclerotic plaques. This question is currently under investigation in a prospective nine-center study in which treatment efficiency will be controlled by coronary angiography of 45 patients treated with HELP over a period of 2 years.

The combination of HELP with a new generation of drugs (HMG CoA reductase inhibitors) offers a new dimension in the treatment of severe hypercholesterolemia and possibly atherosclerosis.

Summary. The HELP procedure provides a new means for the treatment of severe hypercholesterolemia with the additional effect of lowering fibrinogen. It utilizes only disposable material, it retains a high degree of specificity with 100% efficiency for LDL and fibrinogen extraction. It has the advantage that the patient is not exposed to foreign proteins or compounds with the attendant immunological problems. It displays a high degree of reproducibility and an almost unlimited capacity, which guarantees a constant therapy independent of the clinic performing the treatment.

We trust the clinical benefits of the HELP system will be substantial.

References

1. Goldstein JL, Brown MS (1983) Familial hypercholesterolemia. In: Stanbury JB, Wyngaarden JB, Frederickson DS, Goldstein JL, Brown MS (eds) The metabolic basis of inherited disease, 5th edn. McGraw Hill, New York
2. Seidel D, Wieland H (1982) Ein neues Verfahren zur selektiven Messung und extrakorporalen Elimination von Low Density Lipoproteinen. J Clin Chem Clin Biochem 20:684-685
3. Eisenhauer T, Armstrong VW, Wieland H, Fuchs C, Scheler F, Seidel D (1987) Selective removal of low density lipoproteins (LDL) by precipitation at low pH: first clinical application of the HELP system. Klin Wochenschr 65:161-168

Very Early Urokinase Treatment in Acute Myocardial Infarction

J. Schofer, D. G. Mathey, and W. Bleifeld

Time Dependence of Myocardial Salvage

From experimental studies it is known that after 40 min of coronary artery occlusion only 60% of ischemic myocardium can be salvaged by reperfusion; after a 3-h coronary artery ligation myocardial infarction had developed completely [6]. A similar relationship between myocardial salvage and the time interval from symptom onset to start of thrombolytic therapy could be found in patients with acute myocardial infarction [4]. For estimation of myocardial salvage after thrombolysis in this study, regional wall motion in the infarct region was measured 2–3 weeks after the acute infarct. A normal or only slightly depressed wall motion was interpreted as a significant limitation of infarct size due to thrombolytic therapy, an abnormal wall motion, in contrast, as irreversible myocardial damage.

In about 80% of patients in whom thrombolytic therapy was started within 2 h after symptom onset, follow-up wall motion in the infarct area was within the normal range. In patients, however, in whom thrombolysis was introduced later than 2 h after infarct onset, a normal follow-up wall motion in the infarct area was only found in half of the cases; in the remaining patients despite reperfusion achieved by thrombolysis the infarct had developed completely. This time dependence of myocardial salvage was not influenced by the infarct location or by whether a subtotal or a total coronary occlusion was found before thrombolysis.

Thrombolysis with Urokinase

Initiation of thrombolytic therapy within such a short time requires a method of thrombolytic therapy safe and easy enough to be performed even before hospital admission. For this purpose, only intravenous thrombolytic therapy appears feasible. As thrombolytic agent we used urokinase, which has several advantages compared to streptokinase. It is nonantigenic, has no hypotensive effect, and can thus be given as a bolus injection [3, 7]. Repeated applications are possible, no neutralizing antibodies are present, and there is a direct dose-effect relationship. The purposes of the study were to assess the influence of an intravenous bolus injection of 2×10^6 U urokinase on the patency rate and on the infarct size and to assess the risk of the therapy. A total of 50 patients with acute myocardial infarction received a bolus injection of urokinase followed by coronary angiography using the Judkins technique which was performed 60 min later. After angiography an intravenous infusion of heparin with an initial dose of 200 U/kg body weight per 12 h was started, and the dose was then adjusted to achieve a threefold increase in thrombin time.

Results of Coronary Angiography

Infarct location was equally distributed over the 50 patients. Thrombolysis resulted in a coronary patency rate of 60% at 1 h after urokinase application. The patency rate was not significantly different between the three infarct vessels. In 24 patients reangiography could be done 2 – 3 weeks after infarction, revealing still patent coronary arteries in 23 of the 24 patients.

Effect of Urokinase on Blood Coagulation and Fibrinolytic System

The effect of the urokinase bolus on blood coagulation is summarized in Table 1. Plasma fibrinogen concentration decreased significantly 2 h after the injection of 2×10^6 U urokinase with no difference between patients with and without successful reperfusion (77 ± 52 versus 84 ± 24 mg%; not significant). At 24 h after thrombolysis the fibrinogen concentration was again in the normal range. At 2 h after injection of urokinase the partial thromboplastin time, the thrombin time, and the prothrombin time were all prolonged significantly.

Serial measurements of plasminogen, plasmin, and fibrinogen were performed in six patients to assess the effect on blood coagulation and fibrinolytic system (Fig. 1). Plasmin activity peaked 15 min after the bolus injection, when the first measurement was performed. At 5 h after injection, a measurable plasmin activity was no longer detectable. Plasminogen decreased to 40% after 1 h and returned to normal after 36 h. The effect on the fibrinolytic system was accom-

Table 1. Coagulation values after an intravenous bolus injection of 2×10^6 U urokinase in 50 patients with acute myocardial infarction

		before urokinase	2 h after urokinase	p	24 h after urokinase
fibrinogen	(mg %)	379 ± 142	79 ± 68	< 0.001	213 ± 90
partial thromboplastin time	(s)	39 ± 8	92 ± 54	< 0.001	54 ± 13
thrombin time	(s)	21 ± 1	171 ± 27	< 0.001	132 ± 61
prothrombin time	(s)	15 ± 1	25 ± 9	< 0.01	17 ± 2

Mean values ± 1 SD

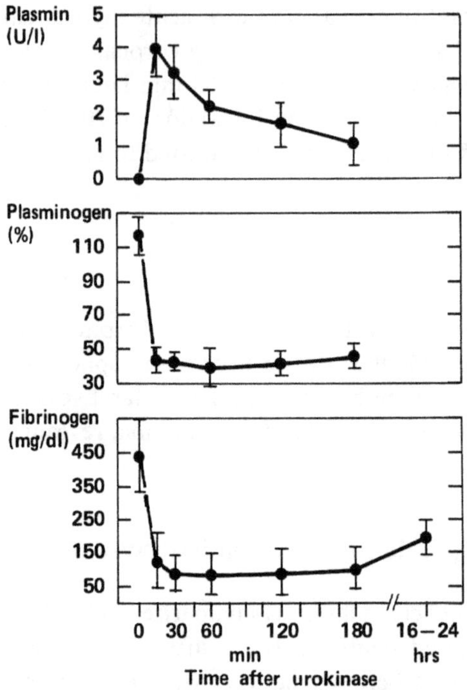

Fig. 1. Serial measurements of plasmin, plasminogen, and fibrinogen after a bolus injection of 2×10^6 U urokinase in six patients with acute myocardial infarction

panied by a drop in fibrinogen concentration to a minimum value of 80 mg% at 60 min after injection.

Regional Wall Motion in the Infarct Area

To study the degree of myocardial salvage in relation to the time from symptom onset to treatment, patients were divided into three groups (Fig. 2). The first group had undergone thrombolysis within 2 h after symptom onset; in the second group urokinase was given 2 – 4 h after symptom onset; and in the third group no reperfusion was achieved. In most patients treated within 2 h after symptom onset follow-up wall motion in the infarct area was within the normal range. Compared to patients without reperfusion, wall motion in this early-treated group was significantly less abnormal. In contrast, wall motion of patients treated later than 2 h did not differ significantly from wall motion of patients in whom thrombolysis failed to open the infarct artery.

Serum CK Measurements

As a measure of infarct size maximal serum creatine phosphokinase (CK) was determined [1]. Peak CK differed significantly between patients who were treated

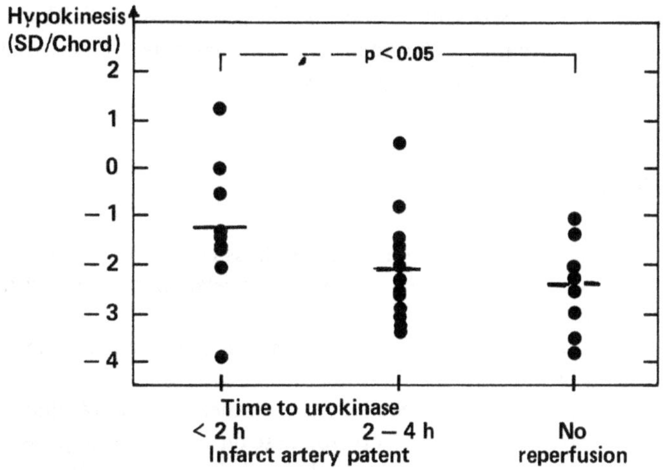

Fig. 2. Wall motion at the infarct site measured in follow-up contrast cineangiograms in reperfused patients who received urokinase within 2 h of symptom onset, after 2 h of symptom onset, and in nonreperfused patients

within 2 h and those in whom reperfusion was unsuccessful (802 ± 763 U/l versus 1973 ± 1061 U/l; $p<0.01$), but not between patients treated later (1848 ± 1655 U/l) and the latter group, confirming that significant myocardial salvage was only achieved if thrombolysis was started very early.

Complications Related to Urokinase Thrombolysis

The bolus injection of urokinase was well tolerated in all patients. No serious bleeding complications occurred despite acute angiography 60 min after urokinase application. There was no fall in blood pressure or anaphylactic reaction. In two patients who underwent emergency bypass surgery within 24 h after thrombolysis fibrinogen had to be substituted. In one patient ventricular fibrillation occurred, which, however, was probably not induced by reperfusion because the ST segment elevation was still present in this patient after sinus rhythm was restored.

Conclusions

Thus, the intravenous bolus injection on 2×10^6 U urokinase seems to be effective, safe, and an alternative to intravenous streptokinase infusion. The patency rate after urokinase of 60% seems to be comparable with the patency rate after 1.5×10^6 U streptokinase infused ofer 90 min [2, 5, 7, 8]. If thrombolytic therapy is initiated within 2 h after symptom onset, a significant limitation of the infarct size can be achieved in more than 80% of reperfused patients. The question remains to be answered whether this method of thrombolytic therapy can be applied in the prehospital phase.

References

1. Bleifeld W, Mathey D, Hanrath P, Buss H, Effert S (1977) Infarct size estimated from serial serum creatine phosphokinase in relation to left ventricular hemodynamics. Circulation 5:303
2. Huhmann W, Nieth H (1983) Was leistet die systemische Lyse beim akuten Herzinfarkt? (Abstract). Z Kardiol 72 [Suppl 1]:67
3. Lew AS, Laramee P, Shah PK, Rodriguez L, Ganz W (1985) The effect of the rate of intravenous infusion of streptokinase on systolic blood pressure and on the time interval to reperfusion (Abstract). J Am Coll Cardiol 5:421
4. Mathey DG, Sheehan FH, Schofer J, Dodge HT (1985) Time from onset of symptoms to thrombolytic therapy: a major determinant of myocardial salvage in patients with acute transmural infarction. J Am Coll Cardiol 6:518
5. Neuhaus KL, Tebbe N, Sauer G, Köstering H, Kreutzer K (1981) High-dose i.v. streptokinase infusion in acute myocardial infarction (Abstract). Eur Heart J 2:144
6. Reimer KA, Lowe JE, Rasmussen MM, Jennings RB (1977) The wavefront phenomenon of ischemic cell death. I. Myocardial infarct size vs. duration of coronary occlusion in dogs. Circulation 56:786
7. Schröder R, Giamino G, von Leitner ER, Linderer T, Brüggemann T, Heintz J, Vöhringer HF, Wegscheider K (1983) Intravenous short-term infusion of streptokinase in acute myocardial infarction. Circulation 67:536
8. Schwarz F, Hoffmann M, Schuler G, Kübler W (1983) Combined intravenous and intracoronary versus intracoronary streptokinase therapy in acute myocardial infarction. J Am Coll Cardiol 1:615

Prourokinase in Acute Myocardial Infarction: Is it Effective?

C. Bode, S. Schönermark, G. Schuler, R. Zimmermann, H.-G. Simanek, F. Schwarz, and W. Kübler

Treatment of acute myocardial infarction with plasminogen activators reduces infarct size and mortality [1]. However, this form of therapy has been attended by significant problems. Urokinase and streptokinase lack fibrin selectivity and promote generalized fibrinogenolysis, at times resulting in severe bleeding [2]. Tissue-type plasminogen activator (TPA) and single-chain urokinase-type plasminogen activator (prourokinase) are both reported to be more clot-specific [3, 4]. In contrast to TPA, relatively few patients have been treated with prourokinase, and therefore experience with respect to the fibrin specificity and thrombolytic efficacy of this drug in a clinical situation is limited [5, 6, 7]. This study was undertaken in order to prove whether or not prourokinase is an effective, clot-selective fibrinolytic agent in patients with acute myocardial infarction.

The plasminogen activator used in this study was prourokinase, highly purified from the transformed kidney cell line TCL 598. The purified protein showed an apparent molecular weight of 55 kD on SDS-polyacrylamide gel electrophoresis. The molecule is physiologically glycosylated. The specific activity after plasmin activation was 130×10^3 IU/mg protein.

For this study patients were eligible who had chest pain typical of myocardial infarction for at least 30 min. Chest pain had to be still present at the time of initiation of therapy. Furthermore, ST-segment elevations of at least 2 mm in at least three leads were a prerequisite for enrollment. The patients had to present within 5 h after the onset of pain. Informed consent had to be obtained. Finally a totally occluded infarct vessel at the time of a first coronary angiogram was required. Exclusion criteria comprised severe illness in addition to coronary heart disease.

Further, patients on oral anticoagulants and those older than 75 years were not included in the study. The usual contraindications against cardiac catheterization and thrombolytic therapy were observed.

After checking the inclusion and exclusion criteria, selective coronary angiography was performed and total occlusion of the infarct vessel confirmed. Thereafter, 0.2 mg nitroglycerin were injected intracoronarily in order to exclude coronary spasm. After these injections, multiple injections into the infarct vessel prior to the end point were omitted in order to avoid an artificial transport of plasminogen activator to the site of the clot. Blood samples were taken prior to the initiation of treatment and after 1, 2, 4, 12 and 24 h. Four patients in group 1

Table 1. Results of treatment with intravenous prourokinase in patients with acute myocardial infarction

Patient no.	Total dose of prourokinase (mg)	Reperfusion after	
		Prourokinase	Additional streptokinase
Group 1			
1	15	0	–
2	15	0	0
3	15	0	+
4	15	0	+
Group 2			
5	48	0	0
6	48	+	–
7	48	0	0
8	48	+	–
9	48	+	–

+, Successful; 0, unsuccessful; –, not attempted.

and five patients in group 2 received a bolus of 4 mg and 7.5 mg followed by an infusion of 11 and 40.5 mg, respectively, over 60 min. Thrombolysis was achieved in no patient in group 1 during intravenous infusion of prourokinase; however, upon subsequent intracoronary infusion of 250×10^3 IU streptokinase, reperfusion was established in two of three patients. In contrast, complete reperfusion occurred in three of five patients in group 2. Subsequent intracoronary infusion of 250×10^3 IU streptokinase was unsuccessful in the two cases in which 48 mg intravenous prourokinase had not achieved thrombolysis. The clinical results are summarized in Table 1.

Treatment with prourokinase did not result in a generalized "lytic state." Plasma fibrinogen at the end of the 60-min treatment period was $92 \pm 8\%$ and $89 \pm 18\%$ of pretreatment values in groups 1 and 2, respectively. In contrast, after treatment with streptokinase, plasma fibrinogen levels fell to $16 \pm 2\%$ of pretreatment values, and a depletion of plasminogen and α2 antiplasmin occurred. In one patient with a history of gastric ulcers, a minor upper gastrointestinal bleeding episode was observed during treatment in group 2. In three patients in group 1 and four patients in group 2 successful percutaneous coronary angioplasty was performed after thrombolytic therapy. All patients survived the myocardial infacrtion and were later discharged.

The study suggests that prourokinase is an effective and safe thrombolytic agent in patients with acute myocardial infarction. Further studies are needed to show the optimal dosage and possibly the optimal combination of other thrombolytic agents with prourokinase [8].

References

1. Gruppo Italiano per lo Studio della Streptochinasi nell' Infarto Miocardico (GISSI) (1986) Effectiveness of intravenous thrombolytic treatment in acute myocardial infarction. Lancet I:397-401
2. Laffel GL, Braunwald E (1987) Thrombolytic therapy: a new strategy for the treatment of acute myocardial infarction. N Engl J Med 311:710-717, 770-776
3. Collen D (1985) Human tissue-type plasminogen activator: from the laboratory to the bedside. Circulation 72:18-20
4. Pannel R, Gurewich V (1986) Pro-urokinase: a study of its stability in plasma and of a mechanism for its selective fibrinolytic effect. Blood 67:1215-1223
5. Van de Werf F, Nobuhara M, Collen D (1986) Coronary thrombolysis with human single-chain urokinase-type plasminogen activator (prourokinase) in patients with myocardial infarction. Ann Intern Med 104:345-348
6. Bode C, Schuler G, Schwarz F, Zimmermann R, Horn A, Kübler W (1987) Usefulness of intravenous thrombolytic therapy with prourokinase in acute myocardial infarction. Am J Cardiol 60:371
7. Van de Werf F, Vanhaecke J, DeGeest H, Verstraete M, Collen D (1986) Coronary thrombolysis with recombinant single-chain urokinase-type plasminogen activator in patients with acute myocardial infarction. Circulation 74:1066-1070
8. Collen D, Stump D, Van de Werf F (1986) Coronary thrombolysis in patients with acute myocardial infarction by intravenous infusion of synergic thrombolytic agents. Am Heart J 112:1083-1084

Recombinant Tissue-Type Plasminogen Activator in the Treatment of Myocardial Infarction

K.L. Neuhaus

Recent studies have reported recombinant tissue-type plasminogen activator (rt-PA) to be more effective in early recanalization of infarct-related coronary artery occlusion than the conventional non-fibrin-specific thrombolytic agents such as streptokinase and urokinase [1 – 3]. Reliable data on the efficacy of thrombolytics with respect to reopening occluded coronary arteries can only be obtained from randomized trials, which are listed in Table 1. Reperfusion rates of about 60% and patency rates of 70% – 75% have been shown both for double-chain and single-chain preparations of rt-PA, when given in appropriate doses of 60 – 80 mg and about 100 – 150 mg, respectively. Usually perfusion data refer to angiographic findings obtained 90 min after the onset of therapy. There is general agreement that early reperfusion must be achieved within 1 – 1.5 h to be of significant importance for the salvage of ischemic myocardium. Thus, rt-PA has the potential of limiting myocardial infarct size when given early and in the appropriate dosage. Data on infarct size limitation, such as have been presented for streptokinase [5, 6], are still lacking for rt-PA. This is also true for a reduction of hospital mortality, which has been demonstrated for streptokinase [7, 8] and for acylated plasminogen-activator complex in a recent British trial which has not yet been published.

The problem of early reocclusion after successful recanalization of the infarct-related artery may be more important for a specific fibrinolytic agent such as rt-PA than for conventional agents. Reocclusion rates of 10% – 20% or even 30% for the in-hospital period have been found (Table 2), which most probably is significantly higher than after intravenous streptokinase or urokinase [3]. More recent data have shown that a maintenance infusion, which had been claimed to prevent reocclusion [9], may be of little effect in this context [11].

The bleeding risk which is a major disadvantage of conventional thrombolytic drugs, was thought to be largely eliminated by fibrin specificity of the new generation of fibrinolytics, namely rt-PA and pro-urokinase. The reason was that fibrinogen breakdown was much less after equivalent doses of rt-PA, being about 30% – 50% with conventional doses of 100 or even 150 mg over 3 – 6 h. In some patients fibrinogen levels fell as much as after streptokinase, and more importantly, the bleeding risk turned out to be only weakly correlated to fibrinogen breakdown. Intracranial bleeding was seen in a similar proportions of patients treated with rt-PA and with streptokinase. As far as can be concluded

Table 1. rt-PA in randomized trials

Study	rt-PA versus	*n*	Angiography	Patency %	Dose at 90 min	Total dose
TIMI	SK	98/115	90′	60/35[a]	50 mg d.c.	80 mg
ECSG I	Plac.	63/64	90′	61/21	55 mg d.c.	55 mg
ECSG II	SK	64/65	75–90′	70/55		
Topol	Plac.	75/25	60, 90, 120′	69/24	70 mg s.c.	
TAMI	Plac.	38/12	60, 90, 120′	71/17	70 mg s.c.	100 mg
GAUS	Urok.	124/121	90′	69/66	70 mg s.c.	70 mg
TIMI	rt-PA (open)	33	60′	82[a]	100 mg s.c.	150 mg
TAMI	rt-PA (open)	386	90′	75	70 mg s.c.	100 mg

s.c., Single chain rt-PA; d.c., double chain rt-PA.
[a] Reperfusion.

Table 2. Reocclusion rate after successful thrombolysis with rt-PA

Study	*n*	Total dose (mg)	Duration (h)	Reocclusion rate (%)	In-hospital reinfarctions (%)
TIMI	21 (59)	80 d.c.	3	33 early and late	(~20)
ECSG	81	~50 d.c.	1.5	–	6
Topol et al.	59	~90 s.c.	3	8.5 early ~30 late	4
Gold et al.	17	~50 s.c.	1–2	35 (1 late)	–
	7	~90 s.c.	5–6	0 (1 late)	–
GAUS	57	70 s.c.	1.5	10 early	9
TIMI II	88	100 s.c.	6	20 early	–

Table 3. Intracranial bleeding with rt-PA

	Total dose (mg)	*n*	Intracranial bleeding	Incidence (%)
TIMI	~80 d.c.	386	1	<0.3
Genent.	40–80 d.c.	341	0	0
Genent.	80–119 s.c.	251	1	0.4
Genent.	120–170 s.c.	406	2	0.5
TIMI	150 s.c.	311	5	1.6
GAUS	70 s.c.	125	1	0.8
	<120 s.c.	1103	3	0.27 (Av.)
	>120 s.c.	717	7	0.98 (Av.)
		1820	10	0.55 (Av.)

from available data (Table 3) a total dose of more than 120 mg rt-PA may be associated with an unacceptably high risk of intracranial hemorrhage, at least when it is given over several hours.

In summary then, there are some important open questions in spite of several thousand treatments concerning the routine use of rt-PA in acute myocardial infarction:

1. There is no real dose-finding study. The proper dose and duration of treatment are not yet defined.
2. Limitation of infarct size and a reduced mortality from acute myocardial infarction have not yet been documented for rt-PA.
3. A reduced bleeding risk could not be demonstrated, because fibrin specificity does not discriminate between intravascular thrombi and hemostatic plugs.

References

1. TIMI Study Group (1985) The thrombolysis in myocardial infarction (TIMI) trial. Phase I findings. N Engl J Med 312:932–936
2. Verstraete M, Bernard R, Bory M, et al (1985) Randomized trial of intravenous recombinant tissue-type plasminogen activator versus intravenous streptokinase in acute myocardial infarction. Lancet I:842–847
3. Neuhaus KL, Tebbe U, Gottwik M, et al. Intravenous rt-PA and urokinase in acute myocardial infarction: results of the German Activator Urokinase Study (GAUS) (submitted for publication)
4. Verstraete M, Bleifeld W, Brower RW, et al (1985) Double-blind trial of intravenous tissue-type plasminogen activator versus placebo in acute myocardial infarction. Lancet II:965–969
5. Schröder R, Neuhaus KL, Leizorovicz A, Linderer T, Tebbe U, for the ISAM Study Group (1986) A prospective trial of intravenous streptokinase in acute myocardial infarction (ISAM). N Engl J Med 314:1465–1471
6. Kennedy JW, Ritchie JL, Davis KB, et al (1985) The Western Washington randomized trial of intracoronary streptokinase in acute myocardial infarction. N Engl J Med 312:1073–1078
7. Gruppo Italiano per lo Studio della Streptochinasi nell' Infarto Miocardica (GISSI) (1986) Effectiveness of intravenous thrombolytic treatment in acute myocardial infarction. Lancet I:397–402
8. ISIS Steering Committee (1987) Intravenous streptokinase given within 0–4 h of onset of myocardial infarction reduced mortality in ISIS-2. Lancet I: 502
9. Gold HK, Leibach RC, Garabedian HD, et al. (1986) Acute coronary reocclusion after thrombolysis with recombinant human tissue-type plasminogen activator: prevention by a maintenance infusion. Circulation 73:347–352
10. Topol EJ, Califf RM, George BS, et al (1987) A randomized trial of immediate versus delayed elective angioplasty after intravenous tissue plasminogen activator in acute myocardial infarction. N Engl J Med 317:581–588
11. TIMI-operations Committee: Announcement of protocol change in TIMI-trial. Letter to the editor. J Am Coll Cardiol 9 [2]:467

Thrombolytic Agents in Early Myocardial Infarction – An Overview in 1987

P. G. Hugenholtz, M. L. Simoons, H. Suryapranata, and F. Vermeer

Introduction

This paper reviews the current status of thrombolysis in early myocardial infarction. It may best be illustrated by an illustrative case. A 60-year-old technician was admitted at night with a 2-h history of persisting chest pain at rest associated with nausea and perspiration. He had been entirely well until 5 months previously, when he developed angina on effort. Despite 200 mg atenolol, 80 mg isosorbide dinitrate, and 40 mg nifedipine daily, anginal attacks increased in frequency and with less provocation, such as effort. They were, however, promptly relieved by nitroglycerin sublingually. On admission to the CCU, the angina pectoris did not respond to nitroglycerin and nifedipine sublingually. Blood pressure was 135/85 mmHg, heart rate 90 bpm and regular. There were no signs of congestive heart failure. The ECG upon admission suggested a large area of acute inferoposterior myocardial infarction. It was decided to attempt immediate and "optimal" reperfusion.

A nitroglycerin infusion (100 µg/min) was started and 500×10^3 U streptokinase (intravenously) was given over 15 min. The patient arrived at the catheterization laboratory without pain before 1 h had elapsed since entry. Lidocaine was given intravenously in a dose of 2 mg/min, and a pacemaker catheter was positioned in the right attrium. Heparin 5000 units was then administered intravenously together with 250 mg acetylsalicylic acid and 100 mg corticosteroid, in order to reduce possible allergic effects of streptokinase and/or the contrast medium (Table 1).

Arteriography of the right coronary artery showed an obstruction of 90% with poor distal run off. Intracoronary streptokinase infusion was carried out at a rate of 400 U/min to a total of 250×10^3 U, diluted in 500 ml physiological solution, at a flow rate of 8 ml/min. Repeat injection after completion of the intracoronary streptokinase infusion showed severe residual stenosis. The coronary artery was dilated in order to provide adequate flow, with four 40-s dilatations with balloon catheter. The gradient decreased from 60 to 16 mmHg; the area stenosis was reduced from 95% to less than 50%. Biplane left ventriculograms demonstrated hypokinesia of the inferoposterior wall with a global ejection fraction of 38%. Upon return to the CCU, it was attempted to achieve an "optimal" hemodynamic state characterized by light sedation, a heart rate between 60 and

Table 1. Response of one patient to "optimal" reperfusion therapy

Time (h)	HR (bpm)	SBP (mmHg)	PCW (mmHg)	CI (l/m^2)	Intervention
0	90	135/85			NTG + nifedipine s.l.
1	70	140/100			NTG 100 μg/min + SK 500×10^3 IU i.v., lidocaine 2 mg/min, heparin 5000 IU i.v., acetylsalicylic acid 250 mg, diadreson F,
2					100 mg i.v., pacemaker, coronary angiography, SK 250×10^3 IU i.c., coronary dilatation,
3					complete coronary + l.v. angiography, thermodilution catheter
4	90	137/82, 102	10		
5	76	91/53, 65			Lidocaine stop
6	75	118/69, 87	6	3.3	Metoprolol 100 mg orally
7	82	128/78, 95			
8	70	118/71, 87	6		NTG infusion 72 μg/min
9					
10	78	125/70, 89	7		
11					Metoprolol 100 mg orally
12	81	131/72, 93	10		
13					
14	74	131/71, 92	9	3.3	NTG infusion 57 μg/min
15					
16	82	128/72, 92	9		NTG infusion 43 μg/min
17					NTG infusion 36 _g/min Metoprolol 100 mg + hydralazine 25 mg orally
18	82	163/92, 120	6		NTG infusion 29 μg/min
19					
20	83	159/84, 113	14	3.8	NTG infusion stop Hydralazine 25 mg orally
21					
22	81	135/75, 96	6		
23					
24	77	134/68, 91	7	3.9	

HR, Heart rate; SBP, systemic blood pressure: systolic/diastolic, mean; PCW, pulmonary capillary wedge pressure; CI, cardiac index; NTG, nitroglycerin; SK, streptokinase.

90 bqm, systolic blood pressure between 100 and 140 mmHg, and pulmonary capillary wedge pressure below 12 mmHg. β-Blockers, diuretics, vasodilators, or inotropic agents were used to the axtent indicated to achieve this state (Table 1).

The maximal creatine phosphokinase and α-HBDH values were 389 IU/l (normal, <50 IU/l) and 327 IU/l (normal, <150 IU/l), respectively. All other blood chemistries and the hemogram were within normal limits. The patient improved throughout the remainder of hospitalization. Before discharge at

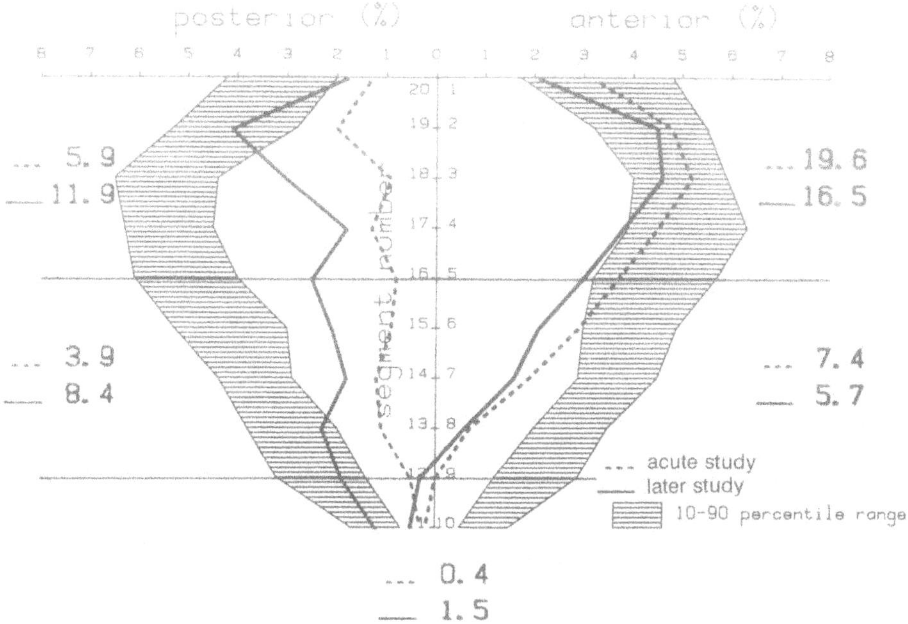

Fig. 1. Sequential change in regional contribution to global ejection fraction from the acute (at admission, *dotted line*) to the chronic (before discharge, *solid line*) stage. *Shaded areas* represent the normal range of the regional contribution to global ejection fraction (anterobasal = segments 1 – 5; anteroapical = segments 5 – 9; apex = segments 9 – 12; inferoapical = segments 12 – 16; inferobasal = segments 16 – 20). The improvement in global ejection fraction was due to significant improvement of the regional myocardial function of the infarct zone (posterior) even after the disappearance of compensatory actions of the initially enhanced function of the noninfarct zone (anterior)

2 weeks, cardiac catheterization was repeated. The right coronary artery showed a residual stenosis of <50%. Despite hypokinesia of the inferoposterior wall, the rest of the left ventricle contracted well; the global ejection fraction was 46%. Although there was significant improvement in global ejection fraction (from 38% to 46%), the question remained whether these difference could be ascribed to salvage of previously jeopardized myocardium in the area supplied by recanalized vessel. In an effort to clarify this, regional left ventricular function was analyzed from the 30° right anterior oblique projection with an automated hard-wired endocardial contour detector. Figure 1 clearly shows the extent of improvement in the regional myocardial function of the infarct zone.

The patient was followed regularly at the outpatient clinic. After 1-year follow-up he remained very well without any complaints.

Table 2. Randomized clinical trials with intracoronary streptokinase

Study	*n*		Treatment delay (min)	Recanalization rate (%)	Limitation infarct size	LVEF (%)			Duration of follow-up (months)	Mortality (%)		
	C	T				C	T	p		C	T	RD (95% CI)
Anderson [7, 8]	26	24	240	75	40%	39	47	0.04	18	19	8	−11(−30, 8)
ICIN [9–15]	264	269	195	79	30%	47	53	0.0001	26	19	11	−8(−13, −1)
Kennedy [1, 2]	116	134	280	69	0	46	46	–	12	15	8	−7(−15, 1)
Khaja [3]	20	20	300	60	–	49	51	–	10	20	5	−15(−35, 5)
Leiboff [4]	18	22	240	69	–	40	43	–	11	6	9	+3(−13, 20)
Raizner [5]	35	29	330	72	–	54	46	–	14 days	6	14	+8(−7, 23)
Rentrop [6]	61	63	350	74	–	–	–	–	6	10	21	+11(−2, 23)

C, Control group; T, thrombolysis group; LVEF, left ventricular ejection fraction; RD (95% CI); risk difference with 95% confidence interval.

Studies with Intracoronary Streptokinase

In order to appreciate the efficacy of optimal lysis it is best to study first the results of intracoronary delivery of the thrombolytic agent. Effects of thrombolytic therapy with intracoronary (Table 2) streptokinase have been carefully investigated in at least seven randomized clinical trials [1 – 8]. Although successful recanalization of an occluded coronary artery was observed in 60% – 80% of patients, the majority of these earlier studies did not demonstrate significant limitation of infarct size, improvement in left ventricular function or reduction in mortality, all of which are criteria to which the optimal study should address itself (Table 2). This discrepancy with the data of the Inter-Universitary Cardiological Institute of the Netherlands (ICIN) study [9 – 15] can be explained by differences in study size (533 patients), shorter treatment delay, and stricter inclusion criteria (patients aged <70 years). In the Western Washington Trial [1, 2], the second largest study with 250 patients, mean treatment delay was 280 min; patients with newly formed Q waves and those receiving maintenance therapy for congestive heart failure were excluded. This study also included many patients who could not benefit much from thrombolytic therapy, according to our current opinion, such as patients with a small ischemic area admitted to the hospital more than 2 h after onset of symptoms, while patients with extensive ischemia leading to new Q waves, who might have benefitted from thrombolytic therapy, were excluded. Also, in the Western Washington Trial no differences in infarct size (measured by thallium imaging in a subset of patients) or in left ventricular ejection fraction were observed between the two treatment groups. Thus, it is difficult to compare these studies. Even so, 1-year mortality was lower in the thrombolysis group (11% versus 19% in the control group; risk difference, –8%) although this difference was statistically not significant ($p = 0.08$). The studies of Khaja [3], Leiboff [4], Raizner [5], and Rentrop [6] included far fewer patients, and it is not surprising that no significant differences in left ventricular ejection fraction or mortality could be observed. On the other hand, in the studies of Anderson [7, 8] 50 patients were included, with a mean treatment delay of 240 min. Intracoronary streptokinase led to higher ventricular ejection fraction compared to controls and a mortality reduction after 18 months follow-up (risk difference, –11%), although the latter difference was not statistically significant due to the small size of the study. It can be concluded from these studies, however, that if reperfusion by lysis is commenced at the right time and with the right dosis, patency rates of ⩾85%, with improvement in overall outcome, can be achieved.

Studies with Intravenous Streptokinase

The intravenous route of administration is obviously the preferred one, although the timing, dose, and action of the lytic agent are of even greater importance. An overview of the outcome of seven trials has been presented by Yusuf et al. [16]. Most of the earlier trials with intravenous streptokinase did not demonstrate a significant reduction in mortality and had less effect on patency rate. Infarct size or left ventricular function were rarely studied. The negative outcome of these earlier trials can best be explained by the fact that patients were admitted up to 48 h after onset of symptoms while the relation between treatment delay and mortality reduction was not properly analyzed. In this overview the authors combined the data from all published randomized trials with intravenous streptokinase and concluded that early mortality might have been reduced by 15% – 20%. However, their conclusions are difficult to interpret, since one cannot expect an identical response to thrombolytic therapy in all groups of patients admitted up to 48 h after onset of symptoms. Thus, their overview does not answer the question as to which patients with acute myocardial infarction are likely to benefit from intravenous streptokinase, as was shown in later studies from our and other centers [9 – 16].

The first convincing results of the efficacy of intravenous streptokinase have come from the GISSI trial [17] (Table 3), in which 11712 patients were enrolled. A significant reduction in early mortality after 15×10^6 U streptokinase to 11% was observed. Hospital mortality was 13% in the control group ($p = 0.0002$). Mortality reduction was only observed, however, in patients with anterior infarction (14% in the streptokinase group versus 18% in the control group; $p = 0.0006$). In patients with inferior or lateral infarction in-hospital mortality was not significantly different between the two treatment groups. In contrast to the ICIN data [9 – 15] no difference in mortality was observed in patients with previous myocardial infarction or in patients with Killip class III or IV at admission. Subgroup analysis revealed that the largest reduction in mortality was obtained in patients randomized within 6 h after onset of symptoms (particularly those within 2 h), while a trend towards a deleterious effect of streptokinase was observed in patients randomized after more than 9 h (Table 3). Nonfatal reinfarction occurred more frequently in the streptokinase group (4%) than in the control group (2%), while the incidence of ventricular fibrillation (7% versus 8% in controls) and of symptoms of pericarditis (7% versus 12% in the control group) was lower in streptokinase-treated patients, findings similar to the observations in the ICIN study. The incidence of major bleeding following streptokinase infusion was very low (0.3%), while cerebrovascular events occurred in less than 1% of the patients, evenly distributed over the two treatment groups as it had been in the ICIN study. Late follow-up data have shown that most of the initial benefits were maintained although no systematic efforts at permanent revascularization were instituted (F. Tognoni 1986, personal communication).

In the ISAM study [18, 19], in which 1741 patients were included, treatment with intravenous streptokinase (15×10^6 U) within 6 h after onset of symptoms resulted in 9% limitation of enzymatic infarct size, measured by the area under the CK-MB curve. Left ventricular ejection fraction, measured by contrast

Table 3. Effects of intravenous (GISSI trial) versus intracoronary (ICIN study) streptokinase on early mortality

GISSI	Time to randomization	In-hospital mortality (%)		
		C	T	RD (95% CI)
	<3 h	12	9	−3 (−4, −1)
	3−6 h	14	12	−2 (−5, 0)
	6−9 h	14	13	−1 (−5, 2)
	9−12 h	14	16	+2 (−4, 8)
	Overall	13	11	−2 (−3, −1)
ICIN	**Time to hospital admission**	**14-day mortality (%)**		
		C	T	RD (95% CI)
	<2 h	11	5	−6 (−12, −1)
	2−4 h	6	6	0 (− 9, 9)
	Overall	10	5	−5 (− 9, 0)

C, Control group; T, allocated to thrombolytic therapy; RD (95% CI), risk difference with 95% confidence interval.

angiography 20−30 days after the infarction, was higher in the streptokinase group (mean, 57%) than in the control group (54%; $p = 0.005$) a difference particularly favoring the larger anterior wall infarctions. Long-term mortality, with an average follow-up of 21 months, was 14% in the streptokinase group and 16% in the placebo group, a difference of the same magnitude as observed in the GISSI trial but not statistically significant due to the smaller size of the study. Significant reduction in mortality by intravenous streptokinase was only observed in patients with first inferior infarction, with the largest differences being observed in patients treated within 3 h after onset of symptoms. Reinfarction rates were equal in the two treatment groups in patients with anterior infarction (5% during 7 months), but nonfatal reinfarction occurred more frequently after treatment with streptokinase in patients with inferior infarction (8% versus 4% in the control group).

Recently, interim results from the Second International Study of Infarct Survival (ISIS-2) [20] were published. In this study 20000 patients with acute myocardial infarction of less than 24 h duration were to be included. In a subgroup of 4000 patients treated within 4 h after onset of symptoms, in-hospital mortality was 12% in the placebo group and 8% in those treated with intravenous streptokinase (1.5×10^6 U). Patient enrollment in the other arms of this trial is still continuing, despite the observed mortality reduction of about 30%.

Table 4. Comparisons between various thrombolytic agents and recanalization procedures

Study	*n*		Thrombolytic agent		Patency rate (%)		In-hospital mortality (%)		Bleeding complications
	I	R	I	R	I	R	I	R	
TIMI [23]	99	115	rt-PA	Sk iv	60	40	5	8	More bleeding in Sk iv group
Verstraete [24]	61	65	rt-PA	Sk iv	70	55	5	5	More bleeding in Sk iv group
Verstraete [25]	64	65	rt-PA	placebo	61	21	1	6	More bleeding in rt-PA group
Williams [26]	47	–	rt-PA	–	68	–	13	–	Significant bleeding in 15
Been [27]	50	–	APSAC	–	88	–	6	–	Severe bleeding in 2
Kaspar [28]	50	–	APSAC	–	64	–	4	–	Minor bleeding in 18
Bonnier [29]	42	43	APSAC	Sk ic	67	67	2	2	No significant bleeding
v.d. Werf [31]	17	–	rsc-PA	–	76	–	6	–	No significant bleeding
O'Neill [32]	29	27	PTCA	Sk ic	83	85	7	4	No bleeding reported

I, Index group, R, reference group; rt-PA, recombinant tissue-type plasminogen activator; Sk, streptokinase; rsc-PA, recombinant single-chain urokinase-type plasminogen activator; APSAC, anisoylated plasminogen-streptokinase activator complex.

Comparing the outcome of these trials, it becomes clear that the intracoronary route is superior to the intravenous one although reserved to those patients who can reach such catheterization laboratories on time. This is best shown by a comparison of the results of the GISSI trial and those of the ICIN study. In the ICIN study in-hospital 14-day mortality was 10% in control group and 5% in all patients allocated to therapy with intracoronary streptokinase, a risk difference of –5%, while in the GISSI trial these figures were, respectively, 13% (control group) and 11% (streptokinase group), a risk difference of –2% (Table 3). These differences are even more favorable for intracoronary therapy when one looks at the subsets treated within 0–2 h. In other words, in-hospital death was prevented in 1 out of 20 patients treated with intracoronary streptokinase and in 1 out of 50 patients treated with intravenous streptokinase. Also, when patients in the GISSI trial, randomized within 3 h after onset of symptoms (risk difference, –3%), are compared to patients in the ICIN study, admitted to the hospital within 2 h after onset of symptoms (risk difference, –6%), larger benefit was derived from treatment with intracoronary streptokinase than from that with intravenous streptokinase.

Studies with Newer Thrombolytic Agents

It is logical, therefore, that many pharmaceutical firms and university research laboratories have searched for better agents to achieve lysis after intravenous administration. Patency of the infarct-related artery can now be achieved with intravenous administration of recombinant tissue-type plasminogen activator (rt-PA) in 60%–70% of patients with acute myocardial infarction, which is considerably higher than the 40%–60% patency rate after intravenous streptokinase [21–'5] (Table 4). Infusion with rt-PA causes less depression of fibrinogen, with a tendency to fewer bleeding complications than intravenous streptokinase, although its occurrence is unpredictable. Furthermore, large-scale investigations presently underway in Europe and in the United States indicate that variations in the dosage (when excessive, such as 100 mg rt-PA or more, associated with increased bleeding) achieve a patency rate close to 80% after intravenous administration.

The efficacy of anisoylated plasminogen streptokinase activator complex (APSAC) in inducing coronary patency has been demonstrated in small trials [26–28], but larger randomized studies are required before its use can be recommended. One of these in England, involving nearly 1000 patients, was ended prematurely when the treated group with acute infarction showed a 44% reduction in 3-month mortality after intravenous APSAC (D. Julian 1987, personal communication). Recently, promising results have also been reported with recombinant single-chain urokinase-type plasminogen activator (PUK) [29–30] and with the combination of PUK and urokinase (70%–80%) patency. Large trials are presently underway to assess the relative value of the various thrombolytic agents and procedures mentioned above, in particular the combination of rt-PA and PTCA, since acute PTCA performed after perforation of the thrombus with a guide wire without use of thrombolytic agents [31, 32] had been shown to be so effective.

Which Patients are Candidates for Thrombolytic Therapy?

It is evident that the interval between onset of myocardial infarction and initiation of thrombolytic therapy mostly determines the efficacy of reperfusion in terms of infarct size, left ventricular function, and mortality. Trials with a large time window (i.e., ≥6 h after onset of symptoms) produced negative results when thrombolytic therapy was compared to conventional treatment (Table 2). Indeed, it can be stated that thrombolytic therapy is not, or is only very rarely, indicated in patients with acute myocardial infarction when treatment delay exceeds 6 h. From all patients admitted within 6 h after onset of symptoms in the GISSI trial and in the ISAM study, major benefits from thrombolytic therapy were observed only in patients treated within 3 h after onset of symptoms. This was also evident in the ICIN study, where the amount of myocardium at risk was also taken into consideration. In fact, all currently designed trials limit the intake of patients to the first 4–6 h after onset of symptoms. The greatest benefit of intracoronary streptokinase on infarct size, left ventricular function, and 3-month mortality is observed in patients admitted to the hospital within 2 h after onset of symptoms and in patients with a large ischemic area (reflected by extensive ST-segment elevation on the admission electrocardiogram) admitted within 4 h after onset of symptoms. However, improvement of long-term survival was most strikingly observed in patients with large, usually anterior, infarctions. In patients with inferior infarction mortality during long-term follow-up appeared to be reduced by thrombolytic therapy only to a minor extent in the ICIN study (9% in the thrombolysis group versus 11% in the control group during 1-year follow-up) and in the ISAM study (10% in the thrombolysis group versus 14% in the control group after a mean follow-up of 21 months). This is most likely due to the reduced area that is salvagable and to the incidence of recurrent infarction after thrombolysis in these patients. Based on these data, the following guidelines are presented for the use of thrombolytic therapy in patients with acute myocardial infarction.

Anterior Infarction

All studies have demonstrated beneficial effects in all patient admitted to the hospital within 2 h after onset of symptoms and in patients with a large ischemic area (total ST-segment elevation of 1.2 mV or more) admitted within 4 h after onset of symptoms. The largest benefit was observed in patients with extensive ischemia admitted within 2 h after onset of symptoms. In patients admitted within 6 h after onset of symptoms it remains unclear whether benefits outweigh the risks of the procedure, although reperfusion could be attempted if clear signs of ongoing ischemia are manifest.

Inferior Infarction

Beneficial effects seem likely in patients admitted within 2 h after onset of symptoms with signs of extensive ischemia, which can be defined as: (a) total ST-segment elevation in leads I, II, III, aVL, aVF, V5, V6 more than 0.6 mV; (b) total ST-segment deviation (total ST-segment depression in leads V1 to V5 added to the total ST-segment elevation) at least 1.2 mV; or (c) presence of at least 0.1 mV ST-segment elevation in lead V4R, indicating right ventricular involvement [33].

In other patients admitted within 6 h after onset of symptoms it seems unlikely that thrombolytic therapy results in major benefit. Furthermore, a minor initial benefit, if present, hardly warrants the risks of the intervention, not to mention costs of acute angiography or subsequent procedures, as these are required in over 50% of all cases at some time in the 1st postinfarction year.

If these current guidelines had been followed in the ICIN trial, thrombolytic therapy would have been offered to 325 patients out of the 533 patients (61%) that were, in fact, admitted to the study. In this subset of patients mean life expectancy was 14.5 years in the control group and 16.3 years in the thrombolysis group. A cost-benefit analysis [13, 34] has shown that total costs per year of life gained by a decision to proceed with thrombolytic therapy with intracoronary streptokinase averaged an extra of NL fl 6000 for those patients in whom thrombolytic therapy was recommended.

Value of Adjuvant Pharmacotherapy

Thrombolytic therapy was accompanied in the present study by supportive pharmacotherapy with platelet-aggregation inhibitors, heparin, oral anticoagulants, lignocaine, and corticosteroids. The exact value of this adjuvant therapy has not been established. The use of lignocaine can be favored in order to prevent ventricular arrhythmias caused either by reperfusion or by the myocardial infarction. The value of the short-term corticosteroid therapy remains debatable, since in the GISSI trial, where no corticosteroids were given, severe allergic reactions after treatment with streptokinase were observed in only 0.1% of patients. The major problem lies in the prevention of reocclusion by pharmacotherapy. Even with the use of platelet-aggregation inhibitors, heparin, and oral anticoagulants, a high incidence of reocclusion and reinfarction was observed in the present trial after initially successful thrombolysis, especially in patients with inferior infarction.

Yet, a recent study with rt-PA given over a prolonged period has shown a low (7%) reocclusion rate, one not matched by any other regimen [36]. Further studies to define the optimal pharmacotherapeutic regiment to prevent reocclusion after successful thrombolysis are urgently needed. The general applicability of thrombolytic agents in patients, particularly those with inferior infarction, depends on the possibilities to prevent reocclusion in these patients.

Coronary Angioplasty

Immediate coronary angioplasty after perforation of the thrombus in the infarct-related coronary artery by a guide wire was proposed as early as 1979 by Rentrop et al. [32] as an alternate approach to the use of thrombolytic therapy in patients with acute myocardial infarction. In a small study reported by O'Neill et al. [31], patency of the infarct-related artery was achieved in 24 out of 29 patients (83%) by this method (Table 3). However, the inevitable longer treatment delay, in setting up the laboratory, etc., restricts this approach to patients in whom intravenous thrombolytic therapy is contraindicated. However, after successful or attempted thrombolysis severe stenosis may remain in the infarct-related coronary artery. This artery may reocclude and abolish the initially beneficial effects of reperfusion. Indeed, reinfarction rates observed in patients with a residual stenosis of 70% or more after successful thrombolysis were as high as 30% during 3-year follow-up, with most of the reinfarctions occurring within 3 months. The additional value of coronary angioplasty in these patients has been confirmed by others [36–40] and was also demonstrated in the ICIN study. Coronary angioplasty appeared to be of value both in patients with anterior and in those with inferior infarction. In patients with anterior infarction reocclusion rates were relatively low (8% at second angiography), but reocclusion might lead to large anterior reinfarctions, while in patients with inferior infarction reocclusion rates were higher (28% at second angioplasty), but the area at risk was on average smaller than in patients with anterior infarction. Consequently, if acute angioplasty after successful thrombolysis is not feasible due to lack of surgical standby, coronary angiography should be carried out within the next few days to assess the suitability for elective PTCA [36–43]. When symptoms and signs of ischemia reappear this intervention should be carried out on a (semi-) urgent basis, as is extensively documented. Quite recently a randomized European study analyzing the need for immediate PTCA after rt-PA in some 200 patients came to the conclusion that no benefit, rather increased risk, was associated with this procedure (M.L. Simoons 1987, personal communication).

Final Recommendations

In patients with acute myocardial infarction in whom thrombolytic therapy can presently be recommended (Table 5), the optimal approach begins with intra-

Table 5. Guidelines for the indications for thrombolytic therapy in patients with acute myocardial infarction

Infarct location	Admission delay	Thrombolytic therapy to be considered in patients with
Anterior[a]	⩽2 h	All anterior infarcts
	2–4 h	Large anterior infarcts, defined as total ST segment elevation (sum of leads I, aVL, V_1 to V_6) ⩾1.2 mV
	4–6 h	Unknown, probably only if total ST-segment elevation ⩾1.2 mV
Inferior[b]	⩽2 h	Large inferior infarcts, defined as total ST-segment elevation (sum of leads I, II, III, aVL, aVF, V_5, V_6) >0.6 mV; or total ST-segment elevation + depression (sum of leads V_1 to V_4) ⩾1.2 mV; ST-segment elevation ⩾0.1 mV in lead V4R
	2–6 h	Unknown if minor benefits outweigh risks
Lateral/posterior	0–6 h	Unknown, minor benefits possible

[a] Anterior infarcts defined as ST segment elevation ⩾0.2 mV in two or more precordial leads.

[b] Inferior infarcts defined as ST segment elevation ⩾0.1 mV in two or more inferior leads.

venous administration of streptokinase (500×10^3 U) – or with rt-PA or other agents when and where available – as early as possible, usually immediately upon hospital admission, followed by acute angiography and intracoronary administration of streptokinase or rt-PA whenever needed. Only when signs of reperfusion have appeared prior to angiography, such as in sudden relief of chest pain with marked decrease of ST-segment elevation, can angiography and subsequent procedure be delayed. When, even after intracoronary thrombolysis, a residual stenosis of 70% or more in the infarct-related artery with poor run-off into the distal coronary bed is seen, immediate PTCA is recommended. When acute PTCA is not feasible or when acute angiography has not been performed following intravenous thrombolytic therapy, coronary angiography within the next days remains indicated to assess the suitability for elective PTCA.

Impact of These Recommendations on Health Care

Following these guidelines, thrombolytic therapy can be offered to 15%–25% of all patients admitted to the hospital with acute myocardial infarction [41]. Even in large hospitals in the Netherlands the number of patients treated with thrombolytic therapy would then not exceed 100 patients per 500-bed hospital per year. When catheterization laboratories are available on a 24-h basis, total workload for their technical staff would be increased only to a moderate extent. The costs for this increased workload were included in a cost-benefit analysis. The apparent benefits from thrombolytic therapy certainly warrant the additional costs (NL fl 6000 per year of life gained) even in the present times when budgets available for health care are limited. However, many patients with acute myocardial infarction are admitted to community hospitals with limited or no possibilities for acute angiography. It is for this reason that Verstraete [42] stated that intravenous thrombolytic therapy would be "the only way." Furthermore, even if thrombolytic therapy is restricted to intravenous administration in those hospitals, the number of subsequent catheterizations to be performed in adjacent large hospitals in order to assess the suitability for elective PTCA, would lead to a further increase in workload in the catheterization laboratories in these hospitals of the new generation of more effective thrombolytic agents (rt-PA, srcu-PA, and APSAC) currently being investigated in large clinical trials, preliminary results have indicated that intravenous use of these leads to successful thrombolysis in a higher percentage of patients than presently can be achieved with intravenous streptokinase (Table 3). Part of these trials have answered the question as to whether PTCA is mandatory after successful thrombolysis. It is now clear that this additional procedure can be deferred for a few days in the majority of cases.

Questions for the Future

In this overview the characteristics have been defined of those patients with acute myocardial infarction to whom early thrombolytic therapy would offer a major benefit. However, this concerns only the 20%–30% of all patients who are admitted to the hospital with acute myocardial infarction within the specified time limit. It is still unclear whether later thrombolytic therapy with the newer agents might offer benefit to other patients with acute myocardial infarction. Presently, it seems unlikely that patients admitted to the hospital more than 6 h after onset of symptoms would benefit from any reperfusion strategy in a major way only. Patients admitted up to 24 h after onset of symptoms with new symptomatic and extensive ischemia (usually located anteriorly) or with signs of cardiogenic shock constitute a group of high-risk patients who might derive further benefit from late reperfusion [43].

It is likely that in the near future the new generation of thrombolytic agents (rt-PA, rscu-PA, and APSAC) will become first choice for the intravenous initiation of thrombolytic therapy. Then, the indications for either acute or delayed angiography might be different from those at present although this is less and less likely. Further cost-benefit analysis will certainly be required to assess the additional value of intracoronary thrombolysis and coronary angioplasty after intravenous administration of rt-PA, rscu-PS, or APSAC. The required capacity of catheterization laboratories and facilities for coronary angioplasty and bypass surgery will depend on the results of those analyses. We expect, however, that the guidelines presented here will change but little with other thrombolytic agents, and that a stepwise approach, including intravenous and possibly intracoronary treatment followed by coronary angioplasty in selected or surgery at some point in selected patients, will ultimately be confirmed to be the optimal strategy.

References

1. Kennedy JW, Ritchie JL, Davis KB, Fritz JK (1983) Western Washington randomized trial of intracoronary streptokinase in acute myocardial infarction. N Engl J Med 309:1477–1482
2. Kennedy JW, Ritchie JL, Davis KB, et al (1985) The Western Washington randomized trial of intracoronary streptokinase in acute myocardial infarction. N Engl J Med 312:1073–1078
3. Khaja F, Walton JA, Brymer JF, et al (1984) Intracoronary fibrinolytic therapy in acute myocardial infarction. N Engl J Med 308:1305–1311
4. Leiboff RH, Katz JR, Wasserman AG, et al (1985) A randomized, angiographically controlled trial of intracoronary streptokinase in acute myocardial infarction. Am J Cardiol 53:404–407
5. Raizner AE, Tortoledo FA, Verani MS, et al (1985) In: Myocardial infarction: a prospective, randomized, controlled trial. Am J Cardiol 55:301–308
6. Rentrop KP, Feit F, Blanke H, et al (1984) Effects of intracoronary streptokinase and intracoronary nitroglycerin infusion on coronary angiographic patterns and mortality in patients with acute myocardial infarction. N Engl J Med 311:1457–1463
7. Anderson JL, Marshall HW, Bray BE, et al (1983) A randomized trial of intracoronary streptokinase in the treatment of acute myocardial infarction. N Engl J Med 308:1312–1318
8. Anderson JL, McIlvaine PM, Marshall HW, et al (1986) Long-term follow-up after intracoronary streptokinase for myocardial infarction: a randomized controlled study. Am Heart J 6:1402–1407
9. Simoons ML, Serruys PW, van den Brand M, et al (1985) Improved survial after early thrombolysis in acute myocardial infarction. Lancet II:578–582
10. Verheugt FWA, van Eenige MJ, van der Wall EE, et al (1985) Bleeding complications of intracoronary fibrinolytic therapy in acute myocardial infarction. Br Heart J 54:455–459
11. Res J, Simoons ML, Verheugt F, et al (1984) Thrombolysis in acute myocardial infarction; hemodynamic effects in the CCU (Abstract). Circulation 70[II]:1318
12. Vermeer F, Simoons ML, Lubsen J (1986) Reduced frequency of ventricular fibrillation after early thrombolysis in acute myocardial infarction. Lancet II:1147–1148
13. Vermeer F, Simoons ML, Bär FW, et al (1986) Which patients benefit most from early thrombolytic therapy with intracoronary streptokinase? Circulation 74:1379–1399
14. Fioretti P, Vermeer F, Simoons ML, et al (1986) Limitation of scintigraphic infarct size and exercise induced ischemia after early thrombolysis (Abstract). Circulation 74[II]:506

15. Serruys PW, Simoons ML, Suryapranata H, et al (1986) Preservation of global and regional left ventricular function after early thrombolysis in acute myocardial infarction. J Am Coll Cardiol 7:729–742
16. Yusuf S, Collins R, Peto R, et al (1985) Intravenous and intracoronary fibrinolytic therapy in acute myocardial infarction: overview of results on mortality, reinfarction and side effects from 33 randomized controlled trials. Eur Heart J 6:556–585
17. Gruppo italiano per lo studio della streptochinase nell' infarcto miocardio (GISSI) (1986) Effectiveness of intravenous thrombolytic treatment in acute myocardial infarction. Lancet II:397–404
18. ISAM Study Group (1986) A prospective trial of intravenous streptokinase in acute myocardial infarction (ISAM). N Engl J Med 314:1465–1471
19. Schröder R, Neuhaus K, Leizorovicz A, et al (1987) A prospective placebo-controlled double-blind multicenter trial of intravenous streptokinase in acute myocardial infarction (ISAM): long term mortality and morbidity. J Am Coll Cardiol 9:197–203
20. ISIS Steering Committee (1987) Intravenous streptokinase given within 0–4 hours of onset of myocardial infarction reduces mortality in ISIS-2. Lancet 9:502
21. Schröder R (1983) Systemic versus intracoronary streptokinase infusion of acute myocardial infarction. J Am Coll Cardiol 1:1254–1261
22. TIMI Study Group (1983) The thrombolysis in myocardial infarction (TIMI) trial: phase I findings. J Am Coll Cardiol 1:1254–1261
23. Verstraete M, Bory M, Collen D, et al (1985) Randomized trial of intravenous recombinant tissue-type plasminogen activator versus intravenous streptokinase in acute myocardial infarction. Lancet I:842–847
24. Verstraete M, Brower RW, Collen D, et al (1985) Double-blind randomised trial of intravenous tissue-type plasminogen activator versus placebo in acute myocardial infarction. Lancet II: 965–969
25. Williams DO, Borer J, Braunwald E, et al (1986) Intravenous recombinant tissue-type plasminogen activator in patients with acute myocardial infarction: a report from the NHLBI thrombolysis in myocardial infarction trial. Circulation 73:338–346
26. Been M, De Bono DP, Muir AL, et al (1986) Clinical effects and kinetic properties of intravenous APSAC – anisoylated plasminogen-streptokinase activator complex (BRL 26921) in acute myocardial infarction. Int J Cardiol 11:53–61
27. Kaspar W, Meinerts T, Wollschlager H, et al (1986) Coronary thrombolysis during acute myocardial infarction by intravenous BRL 26921, a new anisoylated plasminogen-streptokinase activator complex. Am J Cardiol 58:418–421
28. Bonnier JJRM, de Swart JBRM, Hoffmann JJML, et al (1987) Intravenous APSAC versus intracoronary streptokinase in the treatment of acute myocardial infarction (Abstract). J Am Coll Cardiol 9:62A
29. Collen D, Stassen JM, Blaber G, et al (1984) Biological and thrombolytic properties of proenzyme and active forms of human urokinase. III. Thrombolytic properties of natural and recombinant urokinase in rabbits with experimental jugular vein thrombosis. Thromb Haemost 52:27–30
30. Van den Werf F, Vanhacke J, de Geest H, et al (1986) Coronary thrombolysis with recombinant single-chain urokinase-type plasminogen activator in patients with acute myocardial infarction. Circulation 74:1066–1070
31. O'Neill W, Timmis GC, Bourdillon PD, et al (1986) A prospective randomised clinical trial of intracoronary streptokinase versus coronary angioplasty for acute myocardial infarction. N Engl J Med 314:812–818

32. Rentrop P, Blanke H, Wiegand E, et al (1979) Wiederöffnung verschlossener Kranzgefäße im akuten Infarkt mit Hilfe von Kathetern. Dtsch Med Wochenschr 104: 1401 – 1405
33. Bär FW, Res J, Braat SH, et al. Location of the coronary lesion and importance of lead V4R to predict success of thrombolytic therapy. Am J Cardiol (manuscript submitted)
34. Vermeer F (1987) Thrombolysis in acute myocardial infarction. Van Gorkum, Assen
35. Verstraete M, Arnold AE, Brower RW, et al (1987) Acute coronary thrombolysis with recombinant human tissue type plasminogen activator: initial patency and influence of maintained infusion on reocclusion rate. Am J Cardiol 60:231 – 237
36. Smalling RW, Nishikawa A, Merhige ME, et al. (1986) Intravenous tissue-type plasminogen activator followed by percutaneous transluminal coronary angioplasty in acute myocardial infarction: acute and follow-up quantitative angiographic analysis (Abstract). Circulation 74[Suppl II]:23
37. Collins GJ, Califf RM, Philips HR, et al. (1986) Quantitative angiographic changes occurring within 24 hours and one week following tretment with tissue plasminogen activator in patients randomized to immediate and late angioplasty (Abstract). Circulation 74[Suppl II]:275
38. Topol EJ, Califf RM, George BS, et al. (1986) A multicenter randomized trial of intravenous recombinant tissue plasminogen activator and emergency coronary angioplasty for acute myocardial infarction: preliminary report from the TAMI trial (Abstract). Circulation 74[Suppl II]:23
39. Serruys PW, Wijns W, Van den Brand M, et al. (1983) Is transluminal coronary angioplasty mandatory after successful thrombolysis? Br Heart J 50:257 – 265
40. Hugenholtz PG (1987) Acute coronary artery obstruction in myocardial infarction: overview of thrombolytic therapy. J Am Coll Cardiol 9:100 – 118
41. Murray N, Lyons J, Layton C, et al. (1987) What proportion of patients with myocardial infarction are suitable for thrombolysis? Br Heart J 57:144 – 147
42. Verstraete M (1985) Intravenous administration of a thrombolytic agent is the only realistic therapeutic approach in evolving myocardial infarction. Eur Heart J 6:586 – 593
43. De Feyter P, Serruys PW, Soward A, et al. (1986) Coronary angioplasty for early postinfarction unstable angina. Circulation 74:1365 – 1370

Is There a Role for Thrombolysis in Non-Q-Wave Myocardial Infarction and Unstable Angina Pectoris?

B. L. Zaret and H. J. Bigham, Jr.

Introduction

The role of thrombolysis in the therapy of acute transmural myocardial infarction has been established. Several large clinical trials have demonstrated that prompt administration of thrombolytic therapy can result in decreased mortality, improvement in ventricular function, and reduction in myocardial infarct size [1 – 5]. To date major trials have involved primarily, if not exclusively, patients with transmural myocardial infarction manifesting ST segment elevation on the electrocardiogram and total coronary occlusion on the coronary angiogram. Relatively little data are available concerning thrombolytic therapy in infarct patients presenting with ST segment depression electrocardiographically as well as those with unstable angina without infarction. The evaluation of such patients is of major importance since it has been estimated that approximately one-third of patients hospitalized with myocardial infarction are subsequently shown to have a non-Q-wave, i. e., presumed nontransmural, myocardial infarction.

Recent studies suggest that acute thrombosis may play an important role in the pathophysiology of both non-Q-wave myocardial infarction and unstable angina pectoris [6 – 13]. In addition, specific types of coronary angiographic lesions have been noted in these unstable coronary syndromes [14 – 16]. Nevertheless, the role of thrombolytic therapy in the management of patients with non-Q-wave infarction and unstable angina remains unclear. This report reviews current evidence concerning the role of thrombosis in patients with both non-Q-wave infarction and unstable angina pectoris. Natural history data as well as initial pilot studies involving thrombolytic therapy are reviewed. An attempt is made to develop a framework in which one can answer the question: "Is there a role for thrombolysis in non-Q-wave myocardial infarction and unstable angina?" In view of differences between the clinical course and consequences of these syndromes in comparison to transmural Q-wave myocardial infarction, end points appropriate for analysis of therapeutic efficacy in non-Q-wave infarction and unstable angina are discussed.

Non-Q-Wave Myocardial Infarction

Non-Q-wave myocardial infarction is defined by (a) ischemic chest pain of at least 30 min duration, (b) the development of ST segment depression and/or new

T-wave inversion in at least two leads, (c) the absence of either development of new Q waves or loss of R wave of at least 50% without Q-wave development, (d) evidence of myocardial necrosis evidenced by elevated plasma creatine kinase. There is indirect evidence suggesting that a likely pathophysiologic scenario in non-Q-wave infarction involves an initial complete thrombotic coronary occlusion at the site of atherosclerotic stenosis, with subsequent early spontaneous reperfusion. Over time there remains a tendency for recurrent occlusive thrombus formation, presumably at the site of the initial obstruction. In the initial phase of the TIMI trial approximately 20% of patients undergoing coronary angiography were noted on admission to have incomplete coronary occlusion [17]. This occurred despite the fact that 1-mm ST segment elevation was an electrocardiographic admission criterion. These patients generally had relatively better preserved left ventricular function [17, 18] and presumably fall into the group destined to develop non-Q-wave infarction. DeWood et al. evaluated coronary arteriographic findings in individuals with non-Q-wave myocardial infarction who were studied within the first week of the event [19]. Total occlusion of the infarct-related coronary artery was noted in 26% of patients within 24 h of the event, in 37% of patients between 24 and 72 h after peak symptoms, and in 42% of patients studied between 72 h and 7 days after peak symptoms. The increasing incidence of total occlusion over time was paralleled by a rise in the incidence of visible collateral vessels, from 27% within the first 24 h, to 34% at 24 – 72 h, and 42% at 72 h to 7 days. These data stand in contrast to those of Q-wave infarction where total occlusion of the infarct-related vessel is the rule in the early hours after infarction, with an increasing frequency of subtotal occlusion over time [20]. These data suggest that although early in the course of events there is often subtotal occlusion of the infarct related vessel in non-Q-wave infarction, the lesion is quite unstable and demonstrates a propensity toward further thrombus formation and recurrent total occlusion.

These angiographic observations are paralleled by clinical observations indicating that non-Q-wave infarction is frequently associated with recurrent myocardial infarction, extension of infarction, or development of progressive unstable angina pectoris [21]. In general, initial non-Q-wave infarctions are smaller than Q-wave infarctions, as evidenced by both magnitude of enzyme release and extent of regional and global left ventricular dysfunction. Although initial mortality of non-Q-wave infarction tends to be lower than noted in Q-wave infarction, this prognostic benefit appears to dissipate over the ensuing 1 – 2 years as a result of both early and late reinfarction. In the recent diltiazem non-Q-wave infarct trial, reinfarction occurred within 14 days in 12.9% of the placebo group [22]. Refractory postinfarction angina occurred in 6.9%. Death within 14 days occurred in only 3.1% of patients. As can be noted, the incidence of in-hospital events following non-Q-wave infarction is relatively low. A mortality study would not be possible when relatively few patients succumb within the study period. Therefore, primary study end points would by necessity involve a combination of coronary events including angina, reinfarction, and death.

There have been no clinical trials to date involving thrombolytic therapy in non-Q-wave infarction. It is of note that in the GISSI study approximately 450 patients entered with ST-segment depression on the electrocardiogram [1]. They were evenly divided between those receiving thrombolytic therapy with streptokinase and placebo. In this relatively small sample there was no difference in mortality. Again, this is not surprising based upon the relatively low mortality rates anticipated in this subset.

Unstable Angina Pectoris

Patients with unstable angina manifest at least one of the following: (a) effort angina of increasing frequency or duration with a clear change from previous patterns, (b) rest angina without provocation by effort or stress, (c) postinfarction angina. By definition, episodes of pain are accompanied by electrocardiographic changes involving ST-segment depression and/or T-wave inversion (although ST-segment elevation also can be seen), absence of newly developed Q waves or loss of R-wave voltage and no major elevation in plasma myocardial creatine kinase. The major distinguishing factor between unstable angina and non-Q-wave infarction involves enzymatic evidence of myocardial necrosis as determined by a rise in plasma creatine kinase. This assessment can only be made after the fact during the 24 h following hospitalization. Therefore, it is not always possible to characterize patients initially into the proper diagnostic group. Clearly, a clinical continuum exists between unstable angina pectoris and non-Q-wave infarction.

From a pathophysiologic standpoint, the occurrence of angina at rest generally is associated with an abrupt decrease in myocardial blood flow. There is mounting evidence from a variety of sources that coronary thrombosis is a frequent concomitant of unstable angina pectoris. Falk demonstrated at necropsy that layered thrombus containing thrombotic material of differing age could be demonstrated in the epicardial coronary arteries of patients with unstable angina pectoris and subsequent sudden death [23]. Of note, there frequently was demonstration of peripheral embolization causing embolic occlusion of smaller coronary arteries and resulting in microinfarction. This was present in 73% of cases [24].

Sherman et al. performed coronary angioscopy at the time of coronary bypass surgery in patients with unstable angina pectoris [12]. A total of 20 patients were evaluated: 10 with unstable angina and 10 with stable coronary disease. Complex plaque formation was seen in four of the ten patients with unstable angina and none of the patients with stable disease. Likewise, thrombus was demonstrated in seven of the ten patients with unstable angina. Of interest, all seven patients with rest angina demonstrated thrombus.

At the time of coronary angiography, coronary thrombus had been demonstrated with a variable frequency in patients with unstable angina [6–13].

Table 1. Coronary thrombosis in unstable angina

Study	Ref.	Thrombus cases/total number of patients	
Holmes 1981	6	6/1202	(1.3%)
Vetrovec 1981	7	8/129	(6.2%)
Mandelkorn 1983	8	4/9	(44%)
Zack 1984	9	10/83	(12%)
Bresnahan 1985	10	24/67	(35%)
Capone 1985	11	44/119	(37%)
Sherman 1986[a]	12	7/10	(70%)
Gold 1987	13	8/11	(73%)

[a] Angioscopy.

Studies performed since 1981 have indicated a frequency of thrombus in culprit coronary arteries ranging from 1.3% to 73% (Table 1). Since the lesion generally involves subtotal occlusion, definition of thrombus angiographically is not as straightforward as in the instance of total coronary occlusion. In addition to obvious thrombus formation, eccentric subtotal occlusions also may be noted. These eccentric lesions are generally asymmetric with a narrow neck and demonstrate irregular borders [14–16]. Such lesions, designated type II eccentric lesions by Ambrose et al., have a high association with the clinical presentation of unstable angina in comparison to stable angina [14]. Such an angiographic appearance is believed to represent ruptured atherosclerotic plaque, partially occlusive thrombus, or both. In contrast to the angioscopic data, these angiographic lesions have been noted in all types of patients with unstable angina, independent of their clinical presentation or duration of symptoms. The most dramatic angiographic demonstration of thrombus formation in patients with unstable angina pectoris was reported recently by Gold et al. [13]. In a placebo group of 12 patients receiving conventional therapy, which included heparin, 8 manifested major filling defects on coronary angiography consistent with thrombus formation.

Can therapy designed to lyse or limit thrombus formation impact favorably on the clinical course of patients with unstable angina? There are several lines of evidence which currently are suggestive. In the prethrombolytic era, Telford and Wilson demonstrated that intravenous heparin was of substantial benefit in preventing the occurrence of acute myocardial infarction in patients presenting with "intermediate coronary syndrome" [24]. The Veteran's Administration cooperative study on aspirin and unstable angina pectoris noted that the administration of aspirin to patients with unstable angina resulted in a 51% lower incidence of death or acute myocardial infarction as compared to placebo [25]. Nonfatal acute myocardial infarction was 51% lower in the aspirin group

Table 2. Thrombolysis in unstable angina

Study	Ref.	*n*	Agent	Success	End points
Lawrence 1981	27	40	IV SK	+	Clin
Rentrop 1982	28	5	IC SK	–	Angio
Ventrovec 1981	29	12	IC SK	+	Angio
Mandelkorn 1983	8	9	IC SK	+	Angio
Ambrose 1987	26	36	IC SK	–	Angio
Gold 1987	13	22	IV rt-PA	+	Angio, clin

Clin, Clinical impression; angio, angiographic evaluation; IV, intravenous; IC, intracoronary; SK, streptokinase; rt-PA, recombinant tissue plasminogen activator.

(3.4% versus 6.9%; $p = 0.005$). Reduction in mortality in the aspirin group was also 51% (1.6% versus 3.3%; $p = 0.054$).

A total of six studies have been published since 1981 involving a role of thrombolytic therapy in unstable angina (Table 2). These studies have been relatively small, each generally involving fewer than 50 patients. Both streptokinase and rt-PA have been employed with varying results. The most dramatic results were noted by Gold et al. [13]. They evaluated 23 patients with unstable angina who were equally divided into a placebo group receiving conventional therapy including heparin and a group receiving rt-PA in addition to conventional therapy. Unstable angina pectoris persisted after completion of the infusion in 6 of 11 placebo patients but in only 1 of 12 patients receiving rt-PA ($p < 0.03$). Coronary angiography performed approximately 1.5 days after completion of infusion demonstrated subocclusive thrombus in 8 of 11 patients receiving placebo but in none of 11 patients receiving rt-PA ($p < 0.002$). Persistence of unstable angina pectoris correlated significantly with the presence of intracoronary thrombus. Others have noted less impressive results with thrombolytic therapy (Table 2). Recently, Ambrose et al. evaluated 36 consecutive patients with subtotal coronary occlusion and unstable clinical presentations who received intracoronary streptokinase. The major end point involved coronary angiographic assessment in both a qualitative and quantitative manner [26]. Angiographic analysis demonstrated no major group changes in the culprit coronary artery following therapy, although five individual patients showed some reduction in the percent of coronary stenosis.

Conclusions

Based upon current data, there appears to be a suggestive role for thrombolysis in unstable angina and non-Q-wave infarction. Nevertheless, at this time that role is by no means firmly established. Clearly, well-designed prospective clinical trials with appropriate patient accession are required to provide definitive results based upon necessary statistical power. It must be emphasized that unstable angina pectoris and non-Q-wave infarction form a clinical continuum, and it may prove difficult at the time of clinical presentation to segregate patients into the most appropriate of the two diagnostic categories. Making a categorization after the fact, based upon plasma enzyme determination, has the potential for introducing bias into the analysis. In view of the relatively low acute mortality in these clinical entities, end points will have to involve pooled ischemic events, that is, recurrent angina pectoris, myocardial infarction, and death. It is unlikely that ventricular function can be a major end point of study in these patients (as compared to studies in patients with Q-wave infarction) since initially there is only a relatively modest impairment in both global and regional left ventricular function. Difficulties may exist in terms of defining thrombus angiographically; the incidence of the thrombus also may be influenced by the timing of angiographic studies in relation to the onset of symptoms [19]. In addition, different presentations of unstable angina (such as postinfarction angina and rest angina) may be associated with different clinical outcomes and may require prospective identification for appropriate subgroup analysis [30]. The role of adjunctive therapy such as antiplatelet agents, conventional anticoagulation and antianginals require detailed study. Independent favorable effects have been noted with these forms of therapy in patients with unstable angina [24, 25, 31]. Finally, this group of patients is frequently referred for subsequent aggressive interventional therapy involving angioplasty or bypass surgery [32, 33]. How these independent therapies may impact upon outcome must be carefully considered in the design of trials assessing thrombolysis.

References

1. GISSI Study Group (1986) Effectiveness of intravenous thrombolytic treatment in acute myocardial infarction. Lancet I:397–422
2. Koren G, Weiss AT, Hasin Y, Appelbaum D, Welber S, Rozenman Y, Lothan C, Mosseri M, Sapoznikov D, Luria MH, Gotsman M (1985) Prevention of myocardial damage in acute myocardial ischemia by early treatment with intravenous streptokinase. N Engl J Med 313:1384–1389
3. ISAM Study Group (1986) A prospective trial of intravenous streptokinase in acute myocardial infarction (ISAM). N Engl J Med 314:1465–1471
4. Simoons ML, Serruys PW, van den Brand M, Res J, Verheugt FWA, Krauss XH, Remme WJ, Bar F, deZwaan C, van der Laarse A, Vermeer F, Lubsen J (1986) Early thrombolysis in acute myocardial infarction: limitation of infarct size and improved survival. J Am Coll Cardiol 7:717–728
5. White HD, Norris RM, Brown MA, Takayama M, Maslowski A, Bass NM, Ormiston JA, Whitlock T (1987) Effect of intravenous streptokinase on left ventricular function and early survival after acute myocardial infarction. N Engl J Med 317:850–855
6. Holmes DR, Hartzler GO, Smith HC, Fuster V (1981) Coronary artery thrombosis in patients with unstable angina. Br Heart J 45:411–416

7. Vetrovec GW, Cowley MJ, Overton H, Richardson DW (1981) Intracoronary thrombus in syndromes of unstable myocardial ischemia. Am Heart J 102:1202–1208
8. Mandelkorn JB, Wolf NM, Singh S, Shechter JA, Kersh RI, Rodgers DM, Workman MB, Bentivoglio LG, LaPorte SM, Meister SG (1983) Intracoronary thrombus in nontransmural myocardial infarction and in unstable angina pectoris. Am J Cardiol 52:1–6
9. Zack PM, Ischinger T, Aker UT, Dincer B, Kennedy KL (1984) The occurrence of angiographically detected intracoronary thrombus in patients with unstable angina pectoris. Am Heart J 108:1408–1412
10. Bresnahan DR, Davis JL, Holmes DR, Smith HC (1985) Angiographic occurrence and clinical correlates of intraluminal coronary artery thrombus: role of unstable angina. J Am Coll Cardiol 6:285–289
11. Capone G, Wolf NM, Meyer B, Meister SG (1985) Frequency of intracoronary filling defects by angiography in angina pectoris at rest. Am J Cardiol 56:403–406
12. Sherman CT, Litvack F, Grundfest W, Lee M, Hickey A, Chaux A, Kass R, Blanche C, Matloff J, Morgenstern L, Ganz W, Swan HJC, Forrester J (1986) Coronary angioscopy in patients with unstable angina pectoris. N Engl J Med 315:913–919
13. Gold HK, Johns JA, Leinbach RC, Yasuda T, Grossbard E, Zusman R, Collen D (1987) A randomized, blinded, placebo-controlled trial of recombinant human tissue-type plasminogen activator in patients with unstable angina pectoris. Circulation 75:1192–1199
14. Ambrose JA, Winters SL, Stern A, Eng A, Teichholz LE, Gorlin R, Fuster V (1985) Angiographic morphology and the pathogenesis of unstable angina pectoris. J Am Coll Cardiol 5:609–616
15. Ambrose JA, Winters SL, Arora RR, Haft JI, Goldstein J, Rentrop KP, Gorlin R, Fuster V (1985) Coronary angiographic morphology in myocardial infarction: a link between the pathogenesis of unstable angina and myocardial infarction. J Am Coll Cardiol 6:1223–1238
16. Ambrose JA, Winters SL, Arora RR, Eng A, Riccio A, Gorlin R, Fuster V (1986) Angiographic evolution of coronary artery morphology in unstable angina. J Am Coll Cardiol 7:472–478
17. Chesebro JH, Knatterud G, Roberts R, Borer J, Cohen LS, Dalen J, Dodge HT, Francis CK, Hillis D, Ludbrook P, Markis JE, Mueller H, Passamani ER, Powers ER, Rao AK, Robertson T, Ross A, Ryan TJ, Sobel BE, Willerson J, Williams DO, Zaret BL, Braunwald E (1987) Thrombolysis in myocardial infarction (TIMI) trial, phase I: a comparison between intravenous tissue plasminogen activator and intravenous streptokinase. Circulation 76:141–154
18. Sheehan FH, Braunwald E, Canner P, Dodge HT, Gore J, van Natta P, Passamani ER, Williams DO, Zaret BL (1987) The effect of intravenous thrombolytic therapy on left ventricular function: a report on tissue type plasminogen activator and streptokinase from the thrombolysis in myocardial infarction (TIMI phase I) trial. Circulation 75:817–829
19. DeWood MA, Stifter WF, Simpson CS, Spores J, Eugster GS, Judge TP, Hinnen ML (1986) Coronary arteriographic findings soon after non-Q-wave myocardial. N Engl J Med 315:417–423
20. DeWood MA, Spores J, Notske RN, et al. (1980) Prevalence of total coronary occlusions during the early hours of transmural myocardial infarction. N Engl J Med 303: 897–902

21. Gibson RS, Beller GA, Gheorghiade M, Nygaard TW, Watson DD, Huey BL, Sayre SL, Kaiser DL (1986) The prevalence and clinical significance of residual myocardial ischemia 2 weeks after uncomplicated non-Q-wave infarction: a prospective natural history study. Circulation 73:1186–1198
22. Gibson RS, Boden WE, Theroux P, Strauss HD, Pratt CM, Gheorghiade M, Capone RJ, Crawford MH, Schlant RC, Kleiger RE, Young PM, Schechtman K, Perryman B, Roberts R, Diltiazem Reinfarction Study Group (1986) Diltiazem and reinfarction in patients with non-Q-wave myocardial infarction. N Engl J Med 315:423–429
23. Falk S (1985) Unstable angina with fatal outcome: dynamic coronary thrombosis leading to infarction and/or sudden death. Circulation 71:699–708
24. Telford AM, Wilson C (1981) Trial of heparin versus atenolol in prevention of myocardial infarction in intermediate coronary syndrome. Lancet I:1225–1228
25. Lewis HD, Davis JW, Archibald DG, Steinke WE, Smitherman TC, Doherty JE, Schnaper HW, LeWinter MM, Linares E, Pouget JM, Sabharwal SC, Chesler E, DeMots H (1983) Protective effects of aspirin against acute myocardial infarction and death in men with unstable angina. N Engl J Med 309:396–403
26. Ambrose JA, Hjemdahl-Monsen C, Borrico S, Sherman W, Cohen M, Gorlin R, Fuster V (1987) Quantitative and qualitative effects of intracoronary streptokinase in unstable angina and non-Q-wave infarction. J Am Coll Cardiol 9:1156–1165
27. Lawrence JR, Shepherd JT, Bone I, Rogen AS, Fulton WFM (1979) Fibrinolytic therapy in unstable angina pectoris: a controlled clinical trial, Thromb Res 17: 767–777
28. Rentrop P, Blanke H, Karsch R, Kaiser H, Kostering H, Leitz K (1981) Selective intracoronary thrombolysis in acute myocardial infarction and angina pectoris. Circulation 63:307–317
29. Vetrovec GW, Leinbach RC, Gold HK, Cowley MJ (1982) Intracoronary thrombolysis in syndromes of unstable ischemia: angiographic and clinical results. Am Heart J 104:946–952
30. Bosch X, Theroux P, Waters DD, Pelletier GB, Roy D (1987) Early postinfarction ischemia: clinical, angiographic, and prognostic significance. Circulation 75:988–995
31. Gibson RS, Young PM, Boden WE, Schechtman K, Roberts R (1987) Prognostic significance and beneficial effect of diltiazem on the incidence of early recurrent ischemia after non-Q-wave myocardial infarction: results from the Multicenter Diltiazem Reinfarction Study. Am J Cardiol 60:203–209
32. De Feyter PJ, Serruys PW, van den Brand M, Balakumaran K, Mochtar B, Soward AL, Arnold AER, Hugenholtz PG (1985) Emergency coronary angioplasty in refractory unstable angina. N Engl J Med 313:342–346
33. Luchi RJ, Scott SM, Deupree RH (1987) Comparison of medical and surgical treatment for unstable angina pectoris. N Engl J Med 316:977–984

Anticoagulants After Thrombolysis

F. Markwardt

Introduction

By the late 1970s the primary role of thrombotic coronary artery occlusion in the aetiology of acute myocardial infarction was established, and it soon became apparent that antithrombotic agents are able to prevent this event [5]. Their possible administration in relation to the different stages of progress of coronary heart disease and their ability to prevent formation and extension of coronary thrombosis and subsequent myocardial ischaemia are illustrated in Table 1.

Above all, it was therapeutic thrombolysis that enriched the concept of antithrombotic treatment of myocardial infarction. From what has already been published it is clear that coronary thrombolysis is being investigated vigorously as a potential initial therapeutic step for patients with evolving transmural infarction. Reperfusion induced by intracoronary or intravenous administration of thrombolytic agents may preserve myocardial function and reduce mortality [16].

However, when an occluded artery is recanalized by fibrinolytic therapy, the lesion which triggered the initial thrombus formation may remain. This may predispose to reocclusion unless anticoagulation is instituted. Therefore, it has been suggested that fibrinolytic therapy may be of worthwhile net benefit only if followed by anticoagulant therapy. At least the latter should be taken into consideration if the anticoagulant effect resulting from the reduction of fibrinogen and the formation of FDP is not sufficient [16]. That is why anticoagulation initiated by immediate injection of heparin with subsequent oral anticoagulation belongs to the management of acute myocardial infarction after coronary thrombolysis.

The rational as well as the clinical evidence of the benefit of this kind of treatment has been repeatedly questioned, and the long-term treatment with oral anticoagulants to prevent reinfarction and cardiac death has been one of the controversial therapeutic approaches. The reason for this is that the effect of such treatment depends on the degree of anticoagulation and the possible haemorrhagic complications during administration. The commonly used anticoagulants, whether coumarin or heparin, have certain disadvantages. Oral anticoagulants prevent formation and extension of a fibrin-rich thrombus by retarding the synthesis of vitamin K-dependent clotting factors. This means an interference in the biosynthesis of clotting enzymes which becomes effective only after 12 – 24 h.

Table 1. Antithrombotic treatment in coronary heart disease

Stage of disease	Aims of antithrombotic treatment	Antithrombotic drugs
Angina pectoris	Primary prevention of occlusive thrombi	Antiplatelet drugs, coumarin
Acute myocardial infarction	Lysis of coronary thrombosis	Streptokinase, urokinase, t-PA, scuPA, APSAC
	Improvement of microcirculation by lowering blood viscosity	Streptokinase, urokinase
	Prevention of cardiogenic arterial thromboembolism and coronary rethrombosis	Heparin, coumarin
Reinfarction	Secondary prevention of occlusive thrombi	Antiplatelet drugs, coumarin

At present, immediate anticoagulation can be achieved only with the aid of the sulphated glycosaminoglycan heparin. However, some problems arise in its use as an antithrombotic agent to prevent reocclusion. Apart from the necessity of parenteral administration, heparin exerts its inhibitory effect on the clotting enzyme indirectly by potentiating the inhibitory function of endogenous antithrombin III and heparin cofactor II. Therefore, its inhibitory effect depends on the blood level of these plasma proteins. Furthermore, heparin interacts with other blood constituents such as platelets, fibrinolytic components, and lipoprotein lipases. Finally, heparin may cause an immunoresponse as well as thrombocytopenia and may induce haemorrhagic side effects.

Therefore, the search for new anticoagulants suitable for prevention of coronary thrombosis has been continued.

Native and Recombinant Hirudin – Selective Thrombin Inhibitors

Our efforts have been directed especially to the pharmacological control of the clotting enzyme thrombin, as it occupies a central position within the coagulation system. This is especially evident if one takes into account that thrombin catalyses not only the formation of insoluble fibrin but also activates clotting factors and platelets. Thus, the inhibition of thrombin represents an effective interference in the coagulation process, and a selective tight-binding thrombin inhibitor is expected to prevent thrombosis or its progression. The lack of such inhibitors for in vivo control of thrombin activity challenged us to develop non-plasmatic inhibitors that block the clotting enzyme directly.

Besides the development of synthetic thrombin inhibitors [7] we attempted to solve this problem by isolation and pharmacological characterization of the naturally occurring inhibitor from medicinal leeches (*Hirudo medicinalis*). This substance was characterized as a selective thrombin inhibitor with polypeptide structure and was named hirudin [3, 4, 5]. The analysis of the isolated agent showed a one-chain carbohydrate-free polypeptide stabilized by three intramolecular disulphide bridges. The establishment of the primary structure elucidated that this polypeptide contains 65 amino acids, for which a molecular weight of about 7000 daltons was calculated. Analysing the anticoagulant effect of hirudin we found that it possesses special affinity for the clotting enzyme thrombin. With thrombin, hirudin forms an inactive enzyme-inhibitor complex with a very low dissociation, whereby the active centre of the enzyme is immediately blocked (Fig. 1). Pharmacological studies have shown that hirudin is well tolerated and is an anticoagulant of high quality [14].

Unfortunately, hirudin is not available in adequate amounts for therapeutic use since medicinal leeches are available in a limited number only. Moreover, they have been placed on the List of Endangered Species. This is why it is very difficult to obtain the starting material for isolating the inhibitor. However, hirudin has been brought into the focus of interest again since advanced methods of genetic engineering allow the obtaining of hirudin in sufficient yield, based on the success of the specialists in cloning and expression of a cDNA coding for the naturally occurring anticoagulant and its variants. The amino acid sequence of recombinant hirudin was similar to that of native hirudin except for the absent sulphate residue in position 63, the disulphide configuration being identical. The recombinant desulphato-hirudin shows the same efficient inhibition kinetics as that of the natural authentic hirudin [11, 15].

Antithrombotic Action of Hirudin

This new development prompted us to resume our pharmacological investigations on hirudin in order to demonstrate its antithrombotic action caused by its pronounced and specific anticoagulant effect and to clarify the special action of native and recombinant hirudin on coronary thrombosis [8, 9].

Since the anticoagulant action of this thrombin inhibitor depends directly on its concentration in blood, we studied the concentration-time course of the inhibitor in experimental animals and in man using various routes of administration [14, 15]. Hirudin given intravenously is relatively rapidly eliminated. After the initial disappearance, which was interpreted as a distribution phenomenon, first-order kinetics followed. An elimination half-life of 1 h and a volume of distribution were calculated indicating extracellular distribution. A large percentage of the polypeptide is excreted through the kidneys in unchanged form. Obviously, it is not metabolized or bound in the organism. Subcutaneous administration of the inhibitor yielded maximum plasma levels after 1 – 2 h, and a comparatively long-lasting inhibitor level was obtained.

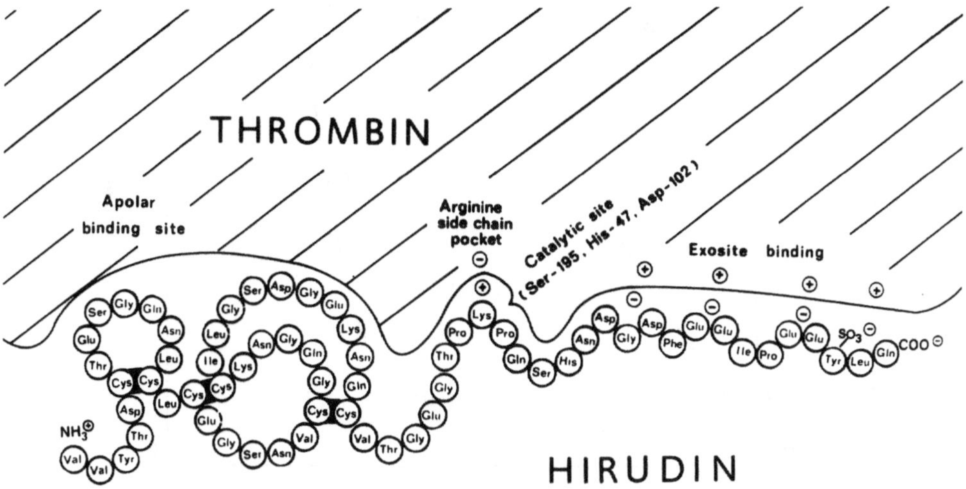

Fig. 1. Scheme of thrombin-hirudin reaction

Table 2. Comparison of effective doses and plasma concentrations of recombinant hirudin in models of experimental thrombosis in rats ($n = 6$ each)

Model of thrombosis	Antithrombotic effect	Dose (μg/kg per minute)	Plasma concentration (μg/ml)
Thrombin-induced DIC	Prevention of microthrombosis	1.0	0.15 ± 0.05
Coronary thrombosis induced by chemical injury of endothelium	Prevention of myocardial ischaemia	2.0	0.35 ± 0.08
Stasis-induced venous thrombosis	Prevention of thrombus formation	8.0	0.62 ± 0.08
Electrically induced arterial thrombosis	Prevention of thrombotic occlusion	20.0	2.15 ± 0.35

We studied the antithrombotic action in various animal models that correspond largely to the pathogenetic mechanism of venous thrombosis or disseminated intravascular coagulation in man [11, 12]. The results, summarized in Table 2, show the antithrombotic effectiveness of the inhibitor. Depending on the dose and the level in blood, hirudin either reduces the size of thrombi or prevents their formation.

As an outstanding effect, the hirudin plasma levels preventing thrombus formation do not prolong bleeding time (Fig. 2). Therefore, in contrast to heparin, no haemorrhagic side effects are observed at antithrombotically effective doses of hirudin [2].

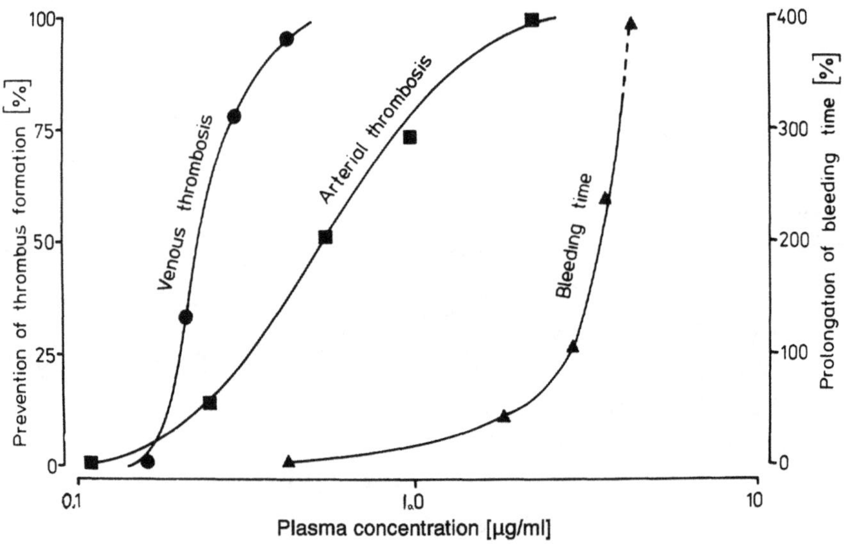

Fig. 2. Plasma concentration-response curves of hirudin for bleeding time and inhibition of thrombus formation in rats

Prevention of Coronary Thrombosis

With respect to the potential use of hirudin for the prevention of coronary thrombosis we studied its preventive effect on thrombotic occlusion of the coronary artery and on reocclusion after intracoronary lysis in animal experiments [1, 8, 9]. At first, the antithrombotic effect was studied in a rat coronary thrombosis model, where a chemical injury of the endothelium formed the thrombus which was induced by the application of silver nitrate solution into the left anterior descending coronary artery. The degree of thrombosis was indirectly estimated as the extent of myocardial ischaemia. Injection of Victoria blue solution into the myocardial circulation allowed the visualization of the extent of ischaemia of the myocardium that was evaluated by a score. This model is of advantage since it requires a simple technique for the induction of coronary thrombosis and renders the possibility of screening antithrombotically efficient substances at a larger scale useful for statistical evaluation of experiments while consuming only small amounts of substance. As a result of subcutaneous injection of hirudin before damaging the endothelium, the myocardial ischaemia was reduced. The score points after administration of hirudin indicated that hirudin prevents the development of coronary thrombosis (Fig. 3).

Within comprehensive studies, coronary thrombosis was induced in mini pigs by a vessel wall lesion caused by direct current. A steel wire electrode was inserted into the right coronary artery via the common carotid artery without opening the thorax. Thrombus formation was recorded by angiography and electrocardiography [10, 13]. In control animals coronary blood flow was reduced, and an occlusive thrombus developed 60 min after electrical stimulation. ECG changes typical of ischaemia occurred, and in some animals a cardiogenic shock

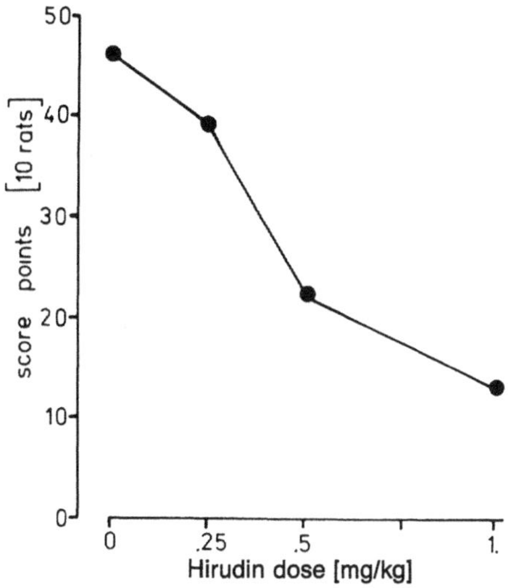

Fig. 3. Prevention of coronary thrombosis (score points) induced by chemical injury of endothelium in rats after s.c. injection of hirudin

developed. As a result of hirudin application 30 min before thrombus induction, thrombus growth was prevented and no signs of myocardial infarction were observed. An example is given in Fig. 4.

Prevention of Reocclusion

Furthermore, we studied the specific role of the thrombin inhibitor hirudin in preventing reocclusion after experimental intracoronary thrombolysis. In previous studies on coronary thrombosis in dogs based on the same method as used with mini pigs we have shown that the occlusion of the right coronary artery could be removed by applying the fibrinolytic activator streptokinase [10]. Intracoronary lysis occurred within a short time after administration of streptokinase. However, early reocclusion due to rethrombosis was found in about 80% of streptokinase-treated animals in these experiments, 4–8 h after terminating streptokinase infusion. On this account, a group of six animals received hirudin infusions (0.5 mg/kg per hour) after recanalization of the coronary artery. During the experiment we found no reocclusion in animals treated with hirudin, in contrast to an 80% reocclusion rate in control animals without anticoagulation (Table 3).

Final Remarks

All in all, there are many comments still to be made on anticoagulation after thrombolysis, but this would lead beyond the scope of the present paper, which was designed to focus attention on some selected aspects connected with pharmacological interference with thrombotic processes in myocardial infarction, especially prevention of reocclusion after coronary lysis by means of hirudin, the anticoagulant agent from medicinal leeches. This naturally occurring specific thrombin inhibitor is an anticoagulant of high quality. The rapid development in the field of genetic engineering will allow obtaining this polypeptide in sufficient

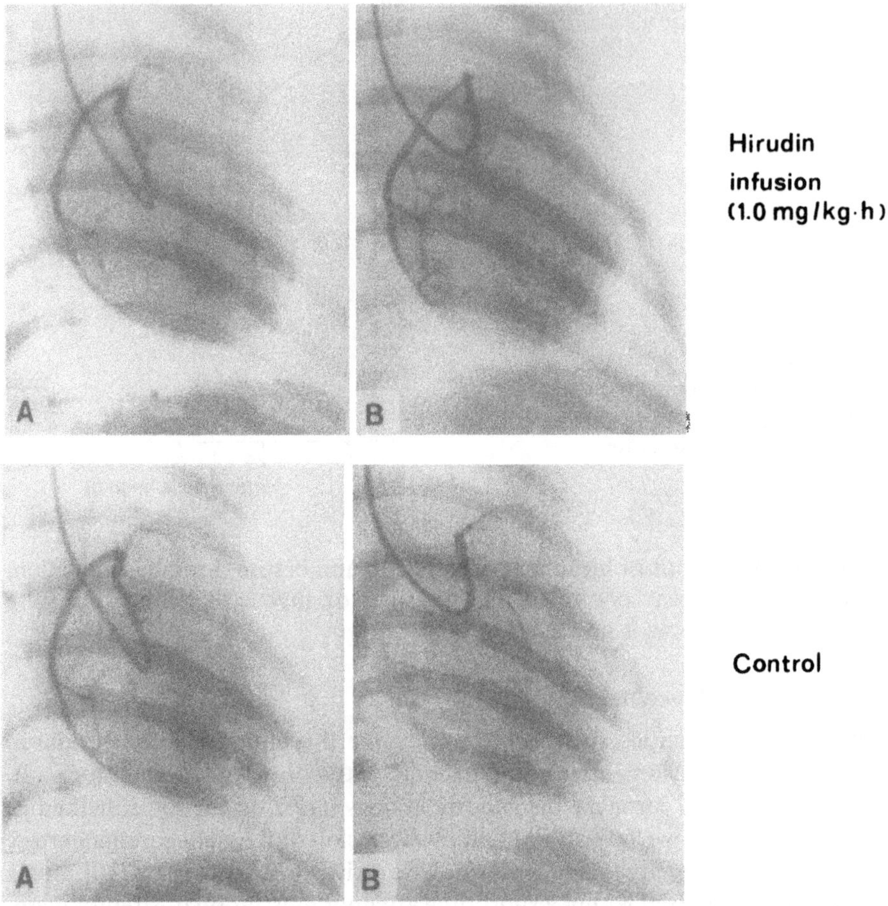

Fig. 4A, B. Preventive effect of hirudin on coronary thrombosis induced by vessel wall lesion caused by electric current (→). Selective angiography of the right coronary pig artery before (**A**) and 60 min after (**B**) induction of thrombosis

Table 3. Experimentally induced coronary thrombosis in dogs

Group	Number of animals with			
	Obstructive thrombosis[a]	Recanalization[b]	Subsequent infusion of	Reocclusion[c]
1	6	5	Saline	4
2	6	4	Hirudin[d]	0

[a] 1 h after thrombus induction.
[b] 3 h after the infusion of 100×10^3 IU streptokinase/kg · h.
[c] 4 h after recanalization.
[d] 1.0 mg/kg per hour.

yield, culminating in revived interest in hirudin, the clinical use of which is at present already taken into consideration. Corresponding clinical studies to confirm its special efficiency in preventing reocclusion after intracoronary lysis, occlusion of coronary bypass as well as PTCA are under way.

References

1. Bucha E, Nowak G, Markwardt F (1988) Prevention of experimental coronary thrombosis by hirudin. Folia Haematol 115:52 – 58
2. Kaiser B, Markwardt F (1986) Antithrombotic and haemorrhagic effects of synthetic and naturally occurring thrombin inhibitors. Thromb Res 43:613 – 620
3. Markwardt F (1957) Die Isolierung und chemische Charakterisierung des Hirudins. Hoppe Seyler's Z Physiol Chem 308:147 – 156
4. Markwardt F (1970) Hirudin as an inhibitor of thrombin. In: Perlmann GE, Lorand L (eds) Proteolytic enzymes. Academic, New York, pp 924 – 932 (Methods in enzymology, vol 19)
5. Markwardt F (1985) Pharmacological control of thrombotic processes for prevention of myocardial ischaemia. In: Szekeres L, Papp J Gy (eds) Proc 4th cong Hung Pharmacol Soc, vol 1, Sect 1. Akademiai Kiado, Budapest, pp 81 – 82
6. Markwardt F (1985) Pharmacology of hirudin: one hundred years after the first report of the anticoagulant agent in medicinal leeches. Biomed Biochim Acta 44:1007 – 1013
7. Markwardt F (1986) Pharmacological approaches to thrombin regulation. Ann NY Acad Sci 485:204 – 214
8. Markwardt F (1986) Antithrombotic action of hirudin in experimental coronary thrombosis (Abstract). European Society of Cardiology, working group "Thrombosis and Platelets", Tours
9. Markwardt F (1987) Prevention of coronary thrombosis by hirudin. In: Papp J Gy (ed) Cardiovascular pharmacology '87. Results, concepts and perspectives. Akademiai Kiado, Budapest, pp 449 – 456
10. Markwardt F, Bernstein K, Drawert J, Eger H, Klöcking H-P, Sedlarik K, Vollmar V, Wilde J (1977) Thrombolytische Behandlung einer experimentellen Koronarthrombose mit Streptokinase. Exp Pathol 14:76 – 88
11. Markwardt F, Fink E, Kaiser B, Klöcking H-P, Nowak G, Richter M, Stürzebecher J (1988) Pharmacological survey of recombinant hirudin. Pharmazie 43:202 – 207
12. Markwardt F, Hauptmann J, Nowak G, Kleßen Ch, Walsmann P (1982) Pharmacological studies on the antithrombotic action of hirudin in experimental animals. Thromb Haemost 47:226 – 229
13. Markwardt F, Klöcking H-P, Sedlarik K, Drawert J (1977) Tierexperimentelle Untersuchungen zur thrombolytischen Wirkung von Ocrase. Acta Biol Med Ger 36:1315 – 1327
14. Markwardt F, Nowak G, Stürzebecher J, Grießbach U, Walsmann P, Vogel G (1984) Pharmacokinetics and anticoagulant effect of hirudin in man. Thromb Haemost 52:160 – 163
15. Markwardt F, Nowak G, Stürzebecher U, Walsmann P (1987) Studies on the pharmacokinetics of hirudin. Biomed Biochim Acta 46:250 – 270
16. Schmutzler R (1983) Die Thrombolyse-Behandlung beim akuten Myocardinfarkt – eine historische Entwicklung. Hämostaseologie 3:52 – 58

Drug Therapy in Coronary Heart Disease, Especially in the Management of Chronic Myocardial Ischemia

P. Lichtlen

This presentation deals with the place of drugs in restoring blood flow to the ischemic myocardium. When we talk about ischemia, we must include all ischemic episodes, both silent and symptomatic ones. Recent technical improvements today allow recording ST-segment changes beat-to-beat continuously over 24 h. Many studies have demonstrated that most ischemic episodes are silent, that is, not accompanied by pain.

In our own study of 58 patients with angiographically documented coronary artery disease, 437 of 580 ischemic episodes (75%) were asymptomatic; they had an average duration of 14.2 min for the asymptomatic and 9.3 min for the symptomatic episodes – hence, total duration of ischemia per day often approached 1 h. Furthermore, there is a circadian variation in ischemic episodes, with a peak in the morning hours around 10:00 a.m. and in the late afternoon around 5:00 p.m. and a minimum of episodes during the second half of the night, between midnight and 6:00 a.m. Most important in patients with stable angina (the majority of cases) is that the ischemic episodes are triggered by a mild increase in heart rate immediately before ST-segment depression, averaging 98 beats/min for the asymptomatic and 100 beats/min for the symptomatic episodes. This signifies that most ischemic episodes are provoked by a mild rise in myocardial oxygen demand and are not due to primary angina – that is, primarily or exclusively to an increase in vasomotor tone.

In order to evaluate the place of anti-ischemic drug treatment in the overall management of ischemic heart disease, we must discuss the pathophysiologic and clinical importance of ischemic events in general. Ischemia is a regional phenomenon, not only with regard to different locations adjacent to each other and distributed over the entire heart, but also with regard to the transmural distribution, where during exercise, ischemia starts in the subendocardial region. Usually it results from a critical impediment to regional flow, a high-grade (>75%) stenosis due to an atherosclerotic plaque, occluding a large epicardial coronary artery to a high degree. Hence, restoration of flow and oxygen delivery must act on this localized impediment either by bypassing, removing, or destroying it by PTCA.

Clinical experience over the past 20 years as well as the study of pathophysiology of ischemic heart disease tell us that the high-grade obstruction in itself is the real danger and risk. Probably all atherosclerotic plaques have the tendency to "grow," but to a very different extent not yet clearly understood (probably depending on cholesterol levels and other risk factors, in addition to local factors). Plaques have a great tendency to rupture their fibrous cap. In stenoses of lesser degree (probably less than 50%) plaque rupture may often occur but go unnoticed and remain clinically silent; the formation of a platelet thrombus, if it occurs, in not occlusive, and may even be integrated into the plaque, leading to a further growth. In stenoses of a high degree (greater than 75%) the thrombus is occlusive, and this results in severe ischemia; low-flow ischemia or even anoxia, acute myocardial infarction, and severe arrhythmias develop, and this may even lead to sudden coronary death. Hence, the obstruction in itself, the atherosclerotic plaque, actually carries the high risk rather than the ischemic episodes.

In recent years we have learned to distinguish between more risky stenoses, so-called complicated stenoses, characterized by a rough surface and overhanging edges, and uncomplicated ones, with a smooth surface. In complicated plaques we often see thrombi sitting at their lower edge, and these are frequently associated with unstable angina or myocardial infarction. I am convinced that this angiographic differentiation between uncomplicated and complicated plaques will play an increasing role in the management of these patients. Of equal importance, especially in terms of medical treatment, is the distinction between eccentric and concentric stenoses. The former type involves a sometimes large normal wall segment with unaltered vascular smooth muscle cells able to contract and relax and thereby to influence the degree of stenoses, especially high-grade stenoses, provoking ischemia. These stenoses can be recognized quite easily in angiograms.

Returning to the management of ischemic heart disease, it therefore becomes obvious that it is important not only to relieve ischemia but to cope with the real threat, the high-grade stenosis, for this is the cause of the actual catastrophy – plaque rupture, thrombotic occlusion and myocardial infarction. Today, to prevent this, either we create a new channel, not affected by a possible plaque rupture, through construction of a bypass, or we deliberately destroy the plaque, inducing a controlled rupture of the plaque – with all its risks – through PTCA. Interestingly, this procedure often leads to a considerable, often angiographically complete regression of the plaque. These two invasive techniques, removal and circumvention of the obstacle, not only abolish the inherent risk of the plaque but at the same time prevent ischemia.

The question arises as to the extent to which drugs are able to reduce the size of these high-risk plaques. It is obvious that not every patient and not all stenoses can be treated invasively, and that a large group of patients must depend on drug treatment alone, or at least in combination with invasive measures. We should therefore expect that these drugs would have at least a certain influence on the obstruction. It has been known for more than 100 years, especially in the case of nitrates, that drugs can successfully interrupt and prevent ischemic episodes. This was shown both for exercise-induced ischemia as well as for spontaneous ischemia occurring during daily life. Today, three groups of drugs with different modes of action are mainly administered: nitrates, β-blocking agents, and calcium antagonists. Their mode of action today, is understood to a great extent and will not be discussed in detail here.

It was long felt that drugs could prevent or interrupt ischemia only by decreasing regional oxygen consumption and demand in the entire heart and thereby in the ischemic area, by reducing those factors having the largest myocardial oxygen consumption: heart rate, contractility, and wall stress (i.e., wall tension). This would decrease myocardial oxygen demand – especially during exercise – to the level of the reduced delivery, by decreasing sympathetic tone through β-blockade, preload through nitrates, and afterload through calcium antagonists. Moreover, and rather surprisingly, it was demonstrated that coronary flow can indeed be raised above the level of ischemia.

Here we must briefly discuss some pathophysiologic aspects. It was demonstrated both in animal studies by Gould (1974), as well as in man by ourselves (Lichtlen 1985), recording regional coronary blood flow, that maximum coronary reserve starts to decrease with obstructions above 50%–60%; at 75% it is decreased by approximately one-third and drops below the "ischemic level." At rest, due to the relatively low oxygen demand, the margin of reserve is preserved up to stenoses of approximately 90% and more. Drugs act by further decreasing the upper ischemic limit and/or by increasing flow above the ischemic level. The latter was long felt impossible, as arterioles in the ischemic zone would be maximally dilated in any case. It was shown, however, that this is possible, especially by administering calcium antagonists (Heusch 1987), but also to a certain extent nitrates. Both calcium antagonists and nitrates relax vascular smooth muscle tone and lead to a considerable dilatation of large epicardial coronary arteries and to eccentric stenoses. They do this, however, by different mechanisms: calcium antagonists block the potential operated calcium channel and by this considerably reduce the calcium influx across the cell membrane, thereby lowering cytosolic calcium. This inhibits smooth muscle contraction. Nitrates, through their NO-group, stimulate cyclic GMP, a strong endogenous smooth muscle relaxant. Alone or in combination they are able to increase the diameter of eccentric, so-called dynamic obstructions by up to 50% (Rafflenbeul and Lichtlen 1982). For high-grade obstructions this signifies a marked improvement of flow – for instance, a decrease from 90% to 80% means an increase in diameter from 1.0 to 1.7 mm.

Furthermore, more recent studies by Aversano and Becker (1985) showed a persistence of coronary vasodilator reserve, especially in the subendocardial region, despite functionally significant flow reduction inducing ischemia, indicating that not all arterioles are maximally dilated in the ischemic zone where coronary reserve is not at its maximum. This was confirmed by Heusch et al. (1987) who demonstrated in instrumented dogs that during exercise-induced ischemia nifedipine was still able to increase flow in this region and was thereby able to abolish or prevent ischemia without lowering afterload. Hence, especially in patients with eccentric obstructions (and these represent approximately 70% of all stenoses) or with subendocardial ischemia, a further improvement of flow, especially by calcium antagonists, is possible. It is important to note that under calcium antagonists this flow behavior is completely different from nitroglycerin or propranolol, where transmural flow decreases following the drop in myocardial oxygen consumption.

Hence, it is not surprising to find a reduction in the number and duration of ischemic episodes during daily life, both under monotherapy with nitrates, calcium antagonists, and β-blockers and under a combination of these drugs. For various reasons, we today prefer a combination treatment. This allows a reduction in the dose of each drug, thereby minimizing side effects, while maintaining or even increasing the anti-ischemic efficacy due to a synergistic action. Furthermore, calcium antagonists, for instance, were shown also to have an antihypertensive and – at least in animal experiments – a certain antiatherosclerotic activity. Therefore, the combinations of β-blockers and nitrates, β-blockers and calcium antagonists, and calcium antagonists and nitrates are widely used. Each combination has its specific advantages and should be employed with regard to the various stages of angina pectoris.

The important question as to whether these drugs also have a prognostic effect, however, remains as yet unanswered, at least with regard to stable angina. It is obvious that these drugs do not and cannot lead to a regression of atherosclerotic plaques. Whether calcium antagonists, e.g., nifedipine and verapamil, are able to reduce the progression of the disease in man, as they have been shown to do in animals, cannot be answered at the present time. A study in man is now under way. Once plaque rupture occurs, the formation of an occlusive platelet thrombus may be prevented by ASA, as has been shown in several studies (Lewis, Veterans' Administration; AMIS, PARIS) that demonstrate a reduction of the events following plaque rupture – myocardial infarction and sudden coronary death. It has also been established that the clot can be lyzed.

Plaque rupture in itself seems to be a random phenomenon. According to Born it may have to be regarded as a kind of fatigue of the material composing the fibrous cap. It is very suggestive to assume that plaque rupture can be provoked by any strain on the plaque, for instance, by a sudden increase in vasomotor tone of the remaining normal smooth muscle cells in eccentric dynamic stenoses. If this is the case then vasorelaxing drugs such as nitrates and calcium antagonists could indeed have a preventive prognostic effect.

Finally, the question arises as to whether prevention of ischemia alone – not only that of the complication of plaque rupture – has a prognostic effect. To answer this question we would have to know whether ischemic episodes have an adverse, irreversible effect on the myocardium or at least have functional effects leading to severe arrhythmias. With regard to severe arrhythmias (VT, VF) we know today from numerous Holter monitoring studies that they occur only in very rarely during ischemia, that is are virtually absent during ischemia as long as there is no scar tissue.

Ischemic episodes, however, seem to be associated with ultrastructural changes and with irreversible cell damage and are clinically often unnoticed. This was demonstrated in animal studies by Schaper and Jennings and in man more recently by Krayenbühl and Schneider (1987). In biopsies taken at the time of bypass surgery, they demonstrated an increased amount of interstitial fibrosis in the poststenotic ischemic region as compared to that in the normally perfused areas.

In conclusion, ischemic episodes occur more often than previously thought, the majority of them being silent. They are a marker for the presence of high-grade, life-threatening stenoses. The risk of ischemia itself seems to be rather low, however the risk of its cause, the advanced atherosclerotic plaque that occludes the coronary vessel to a great degree, is very high, especially in the case of so-called complicated plaques which have already ruptured and are often accompanied by platelet thrombi. Drug treatment, therefore, should not only aim at preventing ischemia and silent episodes only, but also at maximum relaxation of coronary vascular smooth muscle tone. This would reduce the degree of obstructions, maintain maximal coronary arteriolar reserve, and prevent complications through a sudden increase in vasomotor tone, which can eventually lead to plaque rupture. Therefore, drug treatment should aim at maximum efficacy, one which is often reached only through a combination of various antiischemic drugs.

References

1. Gould KL, Lipscomb K (1974) Effects of coronary stenoses on coronary flow reserve and resistance. Am J Cardiol 34:48 – 55
2. Lichtlen PR (1985) Pathophysiology of coronary and myocardial function in angina pectoris: important aspects for drug treatment. Eur Heart J 6 Suppl F:11 – 25
3. Lichtlen PR (1988) The combination of antianginal drugs: effects and indications. Cardiovasc Drugs Ther (in press)
4. Heusch G, Guth BD, Seitelberger R, Ross J (1987) Attenuation of exercise-induced myocardial ischemia in dogs with recruitment of coronary vasodilator reserve by nifedipine. Circ 75:482 – 490
5. Rafflenbeul W, Lichtlen PR (1982) Zum Konzept der „dynamischen“ Koronarstenose. Z Kardiol 71:439 – 444
6. Schaper J, Alpers P, Gottwick M, Schaper W (1985) Ultrastructural characteristics of regional ischemia and infarction in the canine heart. Eur Heart J 6 Suppl E:21 – 31
7. Reimer KA, Jennings RB (1985) Effects of calcium-channel blockers on myocardial preservation during experimental acute myocardial infarction. Am J Cardiol 55:107B – 115B
8. Lewis HD, Davis JW, Archibald WE et al. (1983) Protective effects of aspirin against acute myocardial infarction and death in men with unstable angina. N Engl J Med 309:396 – 403
9. Krayenbühl HP, Hirzel H, Hess OM, Schneider J, Turina M (1987) Hemodynamics of painless ischemia. In: von Arnim T, Maseri A (eds) Silent myocardial ischemia. Steinkopff, Darmstadt, Springer, New York, pp 147 – 151
10. Aversano T, Becker LC (1985) Persistence of coronary vasodilator reserve despite functionally significant flow reduction. Am J Physiol 248:H403 – H411

Discussion: Session II – Thrombolysis in Acute Myocardial Infarction

Chairman: M. Verstraete

Dr. Pitt: I would like to make one comment to Dr. Zaret's presentation on unstable angina. We have just finished a small randomized trial of t-PA in 40 patients with unstable angina pectoris. Dr. John Nicklas in our group found that administration of t-PA to patients with unstable angina results in a significant increase in pacing threshold to angina and a trend toward an increase in vessel diameter secondary to clot lysis. The improvement in the t-PA group was, however, confined to those patients who had angiographically visible clot. As I recall, only half of our patients had visible clot even though angioscopic data suggest that almost everyone with unstable angina has some evidence of thrombus formation. I therefore believe that there is a potential for t-PA in patients with unstable angina pectoris, but only in the subset of patients with angiographically visible thrombus.

Dr. Rapaport: I would like to ask Dr. Schröder if he would clarify his reasons for recommending the use of thrombolytic therapy within 4–6 h in all infarcts that show ST segment elevation. Specifically, when you look at the various mortality studies and the various trials such as the Western Washington Intracoronary Trial, the Western Washington Intravenous Trial, the GISSI trial, and, I believe, your own ISAM Trial, inferior infarcts were not benefited in any of those trials in terms of mortality as the end point. Now, I do understand that in the ISAM Trial left ventricular function was improved among inferior infarcts. In light of the data, is it not reasonable to limit thrombolytic therapy in acute inferior infarcts at the moment to cases seen extremely early, within the first 3 h, and to those inferior infarcts where there is a clinical suggestion of significant right ventricular infarction?

Dr. Schröder: The use of streptokinase therapy to treat patients with inferior myocardial infarction has been controversial. In the ISAM study, significantly reduced long-term mortality has been shown in patients with inferior myocardial infarction of small or moderate enzyme infarct size. The Western Washington Intravenous Streptokinase Trial, on the other hand, showed a strong trend towards reduced mortality in the treated patients with anterior myocardial infarction, but not so in those with inferior myocardial infarction. The total sample size of 368 patients was relatively small in this trial. However, the GISSI trial seems strongly to support the suggestion of little or no benefit of thrombolytic therapy for patients with inferior myocardial infarction. In 4013 patients there was no significant difference in mortality between streptokinase and conventionally treated patients. However, the GISSI trial has the peculiar and unexpected finding of a higher mortality in the first 48 h in the streptokinase group, mainly by a higher incidence of death within the first 6 h after inclusion into the study. Within the latter time limit, 120 streptokinase patients died as compared with only 76 conventionally treated patients. This is in contrast to the ISAM study, where 16 streptokinase and 24 placebo patients died within the first 24 h, and the Dutch ICIN study, where in the first 3 days eight deaths occurred in the streptokinase group as compared with 22 deaths in the control group. The higher early mortality in streptokinase-treated patients in GISSI was to a large extent related to patients with inferior myocardial infarction. This surprisingly high mortality within 6 h of initiation of streptokinase treatment probably had a major influence on the less favorable outcome in patients with inferior myocardial infarction localization in this trial.

The major predictor of survival after myocardial infarction is the status of left ventricular function. Since significant limitation of the infarct size by thrombolytic therapy has been shown in several studies also for inferior myocardial infarction localization (although less pronounced than in patients with anterior myocardial infarction), on the basis of present information I think it would be unjustified to deny patients with inferior myocardial infarction this effective therapy.

Dr. Bode: I would like you to comment on the inhibitor that you postulate for prourokinase. Are there any data on this inhibitor concerning molecular weight or some of its properties?

Dr. Verstraete: It is a weak one. It has not really been characterized yet. It is more a functional than pure characterization. And I can't expand on the clinical relevance of it at this moment. So I have to keep it short here. – Next question?

Dr. Schmutzler: Before I ask a question, I would like to add something to Dr. Rapaport's question to explain why we did not exclude inferior infarction. First, I think it is worthwhile to reopen a vessel. Second, I think there are discrepancies between multicenter and randomized studies and individual cases. If you had the opportunity to perform coronary angiography prior to treatment in patients with a dominant right coronary artery, then I think it would be reasonable to reopen it. It depends on the anatomy and the location, since you might need this right coronary artery years later for collateralization of a subsequently occluded left coronary artery. In general I wouldn't be so strict as to exclude inferior infarction per se, but would make decisions on an individual basis. My question to Dr. Verstraete concerns heparin in combination with t-PA, which I mentioned in my presentation. You and the other aggregation specialists told us to add heparin concurrently to t-PA at the beginning of our t-PA study. However it may be that some of bleeding complications are due to heparin and not to the dosage of t-PA. I would like to ask you your opinion. Should we do this in the future, or should we reduce heparin dosage?

Dr. Verstraete: It is correct that in spite of the fibrinogen-sparing properties of t-PA, bleeding complications remain common in patients with myocardial infarction treated with this drug (26% – 43% of the patients). In most patients bleeding is limited to arterial and venous puncture sites. It is unknown to what extent the combination of t-PA and heparin is responsible for the bleeding complications. Moreover, most patients also received aspirin, a potent inhibitor of platelet function well known to prolong the bleeding time when used alone. No one knows for certain whether we really need heparin and aspirin to prevent reocclusion of the atherosclerotic and still stenotic infarct-related coronary artery. The TAMI group recently completed a trial in which patency at 90 min after t-PA was assessed in 144 patients with and without pretreatment with 10000 IU heparin. No difference in patency rates was found. Heparin was then started after the 90 min angiogram. Thus, no data on the influence of heparin on bleeding and reocclusion are available from this trial.

Therefore, the European Cooperative Study Group will start a randomized trial of patients with myocardial infarction treated with t-PA with and without heparin, and the coronarography will be repeated after 48 – 96 h. This study will provide an answer to following questions: (a) What is the patency after 48 – 96 h after rt-PA with and without heparin. Taking into account the recent TAMI study group data, these patency figures will reflect reocclusion as well as late opening of the infarct related segment in patients treated with and without heparin. (b) What is the incidence of bleeding after rt-PA with and without heparin during the first 48 – 96 h. Since early angiography (90 min) is omitted, there will be no bleeding from arterial puncture sites, thus the "true" picture of bleeding complication can be reviewed.

Dr. Rapaport: I don't have an answer, but I wanted to make a comment. I hope that in the European trial which you are discussing that you not only compared rt-PA to heparin but to heparin plus aspirin. I think we are dealing with a situation that is analogous to the patient with unstable angina, and probably non-Q-wave infarction as well. That is, we seem to be dealing with the same underlying pathogenesis of a plaque rupture where you now have exposed damaged endothelium. Presumably, the situation is present for collagen-induced thromboses that will not necessarily be protected by heparin administration but would presumably be protected with aspirin administration. Certainly, the benefit in the unstable angina trial with aspirin was very dramatic. The Veterans Administration trial showed, some 12 weeks later, over a 50% reduction in mortality and myocardial infarction rates. It suggested that aspirin may well be very important in preventing progression to complete thrombosis after plaque rupture resulting in subsequent myocardial infarction and/or sudden death. Thus, I wonder whether the large reocclusion rates we are seeing after thrombolytic therapy of roughly 20% without PTCA and maybe 12% or so following PTCA may reflect the fact that one is not getting protection against collagen-induced thrombosis. You are a distinguished expert in thrombosis, and I would defer to your judgment in this area.

Dr. Lucchesi: We have been interested in the rethrombosis problem particularly after streptokinase or t-PA, and also prourokinase, which we use in an animal model of coronary thrombosis. One of the best agents till today has been prostacyclin, and I know in Europe you have availability of a prostacyclin analogue, known as iloprost. Do any of you have any experience with this agent in man, since I think it would be similar to prostacyclin in preventing rethrombosis?

Dr. Verstraete: Well, I know the agent. Experience in man in the context that you mean does not exist yet, but several trials are beginning to be developed or designed now. So essentially there is no real evidence now. You do know that that agent has to be given parenterally, unfortunately. We are looking for agents that could be given orally.

Session III
Percutaneous Transluminal Coronary Angioplasty

Chairman: E. Rapaport

Recommendations of the Joint International Society and Federation of Cardiology/World Health Organization Task Force on PTCA

E. Rapaport

A decade has passed since Grüntzig performed the first coronary angioplasty in Zurich. As the initial reports of that experience became widely known, they were greeted with both wonderment and scepticism. Wonderment because the angiographic changes and the pressure gradient measurements established that a remarkable reduction in the degree of obstruction could be produced. Scepticism because initially the mechanism through which this was accomplished was obscure. Furthermore, there were fears of all sorts of disastrous complications. These included downstream embolization, large coronary dissections that would lead to closure or even rupture of vessels, immediate thrombosis or spasm with resultant myocardial infarctions, episodes of late spasm, and even fear that splitting of the fibrous cap of the atherosclerotic lesion would result in accelerated atherogenesis in the future. There were also concerns regarding the likelihood of restenosis. These latter have proven to be justifiable and serve to limit the benefits of the procedure. Nevertheless, as experience accumulated, initially by Grüntzig and his early collaborators, Kaltenbach in West Germany, Stertzer in New York, and Myler in San Francisco, it became evident that the procedure was an innovative and important therapeutic intervention.

Around this time, a conference was held in the United States by the National Heart, Lung, and Blood Institute, following which the decision was made to initiate a registry that would incorporate subsequent experience with PTCA. With the cooperation of the manufacturers, most of the angioplasties performed in the next several years were registered and a considerable amount of data accumulated. Thousands of patients were entered in this registry, and some of this data is presented in this conference.

Originally, angioplasty was performed primarily in the symptomatic patient with exertional angina pectoris, good left ventricular function, and a single, proximal, discrete, concentric, noncalcified lesion. As more experience was gained, it became evident that mortality was quite low, approximately 1%. Furthermore, major complications that required emergency bypass surgery were around 5%. These low complication rates led to a natural extension of the indications. The registry began to incorporate patients with unstable angina, multivessel disease, bypass grafts that were obstructed, and other kinds of cases above and beyond the single-vessel patient. The registry data still dominantly reflects single-vessel disease, but today, as a result of the explosion of angioplasty across the world, there are now more cases done for multivessel coronary disease than for single-vessel coronary disease. This has led, in turn, to confusion as to the relative roles of surgery and angioplasty in the management of patients with chronic stable angina pectoris as well as unstable angina. We have also seen extension of PTCA to patients with acute myocardial infarction, and some of these data are to be discussed in this meeting.

Unfortunately, there are no large-scale randomized clinical trials comparing bypass surgery to angioplasty in patients in whom either procedure might appropriately be used. As a result, most of the data are observational in nature. The liberalization of indications for PTCA combined with the absence of clinical trials have led to a need to set some uniform guidelines in a number of areas connected with angioplasty. In response, the Council on Clinical Cardiology of the International Society and Federation of Cardiology (ISFC), together with the World Health Organization (WHO), appointed a joint task force in late 1984 to attempt to set some guidelines and standards in this area. This task force met between 1985 and 1987 and has completed its work. The Task Force report has now received formal approval by the ISFC and WHO and is presently in press in several national cardiology journals.

I would like to present a brief summary of the findings of that task force. I want to emphasize that this is a condensed summary of findings, and I shall only present some of the highlights of the report.

The task force was chaired by Dr. Martial G. Bourassa of Canada and included the following members:

Edwin L. Alderman, USA
Michel Bertrand, France
Luis de la Fuente, Argentina
A. Gratsianski, USSR
Martin Kaltenbach, FRG
Spencer B. King, USA
Masakiyo Nobuyoshi, Japan
Paul Romaniuk, GDR
Thomas J. Ryan, USA
Patrick W. Serruys, The Netherlands
Hugh C. Smith, USA
Jose Eduardo Sousa, Brazil
Siegfried Bothig, FRG, ex officio
Elliot Rapaport, USA, ex offico

Task force members looked at the frequency of PTCA in their own countries, and rather startling statistics were uncovered. In the United States, where in 1984 some 63000 angioplasty procedures were performed, almost 160000 procedures were performed in 1986. There were approximately 279000 bypass operations in the United States the same year. In other words, for every three cases that went to bypass surgery, there were almost two cases where PTCA was performed. In a very short period of time, angioplasty has become a frequently performed procedure in the United States. Similarly, in many other countries one can see an increasing use of the technique. Nevertheless, there is often a significant variability in the use of PTCA among different countries. For example, in 1986 there were approximately twice as many procedures done in Canada per 100000 adult population as in West Germany. Part of this variability may reflect differences in the prevalence of coronary artery disease among countries. But, even correcting for this variable, it is clear that the technique is at times overutilized in some countries and underutilized in others. Similar types of data exist for bypass surgery. For example, bypass surgery is used considerably more frequently in the United States per 100000 population than it is in any other country in the world.

The task force examined the issue of training requirements for invasive cardiologists performing PTCA. Aside from the usual exposure that all clinical cardiology trainees should have to the cardiac catheterization laboratory, those who wish to become invasive cardiologists need a minimum of 12 months training in the catheterization laboratory. During this time, the task force feels that a trainee should be involved in at least 300 procedures, including 200 as a primary operator. On top of this, however, those who wish to perform angioplasty need additional training. We believe that this must not only include knowledge on the indications, limitations, and complications of angioplasty but also involve an additional year of training during which the trainee must perform at least 75 cases as the primary operator and be involved in at least 125 cases.

It is true that many people doing angioplasty today learned the procedure through a 3-day course and/or visits to another laboratory where they spent days to weeks getting hands-on training. Despite the fact that many cardiologists doing PTCA today learned through on-the-job training, it is now generally agreed that this is no longer an acceptable approach. The task force agreed that there must be a formal training program with at least 1 year of additional experience in the angioplasty laboratory above and beyond that acquired with normal cardiac catheterization laboratory training.

Continuing education after training is important as well. Just as a surgeon must continue to do a minimum number of cases over time in order to maintain skills, the invasive cardiologist doing angioplasty needs a minimum case load of about one case per week. Continued performance of PTCA requires that complication and success rates stay comparable to international standards.

The issue of surgical backup and coverage was addressed in detail. It was agreed that consultation with a cardiovascular surgeon and appropriate arrangements for backup are necessary prerequisites for angioplasty, and that surgical backup coverage could vary in relation to discussions as to the potential high, low, or medium risk of that patient. However, it is recognized that all patients, even so-called low-risk ones, have the potential of developing a catastrophic complication. The level of standby may be varied somewhat depending upon the perceived risk, but there must always be an operating room and a surgical team available to ensure that the patient can be rushed to surgery if the situation demands. As a minimum, there should be arrangements in advance for appropriate surgical coverage. Ideally, prior to the procedure there should be a discussion about the patient between the person doing angioplasty and the cardiovascular surgeon. Agreement should be reached as to the level of standby – whether an actual operating room will be kept open and the team available right at that point in time, or whether standby simply reflects an arrangement that the operating room schedule will be coordinated with the angioplasty schedule to ensure an early available room should an emergency arise. It was recommended by the committee that PTCA should not be performed in catheterization laboratories not physically connected with hospitals having a cardiac surgical program. This recommendation is made despite the fact that there are places in the world where arrangements have been made for helicopter systems and other ways of transporting emergency patients from catheterization laboratories doing PTCA to operating rooms in a nearby hospital. However, the task force believes that that is not an appropriate solution.

One of the problems in evaluating PTCA data is the definition of what constitutes a successful PTCA. The task force recommends that there be at least three major criteria to the definition of a successful PTCA. One is that there are no major complications. The second is that there be an absolute decrease of 20% or more between the initial and the post-PTCA diameter stenosis. Finally, a 50% or greater pre-PTCA diameter stenosis should be reduced to less than 50% immediately after PTCA.

Similarly, there is a need for conformity in defining what constitutes restenosis. Restenosis has turned out to be a significant complication, occurring anywhere from approximately 20% to as high as 30% – 33% of patients after angioplasty. With increasing use of PTCA in multivessel coronary disease it is possible that the figure will be even higher. The task force recommends that restenosis be defined as an immediate post-PTCA diameter stenosis of less than 50% that increases to 50% or greater at follow-up. To accommodate borderline situations, it is recommended that there should be a minimum change of 20% in diameter of stenosis when angiograms are visually assessed or an increase in diameter of stenosis of at least 10% when serial angiograms are assessed by computer.

There were several recommendations regarding postangioplasty management. Heparin should be administered during the procedure. This is generally discontinued immediately after PTCA although some protocols call for routine administration for the next 24 – 48 h. Additional administration for 24 – 48 h is specifically recommended when there is prior evidence of an intraluminal thrombus. Generally it is advised not to use protamine to try to reverse the heparin effect, since there is an increased likelihood of abrupt thrombosis. There is general agreement that antiplatelet agents should be started immediately. The appropriate doses are under study in randomized trials. Currently, dipyridamol is being used in doses ranging from 75 mg to 400 mg together with aspirin varying in dose from 100 mg to 1500 mg. Anticoagulation with coumadin is not felt to be more effective than antiplatelet agents alone.

In addition, patients should be on long-acting nitrates, calcium antagonists, or both. The task force recommends that, whenever possible, β-blockade be reduced or withdrawn prior to PTCA since they may increase the potential for coronary artery spasm.

The heart of the task force report is its recommendation on the indications for PTCA. It was decided to classify current indications into three broad categories:

(a) accepted indications, (b) evolving indications or those indications for which the data base is incomplete, but where it is reasonable and prudent at this time to offer patients the procedure, and (c) relative contraindications. Listed below are the Current Indications for Coronary Angioplasty as recommended in the task force report.

Class I: Accepted Indications

Chronic stable angina unresponsive to medical therapy or unstable angina:

1. Preferably with objective evidence of myocardial ischemia.
2. With good left ventricular function.
3. With a single significant coronary stenosis suitable for PTCA.

Class II: Evolving Indications

1. Chronic stable angina or unstable angina in patients with multivessel disease.
2. Angina in patients with recent coronary occlusion (less than 3 months).
3. No or mild angina following medical therapy with a strongly positive exercise stress test.
4. Documented variant angina with significant fixed lesions.
5. Acute myocardial infarction.
6. Angina after coronary bypass surgery.
7. Angina in inoperable/high-risk patients.
8. Angina in elderly patients ($\geq$75 years).

Class III: Relative Contraindications

1. No or mild angina without evidence of myocardial ischemia.
2. Severe left ventricular dysfunction (EF <25%).
3. Significant left main coronary artery stenosis.
4. Patients in whom the only lesions are chronic coronary occlusions (older than 3 months).

These recommendations represent a great deal of work by members of this international committee, and I hope you will agree with me that they present some important guidelines that will be helpful to everyone in the future in attempting to bring some standardization to how we progress in this field.

The Changing Role of PTCA in Patients with Acute Myocardial Infarction

B. Pitt, E. Topol, and W. O'Neill

Several years ago our group performed a random trial in which we compared the results of percutaneous transluminal coronary angioplasty (PTCA) to intracoronary streptokinase in patients with acute myocardial infarction [1]. The trial showed that we could achieve reperfusion in approximately 85% of patients with either of these strategies, but that there was a significant advantage to the PTCA strategy. The group who received PTCA had, as expected, less residual stenosis of the infarct-related artery than the group who received intracoronary streptokinase. The PTCA group had a significant improvement in both regional and global ventricular function compared to the lytic group. There was also less postinfarction angina pectoris and less exercise-induced myocardial ischemia in the infarct zone, as judged by tomographic thallium 201 myocardial imaging, than in the lytic group. We were, however, somewhat disappointed since one of our hypotheses was that we would achieve less bleeding in patients who received PTCA alone compared to those who received intracoronary streptokinase alone. However, this was not the case, possibly because our patients undergoing PTCA were treated with high-dose heparin therapy. The reocclusion rate in the PTCA group was somewhat lower than in the streptokinase group, but due to the small number of patients studied this was not significant. Similarly, the number of deaths was too small to reach any conclusions concerning the relative effectiveness of these two strategies on mortality.

Based upon this experience and the data by Hartzler [2] and Meyer et al. [3], we felt that there was a role for PTCA in acute myocardial infarction. However, since only few centers could perform emergency PTCA in patients with acute myocardial infarction we next explored the role of sequential therapy with intravenous thrombolytic therapy using streptokinase, followed by PTCA [4]. This strategy allows administration of a thrombolytic agent in the community hospital with subsequent transfer by helicopter [5] or ambulance to a regional center. Our initial experience with this strategy of sequential thrombolysis and PTCA suggested that it would be possible to achieve reperfusion in over 95% of patients and to improve ventricular function in those patients who failed thrombolysis and those with successful thrombolysis but a residual stenosis of the infarct-related artery.

We next set out to determine the proper strategy for PTCA in patients with acute infarction who were initially treated with an intravenous thrombolytic agent such as tissue plasminogen activator (t-PA). Should PTCA be done urgently after thrombolysis or should it be done electively only if indicated by recurrent symptoms of ischemia and/or a positive exercise thallium 201 stress test prior to hospital discharge?

In the thrombolysis and angioplasty trial in myocardial infarction (TAMI [6]) we administered intravenous t-PA to patients seen within 4 h of onset of symptoms of acute infarction or up to 6 h in those with persistent pain. The patients then underwent urgent coronary angiography. If they had an occluded vessel, they underwent PTCA. If they had a patent infarct-related vessel and were suitable candidates for PTCA of their infarct-related vessel, they were randomized to the strategy of urgent PTCA or elective PTCA only if clinically indicated by recurrent symptoms of ischemia or a positive predischarge exercise thallium 201 myocardial stress test.

Both the urgent and elective PTCA groups had a significant improvement in regional ventricular function, but there was no significant difference between the two strategies in regard to ventricular function. Furthermore, there appeared to be a tendency for increased risk of bypass graft surgery and death in those who underwent urgent PTCA.

The group who failed intravenous thrombolysis with t-PA, approximately 25% of patients, who underwent obligatory PTCA had a difficult course. There was a higher in-hospital mortality rate in this group of 10% compared to 2.5% in those with a patent vessel after intravenous thrombolysis. There was a lower success rate for PTCA and a higher complication rate in those who failed intravenous thrombolysis than in those with successful thrombolysis. Of those who had PTCA after failed intravenous thrombolysis 29% had reocclusion when reexamined at 1 week.

This experience in the TAMI trial with urgent PTCA was disappointing and has made us rethink the role of PTCA in patients undergoing intravenous thrombolysis after an acute myocardial infarction. We now believe, given currently available techniques, that in patients with a patent vessel after intravenous thrombolysis PTCA should be performed on an elective basis in response to current symptoms of ischemia, ECG evidence of reocclusion, or those with a positive exercise thallium 201 stress test prior to hospital discharge. Before reaching a final conclusion as to the role of PTCA in patients with acute infarction it may, however, be worthwhile to review some other recent data.

In a recent trial carried out at the Johns Hopkins Hospital [7] patients seen within 4 h of onset of symptoms of acute infarction were randomized to placebo or intravenous t-PA. They underwent an initial cardiac catheterization after IV thrombolysis, were rerandomized to PTCA or no PTCA at 48 – 72 h and then had rest and exercise radionuclide ventriculograms at 7 – 10 days. The trial confirmed the effectiveness of t-PA, in that those who received t-PA had a significantly higher patency rate and better ventricular function that those who received placebo. The interesting finding in regard to the present discussion is the effect of PTCA performed at 48 – 72 h from onset of symptoms on ventricular function. The group who underwent PTCA had a significantly better improvement in global left ventricular ejection fraction during exercise compared to those who did not undergo PTCA. This study suggests that PTCA performed electively after 48 – 72 h can be effective in improving ventricular function. Performance of PTCA 48 – 72 h after infarction can likely be accomplished at a lower complication rate than when it is performed urgently. Early after intravenous thrombolytic therapy clot lysis is still incomplete, platelets activated with the greatest tendency toward reocclusion. These factors increase the risk of urgent PTCA. After several days clot lysis is more complete, platelet activation and the tendency for restenosis less.

Having stated, on the basis of the TAMI trial, that urgent PTCA should not be performed given our current techniques and experience, it is possible that improved techniques may in the future make it possible to more effectively and safely carry out urgent PTCA. This is suggested by a recent study carried out by the TAMI group [7]. This trial, in which the synergistic effects of t-PA and urokinase were explored, was based upon the observations of Colleen et al. [8]. They showed in a rabbit model that there was a synergistic effect on thrombolysis when they administered half of the dose of t-PA and half the dose of urokinase or prourokinase than when they administered full doses of either t-PA or urokinase. We felt that a thrombolytic rate of approximately 75% after intravenous t-PA was in the long run not acceptable. If we could achieve a thrombolytic rate of greater than 90%, the impetus for early coronary angiography and PTCA would be decreased. We therefore carried out a pilot trial to determine whether or not there was a synergistic effect on thrombolysis when t-PA and urokinase were administered together. In this pilot trial [7] increasing doses of t-PA and urokinase were administered to a small group of patients in order to examine the safety and efficacy of each dose combination before proceeding to the next higher and eventually full doses of t-PA (1 mg/kg) and urokinase (2×10^6 U).

The results from this study, in which full doses of t-PA and urokinase were compared to the original TAMI study, in which t-PA alone was used in a dose of 150 mg, did not suggest any evidence for synergism in regard to thrombolytic effectiveness. There was, however, a significant reduction in the reocclusion rate. In the original TAMI trial in which t-PA alone was administered the reocclusion rate was approximately 13%. When urokinase was added to t-PA in the second TAMI trial, resulting in systemic fibrinolysis, the reocclusion rate was significantly reduced to 5% – 6%. This was accomplished without any increased risk of bleeding compared to administration of t-PA alone. These results are of interest in that they show the potential to reduce the reocclusion rate, which is one of the major detriments to urgent PTCA. We believe that the reason for this reduction in reocclusion rate is the occurrence of systemic fibrinolysis associated with urokinase administration. Of further interest were the results in the subset of patients who failed initial thrombolysis with both intravenous t-PA and urokinase, and who subsequently underwent urgent PTCA. In the original TAMI trial the reocclusion rate after PTCA in this subset was 29%. In the more recent trial with both t-PA and urokinase the reocclusion rate after urgent PTCA was only 7% in this subset. The lower incidence of reocclusion was associated with a significant improvement in regional myocardial wall motion in the infarct zone and global left ventricular function at 7 – 10 days compared to the results in the original TAMI trial in which t-PA alone was administered. While the number of patients studied in this pilot trial was relatively small and the results need to be confirmed in a large prospective randomized trial, the data suggest that it is feasible to reduce the reocclusion rate after intravenous thrombolysis and that reduction in the reocclusion rate after intravenous thrombolysis results in improved regional and global ventricular function in the subset of patients who undergo PTCA after failed thrombolysis.

In conclusion, the results of the original TAMI trial with t-PA alone [6] suggest that PTCA should be performed electively. If one carries out urgent PTCA in patients who have undergone successful intravenous thrombolysis, there may be increased risk without significant benefit compared to those who undergo PTCA electively if needed. Furthermore, if PTCA is carried out urgently, it may in some instances be done unnecessarily. Since clot lysis is not complete for several days, an initial high-grade residual stenosis consisting of the underlying atherosclerotic lesion and the incompletely lysed thrombus may on restudy several days later not be significant due to further clot lysis. However, as suggested by the more recent TAMI trial in patients receiving both t-PA and urokinase [7], it is possible to reduce the reocclusion rate and improve the results of PTCA, especially in the subset of patients who failed intravenous thrombolysis and who undergo urgent PTCA. It is possible, as our techniques for performing PTCA and our ability to reduce the incidence of reocclusion improve, that if we reexamine the role of urgent PTCA we would find that it could be performed more safely with greater benefit. Further prospective trials will, however, be necessary to examine this possibility. Until that time, the data suggest that there is no advantage and possibly an increased risk of performing urgent PTCA in patients who have undergone successful intravenous thrombolysis. If PTCA is to be done acutely, it should be performed as sole therapy or in patients receiving a systemic lytic drug, not with t-PA alone.

References

1. O'Neill WW, Timmis GC, Bourdillon PD, et al. (1986) A prospective randomized clinical trial of intracoronary streptokinase versus coronary angioplasty for acute myocardial infarction. N Engl J Med 314:812 – 818
2. Hartzler GO, Rutherford BD, McConahay DR, et al. (1983) Pertcutaneous transluminal coronary angioplasty with and without thrombolytic therapy for treatment of acute myocardial infarction. Am Heart J 106:965 – 973
3. Meyer J, Merx W, Schmitz H, et al. (1982) Percutaneous transluminal coronary angioplasty immediately after intracoronary streptolysis of transmural myocardial infarction. Circulation 66:905 – 913

4. Fung AY, Lai P, Topol EJ, et al. (1986) Value of percutaneous transluminal coronary angioplasty after unsuccessful intravenous streptokinase therapy in acute myocardial infarction. Am J Cardiol 58:686–691
5. Topol EJ, Fung AY, Kline E, et al (1986) Safety of helicopter transport and out-of-hospital intravenous fibrinolytic therapy in patients with evolving myocardial infarction. Cathet Cardiovasc Diagn 12:151–155
6. Topol EJ, Califf RM, George BS, et al (1967) A randomized trial of immediate versus delayed elective angioplasty after intravenous tissue plasminogen activator in acute myocardial infarction. N Engl J Med 317:581–588
7. Topol EJ, Califf RM, O'Neill WW, et al (1987) Synergism of tissue-type and urokinase plasminogen activators for acute myocardial infarction: results of the multicenter TAMI-2 trial. Circulation 76[IV]:307
8. Collen D, Stassen J-M, Stump DC, et al (1986) Synergism of thrombolytic agents in vivo. Circulation 74:838–842

Thrombolytic Therapy and PTCA

R. Erbel, T. Pop, and J. Meyer

With intravenous administration of streptokinase, reperfusion in 50% – 55% of patients with acute myocardial infarction can be expected [1 – 3], and with intracoronary administration of streptokinase in 70% – 75%. This rate can even be increased up to 90% by additional mechanical recanalization [5]. A reperfusion rate of 65% – 70% has been reported for intravenous application of tissue plasminogen activator (rt-PA) [6 – 8]; single-chain prourokinase also seems to be a promising thrombolytic agent [9, 10].

Two controlled randomized studies with intracoronary streptokinase have been published. Kennedy et al.[10] reported of the Western Washington trial a reduction in mortality from 11.2% to 6.7% and Simoons et al. [19] for the Dutch Inter-University trial a reduction from 16% to 8.5%. Both differences were significant. Despite these proven positive results, follow-up of patients with thrombolytic therapy demonstrated an increased rate of angina pectoris, positive stress test and positive thallium-201 scintigrams [11 – 13].

These observations seem to be related to the effet of residual coronary luminal narrowing in limiting coronary blood flow. Already in 1982 Rutsch et al. reported for four West German centers that in 76% of the patients coronary lesions were found of more than 75% and in 94% lesions of more than 50% [14]. Schmidt et al. [15] studied the effect of residual coronary artery stenosis on the size of myocardial infarction in an open-chest canine preparation of coronary occlusion and reperfusion. Animals were randomized to one of the three groups: group 1 ($n = 6$) had a 6-h circumflex occlusion; group 2 ($n = 6$) had a 2-h occlusion, followed by 4 h of partial reperfusion through a residual stenosis adjusted to 30% of baseline flow; and group 3 ($n = 6$) had full reperfusion for 4 h after a 2-h occlusion. At 6 h the area of risk and infarction was determined. Infarction as a proportion of the risk area was $96 \pm 1\%$ in group 1, $90 \pm 2\%$ in group 2, and $79 \pm 4\%$ in group 3 ($p < 0.001$); the differences between the groups were significant (Fig. 1). Thus, a residual stenosis may lead to a deleterious effect on the outcome of coronary reperfusion. Full revascularization after reperfusion seems to be necessary to maximize salvage of myocardium.

Therefore, Meyer et al. [16] introduced percutaneous coronary angioplasty (PTCA) in addition to a transluminal thrombolytic therapy in order to eliminate residual coronary luminal narrowing. It could be demonstrated that PTCA is possible with a low risk and high success rate. Other authors (Table 1) confirmed

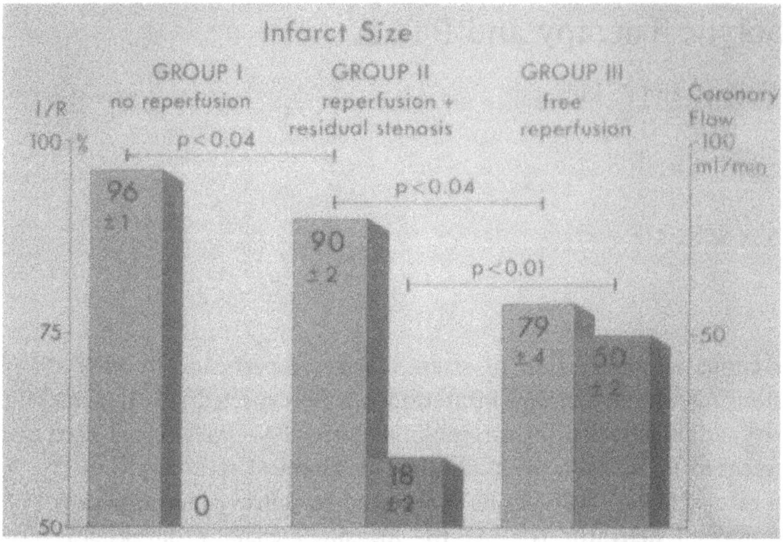

Fig. 1. Ratio of infarct size to area at risk in dogs after 6-h occlusion ($n = 6$), after 2-h occlusion and 4-h reperfusion with flow reduced to 30% of baseline ($n = 6$), and after 2-h occlusion and free flow ($n = 6$). (With permission of the American Heart Association; from Schmidt et al. [13])

their results [17–22]. Residual luminal narrowing was reduced below 50% (Table 1). In a prospective randomized study of patients with acute myocardial infarction the effect of thrombolytic therapy with and without additional PTCA on left ventricular function and rate of reocclusion was studied [25].

In 162 patients with acute transmural myocardial infarction, combined intravenous and intracoronary thrombolytic therapy with streptokinase was initiated. In vessels that remained occluded, mechanical recanalization was performed with a 3F recanalization catheter (group 1; $n = 79$) or 4F Grüntzig balloon catheter (group 2; $n = 83$). After recanalization, intracoronary streptokinase was administered superselectively. After termination of streptokinase infusion (total intravenous and intracoronary dose of 250000 IU), angioplasty was performed only in patients in group 2. There was no difference between the groups in relation to sex, age, infarct location, creatine kinase levels or time between onset of symptoms and start of treatment. A typical example is demonstrated in Fig. 2. Initial coronary angiography showed an open vessel in 27 (34%) of 79 patients in group 1 and in 21 (25%) of 83 patients in group 2. The final reperfusion rate was 90% (71 of 79) in group 1 and 86% (71 of 83) in group 2. Angioplasty as attempted in 69 of the 71 patients in group 2, with a success rate of 65% and an occlusion rate of 3%.

During the hospital stay, reocclusion occurred in 14 (20%) of 71 patients in group 1 (Fig. 3). After thrombolytic therapy, coronary luminal narrowing in group 1 was 75 ± 17% in patients without and 87 ± 6% in patients with reocclusion ($p < 0.05$). In group 2 (Fig. 4) reocclusion was found in 10 (14%) of 71

Table 1. Studies on thrombolytic therapy and PTCA

Author	Year	*n*	Success rate	Coronary stenosis		Reocclusion rate		Complications
				Before	After PTCA	PTCA	Control	
Meyer [16]	1982	21	81%	90%	59%	22%	22%	–
Serruys [17]	1983	18	–	59%	30%	7%	17%	2/18 (13%) occlusion
Hartzler [21]	1983	41	86%	–	30%	15%		2/41 (5%) CABG, 5% occlusion
Gold [20]	1984	28	75%	–	–	14%	6%	1/12 (8%) occlusion
Yasuno [18]	1984	25	72%	–	–	33%	–	2/25 (8%) VF
Papapietro	1985	18	72%	91%	27%	35%	–	1/13 (8%) dissection
Topol [22]	1985	9	78%	84%	29%	0%	67%	2/9 (22%) occlusion
Erbel [5]	1985	46	74%	78%	48%	3%	33%	2/46 (4%) occlusion
Kitazume [23]	1986	21	91%	94%	23%	10%	–	2/22 (9%) occlusion
O'Neill [24]	1986	56	83%	99%	43%	7%	15%	
Erbel [25]	1986	162	65%	82%	51%	14%	20%	2/69 (3%) occlusion, 7% successful PTCA, 32% unsuccessful PTCA

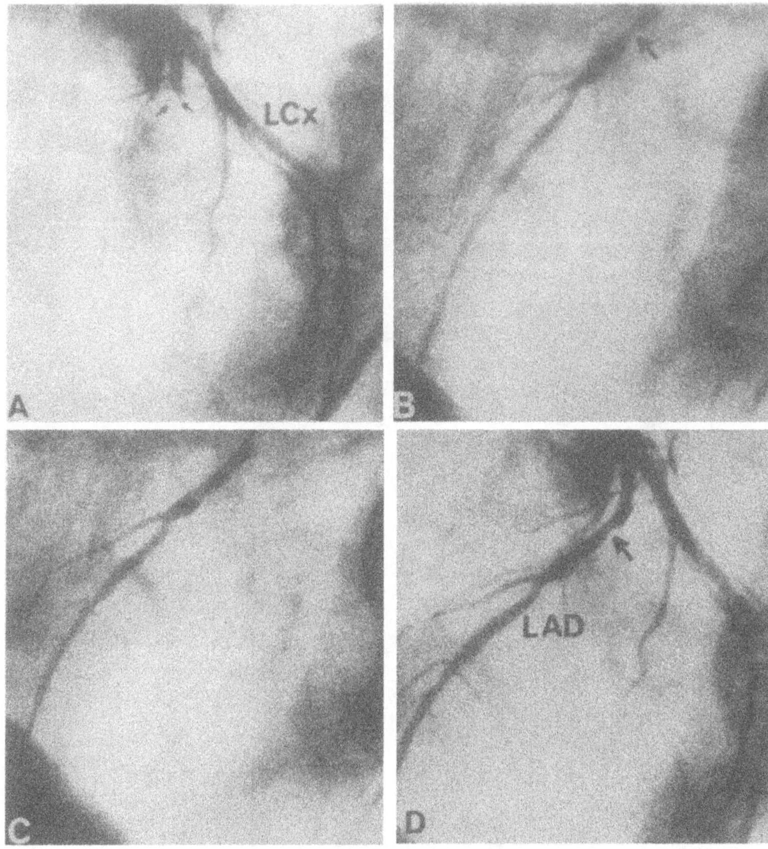

Fig. 2A – D. Acute anterior myocardial infarction. **A** Occlusion of left anterior ascending coronary artery (*LAD*). **B** Mechanical recanalization with 4F balloon catheter. **C** During angioplasty and distal filling of the vessel. **D** After successful angioplasty. *LCx*, left circumflex coronary artery

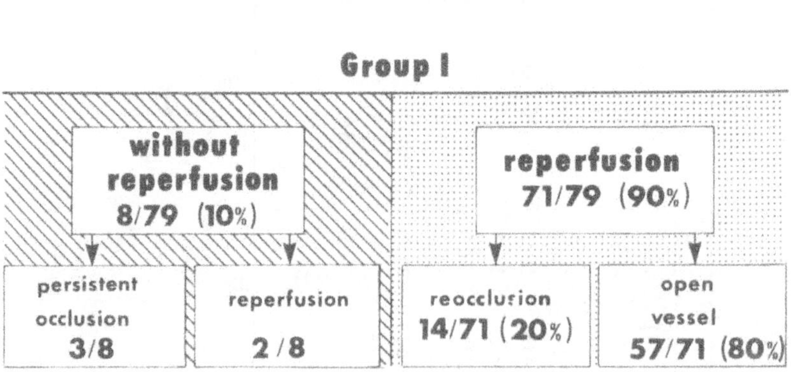

Fig. 3. Follow-up results of patients in group 1 with thrombolytic therapy without PTCA. (With permission of the American College of Cardiology; from Erbel et al. [25])

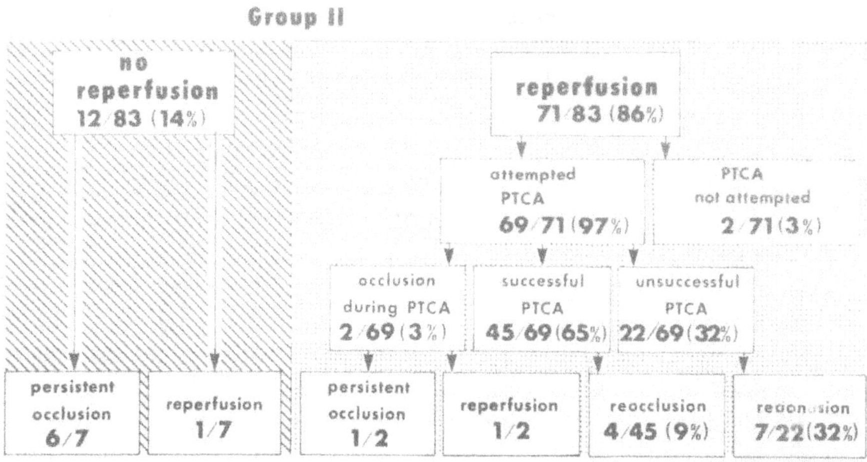

Fig. 4. Follow-up results of patients in group 2 with thrombolytic therapy with PTCA. (With permission of the American College of Cardiology; from Erbel et al. [25])

patients. After angioplasty, the degree of coronary stenosis in group 2 was reduced from 82 ± 12% to 51 ± 30% ($p < 0.001$). Reocclusion was found in 3 (7%) of the 45 patients with successful angioplasty and in 7 (32%) of the 22 patients with unsuccessful angioplasty ($p < 0.01$) [25].

Other investigators described similar reocclusion rates of 17% [27] and 18% [18]. According to other reports [17, 21, 26], reocclusion was dependent on the degree of luminal narrowing after reperfusion. Coronary stenoses were significantly higher in our patients in group 1 with reocclusion compared with those without reocclusion. These results are in accordance with the work of Schwarz and Kübler [25], who reported a reocclusion rate of 8% in patients with less than 70% coronary luminal narrowing and of 26% in those with greater than 70% narrowing. Serruys et al. [17] recorded a reocclusion rate of 17% in 42 patients after attempted thrombolysis and of 5.5% in 18 patients after additional angioplasty using anticoagulant therapy during the hospital stay. Others, using antiplatelet agents or low-dose heparin therapy, reported reocclusion rates of 35% [19] and 33% [18]. Rates of reocclusion after PTCA in addition to thrombolytic therapy are listed in Table 1.

Treatment of the stenosis by PTCA is necessary and should not be postponed because perfusion would be reduced during a waiting period. Our results indicate that 60% of reocclusion occur during the first 5 days after thrombolytic treatment [25].

Besides coronary luminal narrowing, reocclusion is also dependent on continuous full heparinization [25]. In 2 of 3 cases of successful angioplasty and 8 of 14 cases without PTCA, an intermittent normalization of thrombin time was observed at the time of reocclusion.

One other factor is the persistence of coronary thrombus, because in these cases the rate of rethrombosis is high, reaching 30% in our study [25]. Prolonged streptokinase infusion should be considered in cases of persistent thrombus.

Regarding global ventricular function, previous reports [5, 30, 31] described only minor changes in ejection fraction after thrombolytic therapy. A significant increase in left ventricular ejection fraction was reported only in certain subgroups, such as those in which the coronary vessel was already open at the time of the first coronary angiogram [23, 33].

Regional wall motion improved significantly with anterior myocardial infarction treated with angioplasty, whereas in the group without angioplasty regional wall motion was almost unchanged. Increased wall motion of the contralateral wall decreased during the hospital stay. These results are in accordance with those of Sheehan et al. [33], who noted a significant improvement only in patients with thrombolytic therapy and subsequent aortocoronary bypass surgery, as another method of improving coronary perfusion.

For patients with inferior myocardial infarction, the observed changes were only slight. In most patients a decrease in motion of the contralateral wall was observed, combined with a slight decrease in global left ventricular ejection fraction, which remained, however, in the lower normal range.

These results correspond to perfusion studies that demonstrate in thallium-201 scintigrams a reduced score for myocardial scan in the anterior myocardial infarction group with PTCA compared to those without PTCA. Also percentages of patients with positive exercise test were lower than those in patients without PTCA [13, 26].

As regards cardiogenic shock, mechanical recanalization and dilation of occluded coronary vessels seem to be of particular value in patients with cardiogenic shock. Mortality in this group of patients ranges from 65% to 95%, according to the literature (Table 2). In cooperation with the University of Michigan in Ann Arbor, data on patients with cardiogenic shock ($n = 27$) treated by PTCA with and without thrombolytic therapy were pooled. Reperfusion was achieved in 24/27 patients. Residual luminal narrowing measured $44 \pm 25\%$. Hospital mortality in patients younger than 65 years could be reduced to 20% and in patients older than 65 years to 57%. In patients with anterior wall infarction 62% were discharged and with inferior wall infarction 80%. Total mortality measured 30%.

Also for patients with inferior myocardial infarction and signs of right ventricular infarction the need for intracoronary treatment has been confirmed [37]. In an uncontrolled study in 47 patients over the past 4 years, mortality in patients with conventional therapy measured 33% and in those receiving intravenous or intracoronary streptokinase 31%. However, among those with additional PTCA no patient died.

Summary. Intracoronary treatment in acute myocardial infarction seems to be useful in order (a) to reach the maximum rate of reperfusion, (b) to reduce rate of

Table 2. Studies on cardiogenic shock and mortality

Author	Year	*n*	Therapy	Mortality
Griffith [38]	1954	161	Sympathicomimetica	80%
Gunnar [39]	1966	12	Sympathicomimetica	92%
Killip [40]	1967	24	Intensive care	81%
Leinbach [41]	1972	87	Intra-aortic balloon pump	83%
Mundth [42]	1973	33	Heart surgery	60%
DeWood [43]	1980	19	Heart surgery	42%
Meyer [44]	1981	20	Vasodilator	70%
Kennedy	1982	44	Streptokinase	67%
O'Neill [36]	1985	27	Streptokinase/PTCA	30%

reocclusion and reinfarction, and (c) to improve coronary blood flow necessary to maximize salvage of myocardium.

Particularly in patients with cardiogenic shock and right ventricular infarction, PTCA in addition to thrombolytic therapy seems to be a major improvement of therapy. Whether intracoronary therapy including PTCA is superior to intravenous thrombolytic therapy with elective PTCA will hopefully be answered in cooperative studies.

References

1. Neuhaus Kl, Köstering H, Tebbe U, et al (1981) Intravenöse Kurzzeitstreptokinase-Therapie bei frischem Myokardinfarkt. Z Kardiol 70:791–796
2. Schröder R, Biamino G, von Leitner ER, et al (1982) Systemische Thrombolyse mit Streptokinase-Kurzzeitinfusion bei akutem Myokardinfarkt. Z Kardiol 71:709–718
3. Schröder R (1984) Intravenous short-term infusion of streptokinase in acute myocardial infarction. Int J Cardiol 5:631–637
4. Kennedy JW, Gensini GG, Timmis GC, Maynard C (1985) Acute myocardial infarction treated with intracoronary streptokinase: a report of the Society for Cardiac Angiography. Am J Cardiol 55:871–877
5. Erbel R, Pop T, Meinertz T, et al (1985) Combined medical and mechanical recanalization in acute myocardial infarction. Cathet Cardiovasc Diagn 11:361–377
6. Verstraete M, Bernard R, Bory R, et al (1985) Randomized trial of intravenous recombinant tissue-type plasminogen activator versus intravenous streptokinase in acute myocardial infarction. Lancet II:842–847
7. TIMI Study Group (1985) The thrombolysis in myocardial infarction (TIMI) trial: phase I findings. N Engl J Med 312:932–939
8. Verstraete M, Bleifeld W, Brower RW, et al (1985) Double-blind randomized trial of intravenous tissue-type plasminogen activator versus placebo in acute myocardial infarction. Lancet II:965–969
9. Van de Werf F, Nobuhara M, Collen D (1986) Coronary thrombolysis with human

single-chain urokinase-type plasminogen activator (prourokinase) in patients with acute myocardial infarction. Ann Intern Med 104:345–348
10. Kennedy JW, Ritchie JL, Davis KB, Fritz JK (1983) Western Washington randomized trial of intracoronary streptokinase in acute myocardial infarction. N Engl J Med 309:1477–1482
11. Simoons ML, van den Brand M. De Zwaan C, et al (1985) Improved survival after early thrombolysis in acute myocardial infarction. Lancet II:578–581
12. Group Italiano per la Studio della Streptochinasi nell Infarto miocardico (GISSI) (1986) Effectiveness of intravenous thrombolytic treatment in acute myocardial infarction. Lancet I:397–402
13. Fung AY, Lai P, Topol EJ, et al (1986) Value of percutaneous transluminal coronary angioplasty after unsuccessful intravenous streptokinase therapy in acute myocardial infarction. Am J Cardiol 58:686–691
14. Rutsch W, Schartl M, Mathey D, et al (1982) Perkutane transluminale koronare Rekanalisation: Methodik, Ergebnisse und Komplikationen. Z Kardiol 71:7–13
15. Schmidt SB, Varghese PJ, Bloom S, et al (1986) The influence of residual coronary stenosis on size of infarction after reperfusion in a canine preparation. Circulation 73:1354–1359
16. Meyer J, Merx W, Schmitz H, et al (1982) Percutaneous transluminal coronary angioplasty immediately after intracoronary streptolysis of transmural myocardial infarction. Circulation 66:905–913
17. Serruys PW, Wijns W, van den Brand M et al (1983) Is transluminal coronary angioplasty mandatory after successful thrombolysis? Quantitative coronary angiography study. Br Heart J 50:257–265
18. Yasuno M, Saito Y, Ishida M, Suzuki K, Endos S, Takahashi M (1984) Effect of percutaneous transluminal coronary angioplasty: intracoronary thrombolysis with urokinase in acute myocardial infarction. Am J Cardiol 53:1217–1220
19. Papapietro SE, MacLean WAH, Stanley AWE, et al (1985) Percutaneous transluminal coronary angioplasty after intracoronary streptokinase in evolving acute myocardial infarction. Am J Cardiol 55:48–54
20. Gold HK, Cowley MJ, Palacios IF, et al (1984) Combined intracoronary streptokinase infusion and coronary angioplasty during acute myocardial infarction. Am J Cardiol 53:713–720
21. Hartzler GO, Rutherford BD, McConahay DR, et al (1983) Percutaneous transluminal coronary angioplasty with and without thrombolytic therapy for treatment of acute myocardial infarction. Am Heart J 106:965–973
22. Topol EJ, Eha JE, Brink P, et al (1985) Applicability of percutaneous transluminal coronary angioplasty to patients with recombinant tissue plasminogen activator mediated thrombolysis. Cathet Cardiovasc Diagn 11:337–348
23. Kitazume H, Iwama T, Suzuki A (1986) Combined thrombolytic therapy and coronary angioplasty for acute myocardial infarction. Am Heart J 111:826–832
24. O'Neill W, Timmis GC, Bourdillon PD, et al (1986) A prospective randomized clinical trial of intracoronary streptokinase versus coronary angioplasty for acute myocardial infarction. N Engl J Med 314:812–818
25. Erbel R, Pop T, Henrichs KJ, et al (1986) Percutaneous transluminal coronary angioplasty after thrombolytic therapy: a prospective controlled randomized trial. J Am Coll Cardiol 8:485–495

26. Schwarz F, Kübler W (1984) Thrombolytische Therapie des akuten Myokardinfarktes. Internist 25:713 – 720
27. Reduto L, Smalling R, Freund GC, Gould KL (1981) Intracoronary infusion of streptokinase in patients with acute myocardial infarction: effect of reperfusion on left ventricular performance. Am J Cardiol 48:403 – 409
28. Timmis GC, Gangadharan V, Hauser AM, Ramos RG, et al (1982) Intracoronary streptokinase in clinical practice. Am Heart J 104:925 – 938
29. Merx W, Dörr R, Rentrop P, et al (1981) Evaluation of effectiveness of intracoronary streptokinase infusion in acute infarction: postprocedure management and hospital course in 204 patients. Am Heart J 102:1159 – 1167
30. Rentrop P, Blanke H, Karsch R, et al (1981) Selective intracoronary thrombolysis in acute myocardial infarction and unstable angina pectoris. Circulation 63:307 – 317
31. Ritchie JL, Davis B, Williams DL, et al (1984) Global and regional left ventricular function and tomographic radionuclide perfusion: the Western Washington intracoronary streptokinase in myocardial infarction trial. Circulation 70:867 – 875
32. Mathey DG, Kuck KH, Tilsner V, et al (1981) Nonsurgical coronary artery recanalization in acute transmural myocardial infarction. Circulation 102:1181 – 1187
33. Sheehan FH, Mathey DG, Schofer J, Krebber HJ, Dodge HT (1983) Effect of interventions in salvaging left ventricular function in acute myocardial infarction: a study of intracoronary streptokinase. Am J Cardiol 52:431 – 438
34. Serruys PW, Simoons ML, Suryapranata H, et al (1986) Preservation of global and regional left ventricular function after early thrombolyses in acute myocardial infarction. J Am Coll Cardiol 7:729 – 742
35. Meyer J, Erbel R, Pop T, et al (1986) PTCA und intrakoronare Lyse bei akutem Myokardinfarkt. Z Kardiol 75[Suppl 5]:83 – 91
36. O'Neill W, Erbel R, Laufer N, et al (1985) Coronary angioplasty therapy of cardiogenic shock complicating acute myocardial infarction. Circulation 72[Suppl III]:309
37. Meyer J, Merx W, Dörr R, et al (1982) Successful treatment of acute myocardial infarction shock by combinated percutaneous transluminal coronary recanalization (PTCR) and percutaneous transluminal coronary angioplasty (PTCA). Am Heart J 103:132 – 134
38. Griffith GC, Wallace WB (1954) Cardiogenic shock. Circulation 9:527 – 533
39. Gunnar RM, Cruz A, Boswell J, et al (1966) Myocardial infarction with shock. Hemodynamic studies and results of therapy. Circulation 33:753 – 762
40. Killip T, Kimball JT (1967) Treatment of myocardial infarction in a coronary care unit. A two years experience with 250 patients. Am J Cardiol 20:457 – 463
41. Leinbach RC, Dinsmore RE, Mundth ED, et al (1972) Selective coronary left ventricular cineangiography during balloon pumping for cardiogenic shock. Circulation 45:845 – 850
42. Mundth ED, Buckley MJ, Leinbach RC, et al (1973) Surgical intervention for the complication of acute myocardial infarction. Ann Surg 1978:379 – 383
43. DeWood M, Sores J, Notske R (1980) Prevalence of total coronary occlusion during early hours of transmural myocardial infarction. N Engl J Med 303:897 – 902
44. Meyer J, Erbel R, Rupprecht HJ, v. Essen R, Effert S (1981) Relation between admission time, haemodynamic measurements and prognosis in acute myocardial infarction. Br Heart J 46:647 – 656

Percutaneous Transluminal Coronary Angioplasty in Unstable Angina

F. Schwarz

The aim of this study was to compare early and late results of percutaneous transluminal coronary angioplasty (PTCA) in patients with unstable angina to results obtained in patients with stable angina. From 1981 to 1984 at the University Hospital of Heidelberg 486 PTCAs were performed in 401 patients with coronary artery disease. Of these, 115 patients suffered from unstable angina while 213 patients suffered from stable angina; 73 patients had an acute myocardial infarction and were excluded from this study. Coronary angioplasty was performed with the Grüntzig catheter, Simpson catheter, or Hartzler catheter. Since 1983 steerable balloon catheters were used. Reangiography was performed 6 months after PTCA in 64% of patients with unstable angina, and in 71% of patients with stable angina. Primary success was defined as reduction of the stenosis of more than 20% diameter reduction. Recurrence was defined if the stenosis at reangiography was less than 20% lower than the stenosis before treatment.

The early results and the clinical data of patients are given in Table 1. The group with unstable angina contained more women than the group with stable angina. An emergency aortocoronary bypass operation was needed in 7% of patients with unstable angina, as compared to 3% of patients with stable angina. Stenosis was reduced from 87% to 29% in patients with unstable angina and from 84% to 27% in patients with stable angina. The results 6 months after PTCA are given in Table 2. The degree of stenosis at 6 months averaged 53% in patients with unstable angina, as compared to 43% in patients with stable angina. The rate of recurrence amounted 38% in patients with unstable angina and 28% in patients with stable angina (difference not statistically significant).

The early and late results after PTCA in patients with unstable angina are thus comparable to results obtained in patients with stable angina. Since coronary artery bypass operation is needed in a high percentage of patients with unstable angina, PTCA offers an alternative therapeutic approach. In recent years the primary success rate in Heidelberg has increased to 90% by use of steerable balloon catheters. Today PTCA can be performed with good therapeutic success in most patients with unstable angina and with a high primary success rate.

The angiographic result immediately after PTCA was better in patients who revealed long-term success (stenosis after PTCA averaged 22%), as compared to patients who developed recurrence of stenosis (stenosis after PTCA averaged

Table 1. Early results after PTCA

	Unstable angina	Stable angina
Patients (n)	115	213
Age (years)	55 ± 8	53 ± 7
Men (%)	77	90*
One-vessel disease (%)	70	74
Two-vessel disease (%)	26	21
Three-vessel disease (%)	4	5
Primary success (%)	72	79
Emergency operation (%)	7	3
Patients with primary success:		
Stenosis before (%)	87 ± 10	84 ± 12
Stenosis after (%)	29 ± 18	27 ± 17

* $p < 0.05$ as compared to patients with unstable angina.

Table 2. Results 6 months after PTCA

	Unstable angina	Stable angina
Patients (n)	53	120
Stenosis before (%)	87 ± 10	84 ± 11
Stenosis after (%)	30 ± 19	29 ± 17
Stenosis after 6 months (%)	53 ± 31	43 ± 31
Rate of recurrence	20 (38%)	34 (28%)

41%). The aim of coronary artery dilatation is therefore to obtain an excellent primary result.

Since the early and late results in patients with unstable angina are comparable to those obtained in patients with stable angina, we feel that PTCA should be considered in each patient with acute symptoms of coronary artery disease.

Drug Treatment after PTCA

R.A. O'Rourke

Introduction

It is well recognized that there is about a 30% restenosis rate in the first 6 months following what has been termed successful PTCA [1 – 11]. This percentage varies depending on the definition used to classify what is and what is not restenosis. The rate is an important consideration economically, since the difference between successful PTCA without restenosis and PTCA followed by coronary artery bypass graft surgery in the United States averages about $ 12000 per patient.

Several types of treatment have been used singularly or combined after PTCA in order to prevent or reduce the incidence [12 – 18]. The approach may differ early after PTCA during the time when acute thrombosis may play a major role in closure of the artery undergoing successful dilatation, as compared to the chronic therapy used during the subsequent 6 – 9 months when proliferation of tissue with or without further thrombus formation may result in restenosis [2, 8, 10, 19].

In addition, risk factor modification is still important in patients who have had successful angioplasty for severe coronary artery stenosis in order to prevent recurrent disease not only in the vessel that has been dilated but also in the other coronary arteries. Chest pain 6 months or longer after angioplasty is not necessarily due to restenosis but may be caused by advanced atherosclerotic lesions in coronary arteries that did not have significant previous lesions. In many patients in whom successful PTCA has been performed, it is necessary and desirable to treat residual or recurrent ischemia. This may require repeated PTCA, coronary artery bypass surgery, or the use of antianginal medications, particularly in patients with diffuse coronary atherosclerosis.

A schematic representation of the sequence of pathophysiologic events occurring after angioplasty in arteries developing restenosis is depicted in Fig. 1 [19]. During the initial injury there is a denudation of the endothelium plus various degree of trauma to media and elastic tissue with some platelet interaction. Smooth muscle cell proliferation may result in some degree of stenosis often causing early occlusion or thrombus organization, or later restenosis with or without the presence of coronary artery spasm. Post-PTCA treatment is aimed at preventing an overproliferation of smooth muscle cells and inhibiting the

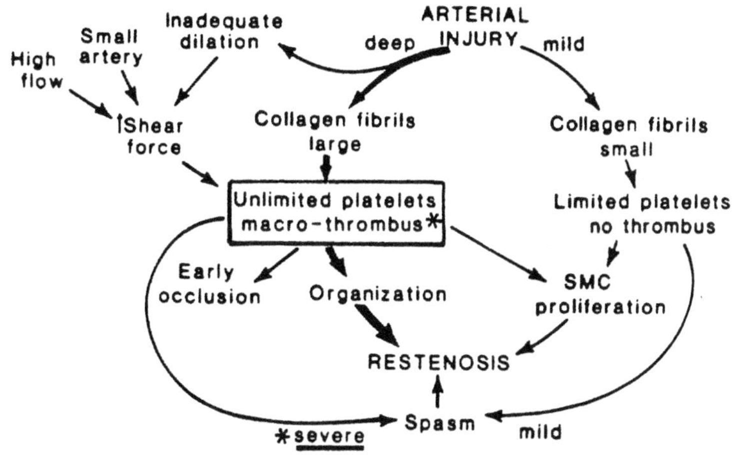

Fig. 1. Proposed pathophysiologic mechanisms of restenosis after arterial angioplasty. The major mechanism of restenosis is probably the one depicted by *broad arrows* that involves organization of mural thrombus. Smooth muscle cell (*SMC*) proliferation via the platelet-derived growth factor probably also contributes but to a lesser degree. Vasoconstriction (*spasm*) is often present proximal and distal to the dilated region after arterial angioplasty in the porcine carotid artery and is directly related to the severity of platelet deposition, but makes an uncertain contribution to restenosis in patients. Mechanisms with an *asterisk* have been reduced or suppressed by platelet inhibitor therapy. (Reproduced with permission from [19])

aggregation of platelets and the subsequent release of substance such as platelet-derived growth factor which promotes tissue proliferation. The goal is to prevent the initial thrombus from occurring in patients undergoing successful dilatation of coronary artery stenosis.

Risk Factors for Restenosis

It is important to review the risk factors favoring restenosis in patients undergoing PTCA (Table 1). There are risk factors that tend to be related to the lesion itself, risk factors related to the procedure being performed to dilate the artery, and risk factors that are patient related. One method of assessing risk factors for restenosis is to study patients with multivessel disease and to observe the natural history of lesions at multiple different sites in different vessels in relationship to a particular factor being evaluated for risk [2]. During follow-up the progression of lesions in nondilated arteries can be compared with one or more areas of restenosis that were dilated. Thus, systemic and local factors can be evaluated as indicators of increased risk for restenosis.

Table 1 includes multiple factors for restenosis that have been identified in many follow-up studies [1–10]. One is the severity of the occlusion prior to

Table 1. Risk factors for post-coronary angioplasty restenosis

1. Lesion-related
Severity
Total occlusions
>90% stenosis
Site
Left main artery
LAD>RCA>LCx
Bifurcation site
Saphenous graft
Prior angioplasty?
Length >10–15 mm
2. Procedure-related
No dissection
>30% residual stenosis
>15 mmHg residual gradient
3. Patient-related
Unstable angina
Male sex
Diabetes
Variant angina
Multivessel disease
Smoking
Hypercholesterolemia

LAD, left anterior descending coronary artery; RCA, right coronary artery; LCx, left circumflex coronary artery. (Modified with permission from [2])

angioplasty, restenosis being particularly more common with greater than 90% arterial stenosis. The site of stenosis is also important, with restenosis more commonly affecting the left anterior descending coronary artery. The results of PTCA also relate to how good the initial dilation was, how small the residual stenosis is, and whether or not dissection was produced (Table 1).

Patient-related factors favoring restenosis are also indicated in Table 1. Restenosis is more common in male patients with unstable angina prior to angioplasty, coronary vasospasm, multivessel disease, continued cigarette smoking, persistent hypercholesterolemia, and diabetes [2, 10, 20].

Early Treatment to Prevent Restenosis

Early post-PTCA treatment usually includes intravenous heparin, and most patients also receive the antiplatelet agents aspirin and dipyridamole. There is

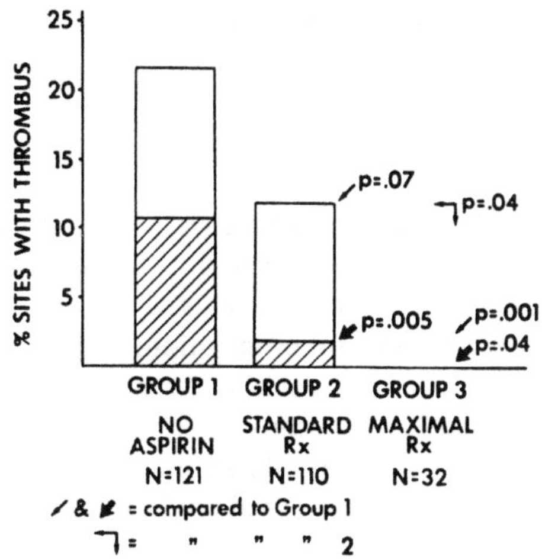

Fig. 2. Effect of increasing antiplatelet pretreatment on the incidence of clinically insignificant thrombus (*nonshaded bars*) and of clinically significant thrombus (*shaded bars*). (Reproduced with permission from [13])

some question whether or not additional benefit is derived by giving them aspirin and dipyridamole before the angioplasty is performed, even before hospitalization. Supporting this approach are animal studies showing less platelet aggregation and less frequent development of thrombus following PTCA in pigs and in rabbits with atherosclerotic lesions when there is pretreatment with a combination of aspirin and dipyridamole [21, 22].

In a retrospective clinical study, Barnathan et al. [13] compared a group of patients (Fig. 2) who were pretreated with aspirin and dipyridamole (group 3) before angioplasty was performed with a group who received no aspirin (group 1) prior to angioplasty. Group 2 patients received aspirin but not dipyridamole prior to angioplasty. The number of sites with thromboses as determined by coronary arteriography 30 min post-PTCA are shown in Fig. 2. Patients with clinically significant complete occlusion (i. e., occlusion with the thrombus resulting in myocardial ischemia) frequently underwent subsequent thrombolytic therapy and/or coronary bypass graft surgery. Consistent with animal studies, there was a significant difference in the incidence of thrombi favoring pretreatment with antiplatelet drugs. In fact, there were no evident thrombi by coronary arteriography in group 3 patients after pretreatment with aspirin and dipyridamole and a >20% likelihood in patients with no pretreatment (Fig. 2). Thus, pretreatment before angioplasty may reduce platelet aggregation and lessen the release of substances that may cause vasoconstriction of the dilated artery after angioplasty. Accordingly, some authors have recommended 24 – 48 h of treatment with aspirin and dipyridamole prior to angioplasty. The trade-off is an increased likelihood of postoperative bleeding in patients who require emergency surgical revascularization after PTCA.

Heparin infusion is often used in patients with complex, technically difficult lesions requiring a lengthy procedure and is usually given for 48 h after the procedure [2]. Nitrate therapy and calcium entry blockers are usually prescribed for the first 2 days after angioplasty to reduce acute injury-related coronary artery spasm [2].

Long Term Treatment to Prevent Restenosis

The long-term medical treatment often used to prevent restenosis includes antiplatelet drugs, calcium-entry blocking drugs, lipid-lowering interventions, and control of diabetes mellitus.

Concerning anticoagulation, Thornton et al. [12] compared anticoagulation with warfarin to aspirin therapy for preventing restenosis after PTCA. Patients received 325 mg aspirin daily during 9 months of follow-up or enough warfarin to maintain the prothrombin time at 2.0 – 2.5 times normal. Of note, no prior prospective randomized study had assessed the efficacy of antiplatelet therapy with aspirin versus no therapy for preventing restenosis; however, such a study is currently in progress comparing no therapy to combined aspirin (975 mg) and dipyridamole (225 mg) daily treatment. Many animal studies suggest that aspirin therapy does decrease the incidence of restenosis following mechanical dilatation [2].

In the study by Thornton and associates [12] 120 patients treated with coumadin were compared with 126 treated with aspirin (Table 2). The two groups of patients were similar regarding the numbers of vessels dilated, the pressure gradient reduction after PTCA, the diameter of the lumen before PTCA, and the extent of residual coronary artery stenosis. Table 3 shows the follow-up total recurrence rate defined in this particular study as a loss by 50% or more of the initial improvement in luminal diameter produced by PTCA. There is a 36% incidence of restenosis in 122 patients followed for 9 months on warfarin therapy as compared to 27% with restenosis while taking aspirin. Interestingly, there was only a 20% restenosis rate in those responding to a follow-up questionnaire who were assigned to the aspirin group, but who did not comply with therapy.

Table 4 from the study by Thornton et al. shows that aspirin tended to be better than coumadin for preventing restenosis in patients with angina of less than 6 months duration prior to PTCA. However, only a total of 248 patients were included in the entire study, a small sample size for making definite conclusions.

Calcium-entry blockers are usually given during the first 2 – 3 days following PTCA, since there is well-documented spasm produced proximal and distal to the area of coronary artery dilatation in such patients [1 – 3, 10]. There are several platelet-derived substances, such as thromboxane A_2, that promote coronary vasoconstriction. However, there has been controversy whether or not calcium-entry blockers should be given long-term to such patients. Calcium-entry blocking drugs frequently are used in post-PTCA patients to prevent restenosis related to spasm and to treat recurrent myocardial ischemia and for secondary prevention in patients who have had angioplasty early or late after acute myocardial infarction.

Table 2. Characteristics of patients and procedures in patients undergoing PTCA

	Coumadin	Aspirin
n	122	126
Age (years)	53	53
	(range 33 – 72)	(range 31 – 77)
Men (%)	81	79
Vessel dilated (%)		
LAD	69	75
RCA	22	20
LCx	3	2
LM	0	1
SVG	6	2
Pressure gradient (mmHg) [a]		
Before PTCA	46.7 ± 17.0	47.9 ± 16.1
After PTCA	15.0 ± 9.3	14.6 ± 8.1
Diameter stenosis (%) [a]		
Before PTCA	72.7 ± 13.8	68.8 ± 14.8
After PTCA	28.9 ± 13.1	27.2 ± 12.4

LAD, Left anterior descending coronary artery; RCA, right coronary artery; LCx, left circumflex coronary artery; LM, left main coronary artery; SVG, sapheous vein graft.
[a] Mean ± SD.
(Modified with permission from [12])

Table 3. Total recurrence rate (R) during follow-up

	Coumadin	Aspirin
Total patients		
n	122	126
R	44 (36%)	34 (27%) (NS)
Total responders to questionnaire		
n	108	102
R	36 (33%)	25 (24%)
Responders on no therapy		
n	28 (26%)	15 (15%) ($p<0.05$)
R	9 (32%)	3 (20%)
Responders on some therapy		
n	80	87
R	27 (34%)	22 (25%) (NS)

(Modified with permission from [12])

Table 4. Duration of anginal symptoms prior to PTCA

	History of angina (months)									
	<3		3–5		6–11		12–23		$\geqslant 24$	
Recurrence	34/100		15/57		12/37		10/23		7/31	
			$\chi^2 = 3.74$, NS (4 df)							
Therapy	C	A	C	A	C	A	C	A	C	A
Recurrence	13/46	21/54	12/33	3/24	9/20	3/17	7/11	3/12	3/12	4/19
		NS	$\chi^2 = 4.08$		$\chi^2 = 3.14$		$\chi^2 = 3.49$		NS	
			$p<0.05$		$p<0.1$		$p<0.1$			

C, Coumadin; A, aspirin; PTCA, percutaneous transluminal coronary angioplasty. (Modified with permission from [12])

Table 5. Baseline clinical characteristics of patients undergoing PTCA

Characteristics	Diltiazem group	Control group
	(*n*) (%)	(*n*) (%)
Risk factors		
Age >60 years	10 (22)	11 (24)
Male sex	36 (78)	35 (76)
Family history of coronary disease	31 (67)	31 (67)
Hypertension	6 (13)	8 (17)
Smoking		
Never	8 (17)	8 (4)
Former	11 (24)	19 (41)
Current	27 (59)	25 (54)
Diabetes	4 (9)	4 (9)
Cholesterol >250 mg/dl	21 (46)	25 (54)
Triglycerides >170 mg/dl	26 (57)	25 (54)
Cardiac history and symptoms		
Prior myocardial infarction	11 (24)	12 (26)
Prior coronary bypass surgery	2 (4)	3 (7)
Prior PTCA (restenosis)	3 (7)	2 (4)
Angina[a]	46 (100)	46 (100)
Class I	1 (2)	3 (7)
Class II	13 (28)	13 (28)
Class III	19 (41)	24 (52)
Class IV or unstable angina	13 28	6 13
Total duration of angina (months)	18 ± 27	20 ± 30
Duration of current level of disability (months)	4 ± 7	5 ± 4

Diltiazem group: $n = 46$; mean age, 51 ± 9 years; control group: $n = 46$; mean age, 50 ± 10. None of the differences is statistically significant.

[a] Classes for severity of angina, after Canadian Cardiovascular Society Classification

Table 6. Baseline angiographic characteristics of patients undergoing PTCA

Characteristics	Diltiazem group		Control group		p
	(n)	(%)	(n)	(%)	
Number of diseased vessels (70%)					
0	5	11	0		<0.05
1	39	85	39	85	
2	2	4	4	9	
3	0		3	7	
Ejection fraction (%)	65±8		63±8		NS
Number of successfully dilated stenoses	50		53		NS
Dilated artery					
LAD	31	62	34	64	NS
RCA	14	28	12	23	
LCX	5	10	7	13	
Site of stenosis					
Proximal	20	40	27	51	NS
Mid or distal	30	60	26	49	
Stenosis					
Single discrete	44	88	45	85	NS
Long or multiple	6	12	8	15	
Stenosis					
Concentric	35	70	34	64	NS
Eccentric	15	30	19	36	
Calcified stenosis	3	6	4	8	NS
Degree of stenosis					
Before PTCA	79±11		77±12		NS
After PTCA	38±15		37±12		NS

LAD, left anterior descending artery; RCA, right coronary artery; LCX, left circumflex artery.
(Modified with permission from [16])

Corcos and associates [16] assessed the effects of daily oral diltiazem on coronary artery restenosis in post-PTCA patients. Forty-six patients received diltiazem (270 mg/day) and an equal number served as controls. The risk factor profile did not differ in the two groups, and the clinical profiles of the two groups were also similar (Table 5). The baseline angiographic findings are included in Table 6. The control group tended to have more multivessel coronary artery disease.

Figure 3 indicates the extent of coronary artery stenosis as determined angiographically after PTCA and at an average of 8.5 months later. There was no difference between the degree of stenosis at any of the three times in patients receiving and not receiving diltiazem. Both groups showed the expected reduction

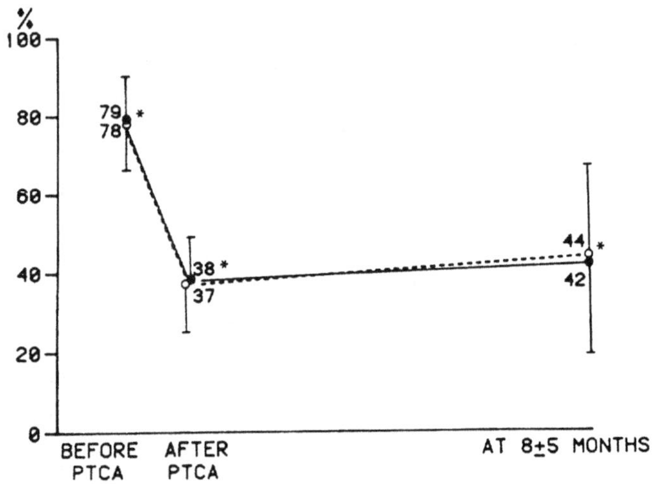

Fig. 3. Mean degree of coronary stenosis before, immediately after, and 8 ± 5 months after PTCA in the control group (*broken line*; $n = 46$) and in the diltiazem group (*unbroken line*; $n = 36$). Difference not significant. (Reproduced with permission from [16])

in coronary artery stenosis after PTCA. Table 7 shows the incidence of coronary restenosis, defined as 70% or greater stenosis at the PTCA site, which averaged 14% in the patients receiving diltiazem and 18% in the control group. This was higher in the small number of patients with multivessel disease as compared to those with single-vessel disease and not different with or without diltiazem. However, all the patients in both groups received daily aspirin therapy.

In a separate study by Whitworth et al. [17] 241 total patients received either 40 mg nifedipine or placebo in addition to 325 mg aspirin daily to determine any difference in the rate of restenosis. Again, the clinical characteristics and extent of coronary artery stenosis were similar in the two groups. As indicated in Table 8 the incidence of restenosis at 6 months and the likelihood of myocardial ischemia during exercise testing did not differ in the two groups.

Tentative conclusions from the two previous studies are (a) that treatment with calicum-entry blockers does not decrease the rate of restenosis after PTCA in patients who do not have characteristic variant angina and (b) that following restenosis in post-PTCA patients occurring after the first 1–2 days angioplasty is probably not related to coronary artery spasm. However, the number of patients in both studies was relatively low, and definitive conclusions would be tenuous.

Since elevated cholesterol and triglycerides and uncontrolled diabetes mellitus are known risk factors for restenosis (see above); patients with elevated serum lipids should be treated with interventions (diet, indications) that normalize the abnormal levels, and diet or medications should be altered to control hyperglycemia.

There are very few data regarding the use of β-blockers after PTCA. β-Blockers have been used primarily for the treatment of myocardial ischemia in

Table 7. Rate of restenosis post-PTCA versus severity of coronary disease

	Diltiazem group ($n = 46$)		Control group ($n = 46$)		Total group ($n = 92$)	
	(n)	(%)	(n)	(%)	(n)	(%)
Restenosis during follow-up						
Single-vessel disease	6/44	14	7/39	18	13/83	16
Multivessel disease	1/2	50	3/7	43	4/8	44
Total	7/46	15	10/46	22	17/92	18
No restenosis during follow-up						
Single-vessel disease	38/44	86	32/39	82	70/83	84
Multivessel disease	1/2	50	4/7	57	5/9	56
Total	39/46	85	36/46	78	75/92	82
Interval between PTCA and repeat angiography (months)						
Mean ± standard deviation	8.24 ± 4.79				8.26 ± 4.91	
Range	1–21				1–21	

(Modified with permission from [16])

Table 8. Incidence of post-PTCA restenosis

	Nifedipine		Placebo	
All patients	(n)	(%)	(n)	(%)
Angiography	28/100	28	29/98	29.5
Exercise stress test	2/11	18	1/12	8
Total	30/111	27[a]	30/110	27[a]
Compliant patients				
Angiography	24/84	29	28/84	33
Exercise stress test	1/8	12	1/8	12
Total	25/92	27[a]	29/92	31.5[a]

[a] p, NS.
(Modified with permission from [17])

post-PTCA patients who do not have lesions that are feasible for dilatation or redilatation, or who are not candidates for coronary bypass surgery, for whatever reason. There are no data indicating whether patients who have had PTCA after myocardial infarction have an additional beneficial effect when β-blockers are used for secondary prevention of recurrent infarction and sudden death.

The risk of restenosis during the first 6 months after initially successful coronary angioplasty remains relatively high despite improved technology and the current use of available drug therapy designed to prevent early or late reoccurrence of stenosis. New drugs or other approaches (low-energy laser remodeling, coronary artery stents, atherectomy) may be useful in reducing post-angioplasty restenosis [3, 23].

References

1. Roubin GS, King SB, Douglas JS (1987) Restenosis after percutaneous transluminal coronary angioplasty: the Emory University Hospital experience. Am J Cardiol 60:39B
2. Blackshear JL, O'Callaghan WG, Califf RM (1987) Medical approaches to prevention of restenosis after coronary angioplasty. J Am Coll Cardiol 9:834
3. Shaw RE, Myler RK, Stertzer SH, Clark DA (1987) Restenosis after coronary angioplasty. Cardiology 1:42
4. Weintraub WS (1987) Design considerations in the study of restenosis after percutaneous transluminal coronary angioplasty. Am J Cardiol 60:3B
5. Faxon DP, Sanborn TA, Haudenschild CC (1987) Mechanism of angioplasty and its relation to restenosis. Am J Cardiol 60:5B
6. Brown BC, Bolson EL, Dodge HT (1987) Percutaneous transluminal coronary angioplasty and subsequent restenosis: quantitative and qualitative methodology for their assessment. Am J Cardiol 60:34B
7. Bussmann WD, Kaltenbach M, Kober G, Vallbracht C (1987) The Frankfurt experience in restenosis after coronary angioplasty. Am J Cardiol 60:48B
8. Val PG, Bourassa MG, David PR, Bonan R, Crepeau J, Dyrda I, Lesperance J (1987) Restenosis after successful percutaneous transluminal coronary angioplasty: the Montreal Heart Institute experience. Am J Cardiol 60:50B
9. Vogel JHK (1987) On passivation and stenosis: restenosis in coronary artery disease and percutaneous transluminal coronary angioplasty. Am J Cardiol 60:68B
10. King SB (1987) A symposium: restenosis after percutaneous transluminal coronary angioplasty. Am J Cardiol 60[3]:1B
11. Kemp HG (1986) Coronary angioplasty and the persistent problem of restenosis. J Am Coll Cardiol 8[6]:1277
12. Thornton MA, Gruentzig AR, Hollman J, King SB, Douglas JS (1984) Coumadin and aspirin in prevention of recurrence after transluminal coronary angioplasty: a randomized study. Circulation 69[4]:721
13. Barnathan ES, Schwartz JS, Taylor L, Laskey WK, Kleaveland JP, Kussmaul WG, Hirshfeld JW (1987) Aspirin and dipyridamole in the prevention of acute coronary thrombosis complicating coronary angioplasty. Circulation 76[1]:125
14. Bettmann MA (1987) Anticoagulation and restenosis after percutaneous transluminal coronary angioplasty. Am J Cardiol 60:17B
15. MacDonald RG, Panush RS, Pepine CJ (1987) Rationale for use of glucocorticoids in modification of restenosis after percutaneous transluminal coronary angioplasty. Am J Cardiol 60:56B
16. Corcos T, David PR, Val PG, Renkin J, Dangoisse V, Rapold HG, Bourassa MG (1985) Failure of diltiazem to prevent restenosis after percutaneous transluminal coronary angioplasty. Am Heart J 109:926
17. Whitworth HB, Roubin GS, Hollman J, Meier B, Leimgruber PP, Douglas JS, King

SB, Gruentzig AR (1986) Effect of nifedipine on recurrent stenosis after percutaneous transluminal coronary angioplasty. J Am Coll Cardiol 8:1271
18. Harker LA (1987) Role of platelets and thrombosis in mechanisms of acute occlusion and restenosis after angioplasty. Am J Cardiol 60:20B
19. Chesebro JH, Lam JYT, Badimon L, Fuster V (1987) Restenosis after arterial angioplasty: a hemorrheologic response to injury. Am J Cardiol 60:10B
20. Vandormael MG, Deligonul U, Kern MJ, Kennedy H, Galan K, Chaitman B (1987) Restenosis after multilesion percutaneous transluminal coronary angioplasty. Am J Cardiol 60:44B
21. Steele PM, Chesebro JH, Stanson AW, Holmes DR, Badimon L, Fuster V (1984) Balloon angioplasty: effect of platelet-inhibitor drugs on platelet-thrombus deposition in a pig model. J Am Coll Cardiol 3:506
22. Faxon DB, Sanborn TA, Haudenschild CC, Ryan TJ (1984) Effect of antiplatelet therapy on restenosis after experimental angioplasty. Am J Cardiol 53:72C
23. Spears JR (1987) Percutaneous transluminal coronary angioplasty restenosis: potential prevention with laser balloon angioplasty. Am J Cardiol 60:61B

Discussion: Session III – Percutaneous Transluminal Coronary Angioplasty

Chairman: E. Rapaport

Question to Dr. Rapaport: I wonder, Dr. Rapaport, whether I understood correctly that your task force has not recommended any secondary preventive measures. I understood that what you recommended was to use aspirin, antiplatelet drugs, and later on calcium antagonists as a possibility to avoid restenosis. But there was nothing said about modification of risk factors.

Dr. Rapaport: This task force was not designed to address the question of secondary prevention per se, but rather what management strategies are undertaken during PTCA and post-PTCA in terms of the intervention itself. For example, the immediate problems of thrombosis and spasm are approached with recommendations for the use of antiplatelet agents and calcium antagonists. However, the long-term management of patients with angina pectoris in terms of secondary prevention is not addressed. There should be no implication that one does not go ahead with appropriate management of the patient, holistically speaking, in relationship to the underlying disease problem. Clearly, the report is not meant to take away from the other aspects of management of the patients including rehabilitation.

Dr. Lichtlen: Dr. Rapaport, if I understood you correctly, the class I, representing the well-accepted indications, also included chronic stable angina and unstable angina with unresponsiveness to treatment. Was this really meant also for stable angina or only for unstable angina? I ask because I think this is not what is usually done in clinical practice; many of these patients have a treatment which reduces their daily episodes of ischemia, but they undergo PTCA because they have a high-grade obstruction which in the long run might be dangerous for their life due to plaque rupture. What is your meaning?

Dr. Rapaport: The approach used was that class I is clear-cut. Class I indications are those where everyone agrees that PTCA is appropriate. There are situations where a patient has one-vessel disease, but there is not an absolute indication for PTCA, for example, a patient made totally asymptomatic with medical management. Thus particular characteristic features are required for patients with one-vessel disease to qualify as a class I indication rather than a class II or evolving indication.

Dr. Lichtlen: I'm sure that Dr. Varnauskas will also discuss single-vessel disease in his presentation. In a study on sudden death, where we have been following patients now for almost 8 years, we have seen that also in single-vessel disease, at least in high-grade obstructions of the left anterior descending branch, the yearly mortality rate is approximately 2%, in contrast to single obstructions of the left circumflex branch and right coronary artery, where yearly mortality amounted to almost zero; therefore, I still think in patients with left anterior descending obstructions, even if there is a good response to medical treatment, patients should undergo PTCA, provided ischemia can be objectivated.

Dr. Rapaport: And what do you think if the patient is totally asymptomatic with high-grade obstruction?

Dr. Lichtlen: No, I think if they have ischemic episodes, independently of whether they are asymptomatical or symptomatical ones, they should be treated.

Dr. Rapaport: I really personally don't have any disagreement. I like to use the criteria of a large area of myocardium at jeopardy. I think if you have a large area of myocardium at risk with one-vessel obstruction, and the patient is asymptomatic, there is little question that that patient can benefit from PTCA. To me, the area of myocardium at risk is a more important indication than symptomatology. On the other hand, there are patients, let's say with a distal RCA single-vessel obstruction where, even with a symptomatic patient, you may not want to go ahead with PTCA.

Dr. Zaret: Question to Dr. Schwarz with respect to unstable angina pectoris. You indicated that three-quarters of the patients had single-vessel disease. I'd like to know more about the remaining quarter who had multivessel disease, and whether the approach was to an angiographically directed, so-called culprit, lesion or total revascularization.

Dr. Schwarz: The rest of the patients had two-vessel disease, and we dilated the more severe lesion and then did an exercise study. When the patient had a severe ischemia of the second lesion, we dilated the second lesion, but in a second session, not in the same session.

Dr. Rapaport: I would like to expand on that question by asking either Dr. Schwarz or Dr. Erbel whether they would agree that in patients with myocardial infarction one attacks only the culprit vessel going to the area of infarction with PTCA, and whether one should not attempt doing multivessel angioplasty in that setting. Is there an agreement on this point?

Dr. Pitt: In our early studies where angioplasty was done acutely it was our policy to attack only the infarct-related vessel. As we shift to elective angioplasty as a result of the TAMI trial, it might be possible to consider the use of multivessel angioplasty in selected patients.

Dr. Erbel: We also attack only the infarct-related vessel, but we take into consideration in patients with multivessel disease coronary bypass surgery, because in patients with myocardial infarction, but reopened vessel of the infarct artery, the bypass surgery can be performed at low risk, as several institutions have demonstrated.

Dr. Rapaport: I think Dr. Messmer plans to address the potential role of bypass surgery in that situation in the session this afternoon.

Dr. Schettler: I think your recommendation to do PTCA only with the availability of heart surgery is very important. In our country more and more units are moving to just the opposite position. They are doing PTCA without any possibility to have heart surgery available. And many of these patients cannot be followed up because of well-known reasons – these teams do not belong to, let's say, well-controlled academic clinics. So I think the risk to the patient is extremely high if there is no surgery available. I have in mind to write a review with the essence of your article in the *Deutsches Ärzteblatt,* a journal for each doctor in about 200000 copies. I think it is absolutely necessary to address this point also with respect to cases of malpractice. You may be sure that if this procedure is being done in a unit which is not well equipped, you can expect that more and more accidents will happen, and this is very important not only for the patients but also for the physicians.

My question is: In our country, most of the cardiologists are prescribing dicoumarol after PTCA, and I see that in your country and in the international field more and more aspirin/persantin is being used. I think this is another point that should be discussed, and we should try to come to an international agreement.

Dr. Rapaport: Thank you. I think we have used the rationale of using aspirin versus anticoagulants in the postinfarct patient, based upon the French multicenter study that showed no real difference in subsequent survival when patients were randomized to oral anticoagulants compared to aspirin.

Dr. Lichtlen: I would like to add a few words concerning the West German situation. The Clinical Commission of the German Cardiac Society published in the last issue of its Journal of Cardiology *(Zeitschrift für Kardiologie)* guidelines on PTCA. There was an extensive discussion among cardiologists performing PTCA as to whether there should be the possibility of an immediate surgical bystand in physical proximity. I was a hard-liner and was turned down in the end; but also the surgeons were quite soft on this point, so that now the formulation about surgical bystand is quite vague, implying only "that the interval between irreversible coronary occlusion and operative revascularization should be kept as short as possible. This includes especially the time of transportation and the way to the operating room." (See: Mitteilungen der Deutschen Gesellschaft für Herz- und Kreislaufforschung); Z Kardiol 76, 382–385 (1987).

Dr. Messmer: I am a hard-liner too, but maybe the soft-line position came out because cardiologists have meanwhile learned how to treat acute occlusion by redilatation of thrombosis, and this may have influenced the soft-line of that paper. Personally, I think because of the law you need immediate standby, because if anything happens and you do not have a surgeon nearby, you are bad off.

Dr. Rapaport: Yes, I think that these techniques of going back and attempting to reopen the vessel in the catheterization laboratory or trying to place an intracoronary reperfusion catheter across the obstruction are temporary measures at best. It does not replace the need for surgery. It is just a way of hopefully postponing the patient from seriously crashing in the catheterization laboratory while emergency surgery is being arranged.

Dr. Pitt: I would like to comment on the use of surgical standby for PTCA in patients with acute myocardial infarction. When we first began to do primary angioplasty in patients with acute infarction and attacked the infarct-related vessel, we did this without surgical standby. We reasoned that if we failed to open an occluded vessel, or if we opened it and it reoccluded, the patient would probably not be worse off than if we had left the vessel alone. However, since we switched to the strategy of sequential therapy with intravenous thrombolysis followed by PTCA, we feel that surgical standby is necessary. Most of the patients undergoing initial IV thrombolysis with t-PA will have an open vessel with viable myocardium. If we perform a PTCA and reocclude this vessel, we risk recurrent episodes of ischemia and infarction. Since the patients could be helped by early bypass graft surgery, we believe that surgical standby should be available.

Dr. Schröder: In the paper of the German Cardiac Society it is said that the surgeon must be nearby but not necessarily in the same hospital. I think this is feasible, if there is a standby in another hospital which can be reached with a delay of about 15–20 min.

Another thing I would like to ask you: In your task force paper, it was also mendioned that each case should be discussed in advance with the surgeon. I wonder how realistic this is. I would like to ask the doctors here who perform PTCAs, whether they discuss each single case in advance with the surgeon and look at the film together. We don't do this.

Dr. Rapaport: I can tell you that at our University Hospital this is an important consideration. The surgeon needs to be familiar with the problem to understand whether it is a high-risk case, to reach an understanding with the cardiologist on a potential management plan, should PTCA fail, and other similar problems. This is the reasoning that led the task force to make this recommendation.

Dr. Schettler: At our clinic, Dr. Kübler's unit always uses the same technique to inform the surgeon. But I think it is not enough to have a surgeon available some kilometers away, because if an accident happens, you have to act within minutes and not later. So I would strictly recommend to be a hard-liner in this sense to protect the patient.

Dr. Rapaport: What we mean is that the surgeon is not just somebody whose name is on a standby list, but that the surgeon really knows who is the patient, what is the problem, why are we doing angioplasty, etc. It doesn't mean that the surgeon necessarily has to see the patient personally. It does mean that the problem has been discussed between the person doing the angioplasty and the one who is going to be the responsible surgeon.

Question: To clarify that, is it in the decision making as to whether the patient should undergo PTCA or surgery?

Dr. Rapaport: No. It is not necessarily a decision-making discussion. The decision has already been made to perform angioplasty.

Dr. Messmer: I don't think that it's really necessary to discuss each and every case in advance, because there are some cases where the cardiologist and the cardiosurgeon agree that it's best to do PTCA, but there are several cases which are questionable, whether it's a good lesion or not, the difficulty, and then the surgeon as well as the patient has some risk factors apart from that lesion. These cases have to be discussed, but I don't think that you have to discuss each and every one. You can't do that in a unit where you have three or four PTCAs per day; that's impossible.

Dr. Rapaport: Well I am not sure that I can agree that it is impossible. It just takes a lot of effort. We're not asking the surgeon to see the patient, we're simply asking that the surgeon understand what is going to be done, and to make sure that the surgeon and his team are available. After that, it takes only another minute or so to discuss what the problem is, and that seems eminently reasonable.

Dr. Pitt: I would like to give you our experience at the University of Michigan. I think we are in agreement with Dr. Messmer. After considerable experience we known the situations that are likely in complications. We go over these cases in detail with our surgeons so that if a complication does occur, they will be prepared to operate. Because in our surgical volume we do not have an empty operating room for these patients, but the surgeons chose a short case for this time slot so that they can quickly complete the case and begin bypass graft surgery of the complicated angioplasty if it is indicated. As Dr. Messmer pointed out, we do not find it practical to discuss what we believe to be routine cases with our surgeons. If however, there is a complication with these patients, the surgeons will do their best to get them to the operating room as quickly as possible.

Dr. Rapaport: What we want is to ensure that there is good communication. We are trying to ensure a level of coverage depending upon the kind of issues that you mentioned. If the patient is a 60-year-old man, let's say, who has a single proximal circumflex lesion with good left ventricular function, it is clearly straightforward and takes only a minute to discuss. It is obvious that other cases are far more complicated. In these situations there has to be a more detailed discussion of the case between the surgeon and the invasive cardiologist.

Dr. Sekiguchi: I want to change the topic to restenonis. I noted in Dr. O'Rourke's presentation that there are no determined factors for restenosis. We have had a nation-wide survey in Japan on the autopsy of patients at a short- and long-term period after PTCA, who died incidently or related to PTCA, and found that cases are overwhelmingly those of hyperplasia of the smooth muscles in the restenosed lumen, and I think it may be a problem to suppress the very active smooth muscle proliferation. It might be related to the release from the platelets or some other reasons. It will be necessary to concentrate on how to suppress the smooth muscle activities.

Dr. Rapaport: Dr. Sekiguchi, do you have any therapeutic suggestions?

Dr. Sekiguchi: Well, this is what I don't know yet, but maybe there are some more factors; some drug may suppress the smooth miscle activity.

Dr. Rapaport: Dr. Schettler, what should we do to suppress smooth muscle proliferation?

Dr. Schettler: I think only with aspirin, because there is a sequence from the platelets releasing a growth factor to the smooth muscles. But I think there are some other drugs on the way, e. g., the prostaglandin series, and I think we have to look forward to what will be done in that field. We already have data about peripheral vascular diseases, but not sufficient for the coronary patient. To start with, I would recommend to take aspirin and maybe persantin, but I think aspirin is the first step in that procedure.

Dr. Rapaport: I think aspirin is already almost universally used in this situation, and quite frequently persantin as well; so, I think it will be necessary for something to be given additionally. Whatever we are doing with antiplatelet agents is obviously not enough. Currently, we are observing a clinically evident restenosis rate in the neighborhood of about 25% – 30%. This is a distinct limiting factor in the benefits that are derived from PTCA. Therefore, whatever efforts can be directed to prevent this high restenosis rate by pharmacological means are certainly desired.

Dr. Broustet: I would like to come back to the surgeons problems. Sometimes the surgeons say, "If you dilate, in no case should I operate this patient later, because I think that the best procedure for this patient is surgery first, or because the status of the patient is not proper for surgery. So in any case, I would not like to operate this patient, if you try to dilate first." This happens sometimes with our surgeon and we are in a very difficult situation.

Dr. Messmer: I think you can't do that, because everyone is an adult, the cardiologist and the surgeon. And if the cardiologist feels that the patient is better for PTCA, or that he can do it, then he is very welcome to do so. And if he runs into troubles, I'm welcome to help him out, but I may make a couple of nasty remarks afterwards, that's true.

Dr. Rapaport: There is of course, the situation which we all recognize where PTCA may be performed in a patient who is not a surgical candidate for various reasons. The procedure is done in that case with the understanding of the surgeon, the patient, and the patient's family that should a complication arise during PTCA, the patient will not be taken to the operating room under any circumstance. This is an exception to the general rules that we have been discussing regarding surgical standby.

Dr. Schwarz: Dr. Pitt, can you summarize your experience with emergency bypass surgery in your cases with evolving myocardial infarction? Who had thrombolysis before and then unsuccessful PTCA? How many patients are in this group, and what were the complications after operation?

Dr. Pitt: That is a very good question. I do not have the data with me, but it has been reported from our TAMI experience. We have had relatively little difficulty with patients who have failed thrombolysis or PTCA in whom we have had to send to surgery. The operative mortality and bleeding complications have been quite low.

Dr. Rapaport: I do think, however, that it should be pointed out that in a number of series in the surgical literature reporting on the results of emergency bypass surgery after failed PTCA, that the patient still is at an increased risk compared to elective surgery. Although the overall operative mortality is still generally quite acceptable, if you really have a patient crashing in the catheterization laboratory and requiring cardiopulmonary resuscitation as he is being taken to the operating room, you are dealing with a serious surgical risk problem, with perhaps as much as a 50% operative mortality.

Dr. Pitt: It is certainly an increased risk compared to elective bypass graft surgery, but not as much as one would have anticipated in a patient with acute myocardial infarction.

Dr. Bode: Dr. Messmer and Dr. Pitt, do you feel that using a fibrin-specific thrombolytic agent decreases the bleeding tendency in emergency bypass operations?

Dr. Pitt: As I pointed out, when we used t-PA, which is a relatively clot-specific agent, we had a high incidence of bleeding mainly at the catheter access site. Our incidence of cerebral bleeding with a dose of 150 mg t-PA was about 1.0% – 1.5%, which I believe is similar to the TIMI group's experience. Now that we have reduced the dose of t-PA to 100 mg, we expect to have a lower incidence of cerebral bleeding. Much of the bleeding in patients receiving t-PA in our trials has been related to the use of high-dose heparin and the performance of cardiac catheterization and PTCA. As our experience increases, the incidence of bleeding at the catheter access site is diminishing. This is pointed out in our experience using full doses of both t-PA and urokinase, in which despite the concomitant use of two thrombolytic agents the bleeding risk actually diminished, reflecting our increasing experience and awareness of the necessity for careful angiographic technique.

Dr. Messmer: Well, I don't think that the thrombolysis therapy per se, either streptokinase, urokinase, or t-PA, has a big influence on bleeding, but that what really makes the patient bleed is the aspirin therapy. And this is what we really fear. We don't fear heparin because that is very rapidly convertible; we don't fear streptokinase or t-PA. But aspirin, that's bad, because it takes days until you have its effect stopped.

Dr. Rapaport: I'm interested to hear you say this, because our surgeons have complained to us that the need to take the patient back to the operating room because of postoperative bleeding with bypass surgery is related to our use of aspirin in patients with coronary disease. In fact, we've altered our management of the patient who enters the hospital with unstable angina associated with rest pain and ECG changes, and we start him only on heparin initially and avoid immediate aspirin until we do our catheterization study. If the patient is going immediately to surgery, we don't start the aspirin at that point but send the patient to surgery on heparin alone. However, if the decision is not to operate, then we will at that point start the patient on aspirin just for the very reasons you mentioned.

Dr. Schröder: I'd like to ask something of Dr. Erbel: You mentioned that the reocclusion after PTCA in patients with acute myocardial infarction was 50% or so, in those where the PTT was not in the therapeutic range. The question then is, what about the other patients who had no reocclusion, what was the percentage of patients with PTT not within the therapeutic range? Is it significantly different from those who had reocclusion?

Dr. Erbel: Most of the patients (60%) who had a reocclusion had a thrombin time not in the therapeutic range. We were very much astonished that we had three reocclusions in patients with successful PTCA. In one of these three patients we could document nearly normal thrombin time, in the other one we had no PTT available at the time of reocclusion. In the two, the thrombin time had dropped to normal, and I think that these facts point to the fact that we have to have a good anticoagulation, particularly if you look at the coronary vessel, where you can see the ruptured plaque without neointima formation even 3 weeks after thrombolytic therapy. New thrombus formation can cover this plaque if the anticoagulation is stopped. And particularly if you look through the literature and look at other papers using PTCA and thrombolytic therapy, there are some with very high restenosis or reocclusion rates, and the studies of Yasuno et al. and Papapietro et al. have reported that they use only low-dose heparin or only antiplatelet agents, and that reocclusion rates of 33% and 35% occurred. So I think these factors demonstrate that anticoagulation is very important.

Summary of Session III

E. Rapaport

There are a number of views which have emerged from this conference that appear to enjoy general agreement among us. The first is that the use of thrombolytic agents does produce an improvement in patients who are seen with acute myocardial infarction, and who are treated early. When I use the term "improved," I refer to two basic types of data. The first is mortality data, and the second is data based on analyses of left ventricular performance or measurements of infarct size, other parameters besides mortality.

Mortality data, of course, are the hardest end points, and we tend to place more emphasis on them. The mortality data are almost exclusively based upon intravenous streptokinase trials. Data from the early trials, which date back into the late 1950s, when pooled, appear to show a benefit in terms of mortality. Because these trials were conducted in patients prior to the use of coronary care units and at a time when hospital mortality was extremely high, and in light of the different protocols and differences in how streptokinase was administered, pooling these data is a somewhat suspect from a scientific standpoint. Nevertheless, it does show some benefit. However, the more modern trials have also tended to confirm these observations. We now have data, primarily from the GISSI trial, which show statistically significant decreases in mortality from the use of streptokinase, and dramatically so within the 1st h. The ISIS-2 trial, where there is preliminary data on some 4000 patients, shows a similiar reduction in mortality. There are other supportive mortality data that can be gleaned from the literature. These include the intravenous and intracoronary data from the Dutch Inter-University Group Trial and the Western Washington Intracoronary Trial.

It is clear from these various trials with streptokinase that there are a number of subgroups of acute myocardial infarct patients in whom benefit was not demonstrated. Except for the GISSI study, the number of patients involved in these trials in insufficient for subgroup analysis to be really productive. In the GISSI trial, the benefit was not seen in patients over the age of 65; in fact, there are some data in the literature suggesting that when patients are getting into their 70s, there is an increased risk of stroke with use of thrombolytic agents, and I question the wisdom of using thrombolytic agents in this group of older patients. There is also evidence from the GISSI trial that reinfarction patients are not benefitted, and that the benefit is primarily in the initial infarct patient. Finally, a reduction in mortality was not demonstrated among inferior infarctions, an observation noted also in the Western Washington Intracoronary and Intravenous Trials. The GISSI trial emphasized the importance of early use of thrombolysis. An approximate 50% reduction in mortality was seen when streptokinase was used in the 1st h. This fell to approximately 25% when streptokinase was given at 1 – 3 h and to close to 15% when thrombolytic therapy was initiated at 3 – 6 h. No benefit was observed when streptokinase was begun 6 h or more after the onset of infarction.

These kinds of subgroup sets still need to be more clearly defined, but it would appear that present data support the routine use of thrombolytic agents in acute myocardial infarction when the patient is seen early, when the infarct is anterior, and when there is evidence of an acute transmural type of myocardial infarction, in other words, when ST segment elevation is present. The benefit in non-Q-wave infarction is suspect since the GISSI trial subgroup of patients presenting with ST segment depression were not shown to benefit from a mortality standpoint. The data presented here by Dr. Zaret suggest that this may be a fruitful area of future investigation, but, at the same time, there is at the moment no convincing data that support the use of thrombolytic agents in the non-Q-wave infarction patient.

There are two other additional issues which I would like to address. The first is, which thrombolytic agent should we use? The data which I have enumerated above were generated primarily through clinical trials using streptokinase. However, both the TIMI-1 Trial in North America and the European Cooperative Trial demonstrated that recombinant tissue plasminogen activator (rt-PA) is a superior thrombolytic agent in terms of its ability to produce early recanalization. This does not necessarily translate into the statement that rt-PA will be a more beneficial agent to use in the patient. One must remember there have been no mortality studies with rt-PA to date. There is also a question as to whether there may be an increased rate of early reocclusion in patients who are receiving rt-PA, because of its short half-life.

This has encouraged examination of combination therapies. Should we use initially an intravenous agent that produces a high rate of recanalization, in the neighborhood of perhaps 60% – 70%, as has been demonstrated with rt-PA, and then follow it with another agent that is likely to have more systemic fibrinolytic activity? Would this enhance or synergize the initial effect seen with the use of rt-PA and lessen the likelihood of early reocclusion?

It is clear that there is increasing interest in combining agents such as rt-PA with urokinase or combining prourokinase with urokinase. We are likely to see an increasing number of studies looking at combination thrombolytic therapy in the future.

The second issue I wish to address is to ask whether having obtained initial thrombolysis, should the patient be left without immediate, definitive management of the residual obstruction? It is clear from the data which Dr. Pitt presented relative to Dr. O'Neill's experiments comparing streptokinase and PTCA that the improvement in residual luminal obstruction seen with PTCA following recanalization is translated into better myocardial function, looking at both regional wall motion and the ejection fraction. One is left feeling that he should do something more than simply open the vessel with thrombolytic therapy and hopefully keep it open with antiplatelet and/or antithrombotic agents. There is an increasing tendency to study these patients after thrombolysis with coronary arteriography with a view toward definitive revascularization. If one decides on angioplasty to decrease the degree of residual obstruction, when should it be performed? Dr. Pitt presented data from the TAMI trial that suggest that there was no demonstrable benefit from an immediate PTCA approach compared to several days later. This suggests a strategy of initial use of a thrombolytic agent followed immediately with heparin, and possibly aspirin and dipyridamol, to try to prevent reocclusion. If the patient demonstrates continuing ischemia either clinically by development of postinfarction angina or by laboratory means such as low-level exercise stress test before leaving the hospital, there is no question but that the patient should be catheterized immediately. PTCA or possibly bypass surgery should be done thereafter, if indicated, as soon as possible. More of an enigma is the patient who becomes totally pain-free and runs an uncomplicated hospital course after thrombolytic therapy. Is immediate angiography necessary before he leaves the hospital, followed by PTCA or surgery if obstructive coronary lesions are visualized? This approach as a routine is yet to be established. I think it will take more experience to see whether this approach is cost-effective and desirable.

Session IV
Coronary Bypass Surgery

Chairman: E. Varnauskas

Coronary Artery Bypass Surgery – State of the Art

E. Varnauskas

Development of coronary artery bypass surgery (CABS) started the era of revascularization, an approach which revolutionized the treatment of obstructive coronary artery disease. With CABS it was first demonstrated that it is possible to relieve ischemia by increasing the energy supply to the myocardium. This is a physiologically more attractive approach than the traditional pharmacological suppression of myocardial energy demand. It soon became evident that CABS works – severe angina is dramatically relieved in the majority of patients after operation. However, only the results of clinical trials eventually provided a reasonable explanation for why it works and when it should be applied. The three major prospective randomized trials – Veteran's Administration (VA), European, and Coronary Artery Surgery Study (CASS) – clearly demonstrated both the advantages and the shortcomings of CABS.

Advantages. There is no doubt that quality of life gradually improves over the first 6–12 months after CABS: (a) angina pectoris disappears in 60%–80% of patients and significantly decreases in an additional 10%–20% immediately after operation; (b) the need of antianginal drugs diminishes markedly; and (c) physical performance increases significantly. Long-term survival improves in selected patient groups. The effect of the improvement is directly related to the risk of premature death, i.e., the greatest benefit of CABS is attained in high-risk patients identified by variables predictive of impaired prognosis.

The noninvasive predictors are (a) signs of ischemia and/or old infarction in the resting electrocardiogram (ECG); (b) a markedly positive exercise test; (c) symptoms and signs of left ventricular failure controlled by medical therapy; (d) symptoms and signs of peripheral arterial disease; and (e) older age. The invasive prognostic predictors include (a) left main disease, defined by >50% reduction of lumen diameter; (b) multivessel disease (>50%) with obstruction in the proximal third of the left anterior descending artery (pxLAD) as one of the diseased vessels; (c) possibly single pxLAD disease defined by >75% stenosis; and (d) left ventricular ejection fraction of less than 0.5 but greater than 0.3. The data suggest that the greater the number of noninvasive predictors, the better is the survival effect of surgery; the efficiency of surgery on 5-year survival reaches 80% in high-risk categories.

The improvement of quality of life and survival rate appears to be related to total or partial relief of myocardial ischemia, as demonstrated, although not invariably, by decreased ischemic response to exercise (ECG, thalium) and improved global and/or segmental left ventricular function postoperatively. It should be noted that the real benefit of surgery is probably greater than the above results of the randomized studies would suggest. The surgical and medical treatments in these studies were compared by the "intention to treat" method. As such, potential effect of CABS is probably diluted by those medically assigned patients who successively were operated on as a result of therapy-resistent angina.

Shortcomings. CABS, like any other major surgery, is associated with operative mortality and perioperative complications. Although it improves symptoms, CABS has no detectable survival benefit in low-risk patients. No convincing evidence exists to suggest that CABS protects the myocardium from new nonfatal infarctions. Although the survival is still significantly improved at 12-year follow-up, as suggested by the European Study, long-term benefit of CABS on cardiovascular function, quality of life, and survival gradually decreases with time. Repeat surgery is required in 7%–10% of patients over a 10-year observation period and carries increased risk of lethal complications. Return to work does not seem to improve significantly. However, this is to a large extent dependent on social and economical factors, which vary between countries. Hospitalization after surgery remains a problem, as it is in patients treated medically.

The above shortcomings are partly explained by early graft closure and partly by a gradual progress of atherosclerotic disease affecting both vein grafts and native coronary arteries. Evolving infarctions and/or cardiac failure are possibly responsible for the accelerated late mortality after surgery.

Applicability of the Results of Randomized Studies. Analysis of results by "intention to treat" is the correct method to avoid biased conclusions, although it contains a risk that the potential effect of surgery is diluted by "cross-overs" resulting in a smaller survival difference between the two treatments.

Although derived from studies of patients with stable chronic angina, the above results of CABS regarding pain relief and other variables related to the quality of life generally apply to other types of symptomatic patients as well. In these other groups, the evidence is equivocal as to the applicability of results regarding survival benefit; a possible exception is the group of patients with unstable angina operated on electively. The survival effect of CABS performed in connection with thrombolysis needs further evaluation to confirm the encouraging results of observational studies.

Technical Improvements of CABS. The results of present-day surgery appear to be improved due to more advanced surgical technique, better postoperative care, and more widespread use of antiplatelet agents to prevent graft occlusion. Recent data indicate that internal mammary artery grafts have a better long-term patency rate than the traditional venous grafts used in the three randomized studies. As a consequence of this patency rate improvement, the long-term survival also appears to be improved in patients with internal mammary artery grafts compared with the historical controls with venous grafts. In addition, other arterial grafts are reportedly being considered which signals an exciting new era for CABS.

Coronary Bypass Surgery After Thrombolysis and Balloon Dilatation

B. J. Messmer, R. Uebis, C. Minale, P. Bardos, and S. Effert

Both thrombolysis for acute myocardial infarction and percutaneous transluminal coronary angioplasty (PTCA) for coronary disease have significantly influenced cardiac surgery.

The Role of Coronary Bypass Surgery in PTCA

For PTCA direct access to an in-house cardiac surgery unit is mandatory. Acute ischemia due to dissection and occlusion of the vessel may still occur in some patients even though better tools have lowered the risk [1]. In addition, cardiologists have learned how to reopen iatrogenic occlusion of a coronary artery either by thrombolysis or by redilatation so that surgery can be done on an urgent and not on an emergency basis. Among the first 1000 PTCAs performed at the University Hospital in Aachen, complications requiring surgery occurred at a rate of 2.5%.

As a result of the steady increase of PTCA, coronary bypass surgery did not decrease at all, but surgical patients changed, especially with respect to the extent of the disease. Surgery for single- and double-vessel disease has markedly diminished while triple-vessel operations continue. In parallel, the average number of bypass grafts per patient has by now increased to four, which means that the surgeon's business is getting harder and harder. The few patients still referred for single bypass operation either have restenosis after PTCA or have had PTCA that has failed or for them PTCA was not advised due to morphologic reasons.

Thrombolysis and Coronary Bypass Surgery in Acute Myocardial Infarct

Acute myocardial infarction has been true challenge for the cardiac surgeon ever since direct coronary bypass surgery was introduced 20 years ago. Immediate revascularization has been tried with variable success [2, 3, 4]. Yet, worldwide only two centers in the United States, in Spokane and Des Moines, have practiced this method to a significant extent. Early and long-term results in the Spokane series published by Berg et al. [5] and De Wood et al. [6] are excellent, but some reservations in regard to the infarct diagnosis early in this series and to the analysis of the results must be made, and the question has been raised as to whether the patients survived because or in spite of immediate surgery [7].

The primary reason why cardiac surgeons did not succeed with primary surgery is certainly the time span necessary to move the surgical apparatus – but also the reservations of many cardiologists who considered treatment of acute myocardial infarction their privilege. In addition, the high costs for a standby surgical team around the clock must also be considered. The recognition that myocardial infarction in the vast majority of patients ultimately results from thrombotic occlusion of a predamaged coronary artery and the clinical introduction of thrombolysis changed the whole scenario [8, 9]. The surgeon's role became secondary, and primary surgery on an emergency basis is hardly ever performed today.

The greatest disadvantage of thrombolysis consists of the high rate of reocclusion which in spite of medical preventions often occurs within a few days after initial success. Recognition of this problem prompted us in 1979 and 1980, respectively, to add PTCA and bypass surgery early after successful thrombolysis [10, 11].

Early and Late Clinical Results After Intracoronary Thrombolysis and Early Bypass Surgery. Since 1980 we have treated 70 patients who after successful intracoronary thrombolysis with streptokinase underwent early aortocoronary bypass operation. The primary requirement for early surgery was documented occlusion of the infarct vessel and reperfusion within 4 h after onset of acute clinical symptoms in patients otherwise suitable for coronary bypass operation. In these patients operation was performed under routine conditions without any special precautions. Timing of surgery depended largely upon the regular operative schedule, but operation was done whenever possible within 10 days and only occasionally thereafter.

One patient (1.4%) died at surgery from intractable heart failure. Significant postoperative heart failure was present in five patients; two of these needed

Table 1. Relation between time of surgery and early complication

Time of surgery (days after lysis)	Patients	Early death	Complications	
			CHF	Bleeding
0–1	11	0	3 (27.0%)	1 (9%)
≥2	59	1	2 (3.5%)	2 (3.5%)
Total	70	1 (1.4%)	5 (7.[illegible]%)	3 (4.3%)

CHF, Congestive heart failure.

support with an intra-aortic balloon pump. This complication was significantly higher in patients who underwent surgery very early after thrombolysis. Whether this was due to reperfusion injury or simply to the heart not having enough time to recover from the initial ischemic damage remains open. Bleeding, however, occurred at the same rate whether surgery was performed within the first 24 h or only later (Table 1).

When compared to other forms of postthrombolytic management, hospital mortality was lowest in patients who underwent early bypass surgery (1.4%). Combination with early PTCA resulted in a mortality rate of 3.1% while follow-up treatment by medical means yielded a rate of 7.8%, which nevertheless is better than the 14.0% in patients with failed reperfusion.

Until now, six late deaths (8.6%) have occurred, but only two of these were of cardiac origin. One of these patients died after 2 months from reinfarction due to graft occlusion to the infarct vessel while the other died after 5 years due to progressive coronary artery disease and reinfarction. Two patients died of cancer and one each of cerebrovascular accident and a car accident. Nonfatal reinfarction was recorded in two patients (2.9%), and among 43 recatheterized patients with a total of 120 bypass grafts, graft occlusion was documented in 15% without any difference between grafts to the infarct vessel and grafts to other areas. Follow-up now extends to 8 years. Actuarial survival is 87% (Fig. 1). The oldest patient of the group has passed his 80s. He has no problem with his heart but may have bronchogenic carcinoma, as tumor cells have been found in a recent sputum cytology although no gross tumor is seen on chest X-ray or computed tomograms.

Ischemic Time Interval of Myocardial Damage and Late LV Function. In order to validate our procedure not only by survival but, more importantly, by late myocardial performance, it is important to know what influence length of ischemia has on myocardial damage and late left ventricular function in patients of this selected subgroup.

In isolated cases we have seen that left ventricular function may recover completely (Fig. 2). The ischemic time intervals ranged from a minimum of 50 min to a maximum of 430 min in a very early patient, who did not profit, however, since he developed a left ventricular aneurysm. The limit of 4 h was exceeded in seven patients, some early in the series and some because of severe persistent pain in spite of reperfusion. The average ischemic time was 3 h (Table 2).

In all, 43 patients had control angiography, at an average postoperative interval of 11 months. Analysis of the results is presented in Table 3. Wall motion at the site of the formerly ischemic area was classified as either normal, + or minimal hypokinesia (which in most instances could only be seen if the site of the area was known by the reviewer), + + or moderate hypokinesia, + + + or severe hypokinesia and akinesia, and aneurysm formation. Furthermore, patients were divided into those who had an ischemic time interval of less than or of more than the average of 3 h. Patients with an ischemia of lesss than 3 h had a

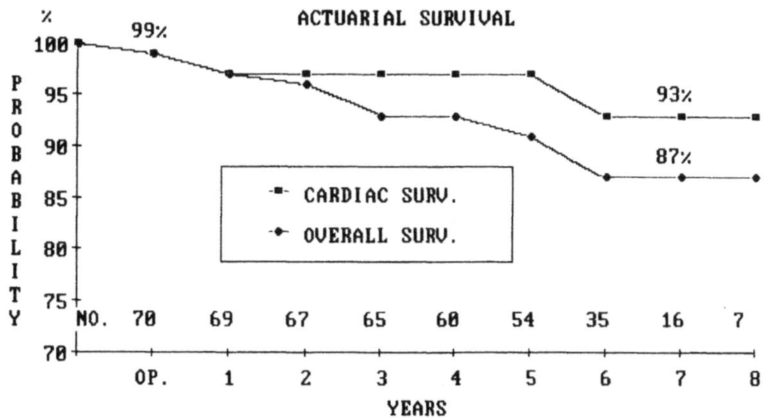

Fig. 1. Overall actuarial survival to 8 years in 70 patients who underwent early bypass surgery after successful intracoronary thrombosis

higher portion of normal left ventricular function or only minimal hypokinesia. Left ventricular aneurysms were not found in this group. On the other hand, moderate and severe hypokinesia and left ventricular aneurysms prevailed after 3 h of ischemia, but much to our surprise minimal damage or normal left ventricular function was still possible even after prolonged ischemia. It should be our aim to recognize this special group of patients at the time of acute hospitalization in order to offer these patients optimal treatment and to prevent possible reocclusion.

In 24 patients transmural needle biopsies from the ischemic and reperfused area were taken at the time of operation. In careful electron-microscopic studies the percentage of myocardial necrosis and, if present, the portion of hemorrhagic necrosis within the specimen was evaluated and correlated to clinical parameters. There was no correlation between ischemic time interval and the extent of necrosis (Fig. 3). This was of some surprise but can be explained by the fact that (a) needle biopsy offers only a punctiform picture and (b) time is only one of several contributing factors. Besides, this finding is supported by the angiographic results of late left ventricular function, which also did not strictly correlate with the ischemic time interval (Table 3).

Likewise no correlation could be found between ischemic time interval and enzyme fallout, neither with regard to the maximum peak ($r = 0.27$) nor to the total enzyme activity ($r = 0.36$), which was calculated according to the method of Shell et al. [12]. A clear correlation was found, however, between levels of creatine kinase (CK) and the amount of necrosis in the biopsies (Fig. 4).

Much has been speculated about the influence of streptokinase or of reperfusion in general on development of hemorrhagic infarction. In 8 of the 24 patients who had biopsies suspicion of a hemarrhagic infarct was expressed by the surgeon at the time of operation because of epicardial purpura. This was confirmed histologically in all patients, but in the remaining 16 patients without

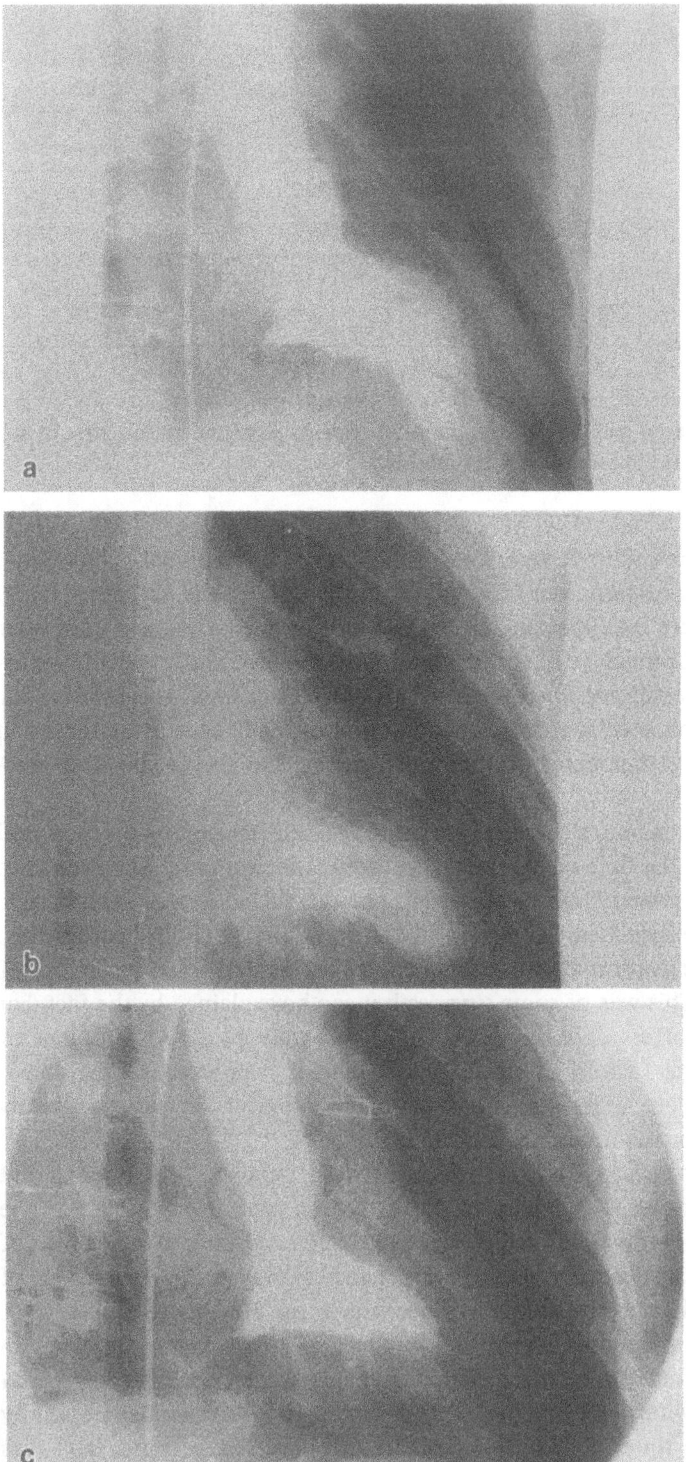

Table 2. Ischemic time interval

Time interval (min)	Patients (*n*)	(%)
<60	2	3
60–119	10	14
120–179	23	33
180–240	28	40
>240	7	10
179 ± 63	70	

Table 3. Ischemic interval and late postoperative LV-function

Ischemic interval	LV-function				
	Normal	Hypokinesia			Aneurysm
		+	+ +	+ + +	
<180 min	9	4	5	1	
>180 min	5	6	2	7	4
Total	14	10	7	8	4
	56%			44%	

$n = 43$; 11 months postoperatively.

◂ **Fig. 2a–c.** Angiographic view of left ventricular endsystolic contraction in a 52-year-old man with acute LAD occlusion before (**a**) and immediately after (**b**) intracoronary thrombolysis and 6 months after early bypass surgery (**c**)

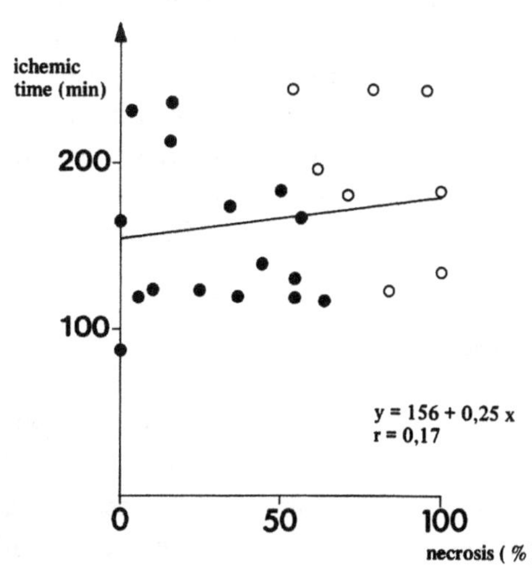

Fig. 3. Relationship between ischemic time interval and percentage of myocardial necrosis in 24 patients with intraoperative biopsy

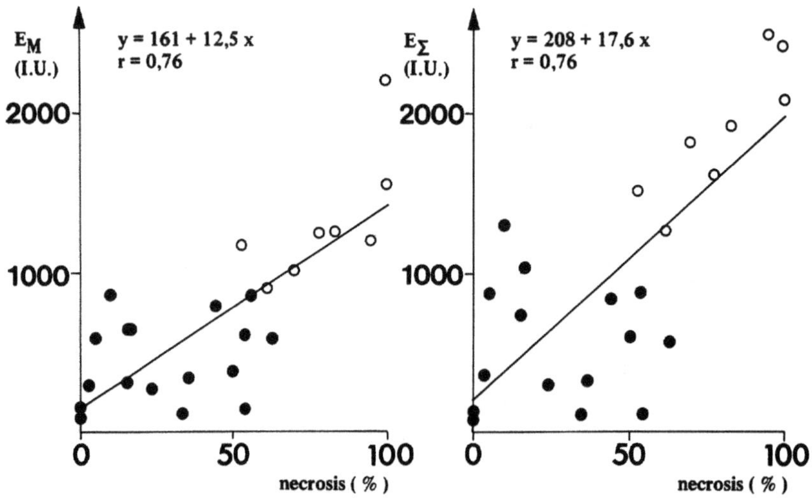

Fig. 4. Relationship between enzyme activity and percentage of myocardial necrosis in 24 patients with intraoperative biopsy

clinical suspicion hemorrhagic necrosis could be detected in 7 although in much smaller portion. Altogether, 15 out of the 24 patients presented hemorrhagic necrosis, ranging from 5% to 100% of the total necrotic area.

The extent of hemorrhagic necrosis, however, did not correlate with the total dose of streptokinase administered nor did it correlate with the ischemic time interval. But a correlation was found between the extent of hemorrhagic infarct and the enzyme levels (Fig. 5).

In 15 of the total of 70 patients we have obtained angiographic results on late left ventricular function as well as histopathologic evaluation of intraoperative biopsy. Comparison of myocardial damage expressed as the percentage of necrosis at the time of operation with late left ventricular function of the corresponding area reveals a correlation of 0.69. This rather modest correlation discloses some of the difficulties with intraoperative biopsis. By inspection and by knowing the infarct vessel and its supply area, the surgeon can take the biopsy more or less from the center of the formerly ischemic area. Yet, every needle biopsy, even with true transmural cylinders, remains limited to the puncture site and may therefore not be fully representative for the whole area.

Conclusion

Aortocoronary bypass surgery after PTCA is nowadays restricted in the vast majority of cases to the rather high number of patients with restenosis. A small minority of patients (in our hospital between 2% and 3%) need urgent, but seldom emergency, surgery because of critical damage to the vessel. Nevertheless,

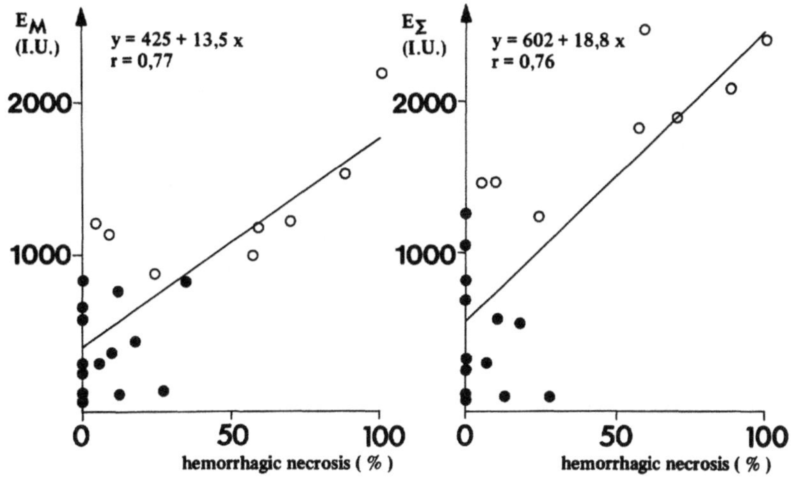

Fig. 5. Relationship between enzyme activity and percentage of hemorrhagic necrosis in 24 patients with intraoperative biopsy

knowledge about the potential risks of PTCA makes surgical standby indispensable, especially in view of legal considerations.

Aortocoronary bypass surgery after successful thrombolysis for acute myocardial infarction can be performed at a low risk, and it can provide excellent long-term results. Because of the relatively high incidence of reocclusion, operation should be performed early, regardless of whether the thrombolytic agent has been given intravenously or by direct application into the occluded coronary artery. Since the ischemic time interval, extent of myocardial necrosis, and late left ventricular function have shown no or only weak correlation in these patients with preexisting coronary artery disease, it is necessary to find reliable selection criteria to identify those patients who would profit optimally from the combined medical and surgical therapy. In this regard, the peak enzyme level and the calculated total enzyme activity may be more predictive than initially anticipated, while modern radionuclide studies may resolve the problem.

References

1. Bredlac CE, Roubin GS, Leimgruber PP, Douglas JS, King SB, Gruentzig AR (1985) In-hospital morbidity and mortality in patients undergoing elective coronary angioplasty. Circulation 72[5]:1044 – 1052
2. Favoloro RG, Effler DB, Cheanvechau C, Quint RA, Sones FM (1987) Acute coronary insufficiency (impending myocardial infarction and myocardial infarction). Surgical treatment by the saphenous vein graft technique. Am J Cardiol 28:598
3. Bolooki H, Kotler MD, Lottenberg L, Desnick S, Andrews RC, Kipnis S, Ellis RM (1975) Myocardial revascularization after acute infarction. Am J Cardiol 36:395

4. Dawson JT, Hall RJ, Hallmann GL, Cooley DA (1975) Mortality in patients undergoing coronary artery bypass surgery after myocardial infarction. Am J Cardiol 33:483
5. Berg R Jr, Selinger SL, Leonhard JJ (1981) Immediate coronary artery bypass for acute evolving myocardial infarct. J Thorac. Cardiovasc Surg 81:493
6. DeWood MA, Spores CR, Berg R, Kendall RW, Grunwald RP, Selinger SL, Hensley GR, Sutherland KI, Sheilds JP (1983) Acute myocardial infarction: a decade of experience with surgical reperfusion in 701 patients. Circulation 68[Suppl II]:8
7. Spencer FC (1983) Emergency coronary bypass for acute infarction: an unproved clinical experiment. Circulation 68[Suppl II]:17
8. Rentrop P, Blanke H, Köstering K, Karsch KR (1979) Acute myocardial infarction: intracoronary application of nitroglycerin and streptokinase in combination with transluminal recanalization. Clin Cardiol 5:354
9. Merx W, Dörr R, Rentrop P, Blanke H, Karsch KR, Mathey DG, Kremer P, Kutsch W, Schmutzler H (1981) Evaluation of the effectiveness of intracoronary streptokinase infussion in acute myocardial infarction: postprocedure management and hospital course in 204 patients. Am Heart J 102:1181
10. Meyer J, Merx W, Schmitz H, Erbel T, Kiesslich R, Dörr R, Lambertz H, Bethge C, Krebs W, Bardos P, Minale C, Messmer BJ, Effert S (1982) Percutaneous transluminal coronary angioplasty immediate after intracoronary streptolysis of transmural myocardial infarction. Circulation 66:905
11. Messmer BJ, Merx W, Meyer J, Bardos P, Minale C, Effert S (1983) New developments in medical-surgical treatment of acute myocardial infarction. Ann Thorac Surg 35:70
12. Shell WE, Kjekshus JK, Sobel BE (1971) Quantitative assessment of the extent of myocardial infarction in the conscious dog by means of analysis of serial changes in serum creatinine phosphate activity. J Clin Invest 50:2614 – 2623

Discussion: Session IV – Coronary Bypass Surgery

Chairman: E. Varnauskas

Dr. Pitt: In the light of Dr. Varnauskas' results, which are most impressive, has he now changed selection of patients for bypass graft surgery? Would you now not take a patient with hypertension for bypass graft surgery?

Dr. Varnauskas: I would like to have these results confirmed in a larger population before making a firm statement regarding surgery in mildly symptomatic patients who have pronounced myocardial hypertrophy. However, it should be emphasized that a treatment of hypertension leading to a reduction of hypertrophy and improvement of coronary reserve appears to be as important as coronary bypass surgery.

Dr. Pitt: Since it is unlikely that there will be any further large scale trials of bypass graft surgery in the near future do you think it might be possible to confirm your observations in regard to hypertension in the CASS study?

Dr. Varnauskas: I don't know. I think that the VA, CASS, and European studies should be analyzed jointly with regard to hypertension and other risk factors.

Dr. Boskis: When you talk about the predictors of the outcome of surgery, you talk about age, stress testing, and hypertension. What about ejection fraction? What is your procedure for risk estimation from ejection fraction?

Dr. Varnauskas: In the last slide I included an ejection fraction of less than 0.50 as a risk factor, simply because the VA study and CASS have demonstrated survival benefit with surgery in these patients. The European study cannot evaluate the risk of reduced left ventricular function because we did not include such patients. This is why I think that the three studies are complementary to each other; they include different populations.

Dr. Messmer: I have a question on your last slide, where you show the internal mammary artery to be so much superior. I would like to be a little bit cautious; one has to know that this patient population where double IMA is possible is generally absolutely different from patients in whom one does four or five vein grafts, because those have generally severe and distal disease, where IMA can't be used. So the internal mammary artery population in general, according to what I have found during the past years, is really different and almost uncomparable.

Dr. Varnauskas: Our experience with internal mammary grafts is limited.

Dr. Messmer: Just one word, because of the right side: a preselection point for stenosis is the bifurcation between the left posterior branch and the intraventricular branch. That's the preselection area. And with the internal mammary artery, the right one, you rarely reach that point; so you generally take for the right internal mammary anastomosis patients who have a stenosis of the proximal part of the right coronary artery, and the rest of the artery is o. k. And that's an absolutely different population.

Dr. Varnauskas: I think you're right. However, our data suggest that the prognostically most important stenosis in multivessel disease is that located in the LAD. And that vessel is frequently very suitable for mammary artery implant.

Question: Did you perform an exercise rest after surgery in the patients of the European study, and was it predictive for the future of the patients after surgery?

Dr. Varnauskas: Yes, we did perform exercise test after surgery. The results have been published, and I have no new data to show you today. The published results demonstrated an improvement in exercise performance and survival.

Question: Did you discuss the late outcome for unstable angina?

Dr. Varnauskas: No, I did not. However, I think that if coronary bypass is done electively in these patients, the present results would probably apply.

Dr. Gotsman: I'd like to ask you a question about quality of life. I think all the studies refer mainly to mortality. And if one thinks of the pathology of the coronary artery graft, we know that after about 10 years the veins occlude. And at this late stage, patients tend to return to a very bad state. But in this interval period, the majority of patients are really very well. And one thing that has concerned us with the three major studies, has been the fact that it really excludes the individual patient who does very well. Many of the patients, for example, with single-vessel disease, who in fact have done very well with coronary artery surgery symptomatically, have shown no change in long-term mortality. For example, a person with a single isolated total LAD obstruction, who today walks around with angina pectoris, in fact had responded for 10 years very well symptomatically to a coronary artery graft. We really look at the question of quality of life.

Dr. Varnauskas: I don't know how to measure the quality of life, and, thus, how to respond to your question. What we have measured (relief of angina, improvement of physical capacity etc.) we have reported. I don't know how well these results relate to your question.

Dr. Gotsman: Let me give you an example. A patient with a total occlusion, the LAD open until the infarct with a good collateral vessel, is usually unsuitable for PTCA. And this kind of patient does very well with a graft. Now, if the graft later closes, say after 10 years, we have in fact given that patient probably 10 years of symptom-free life. My question is not just an example, but the question really is the quality of life; this is the thing that's concerned.

Dr. Schröder: I have two questions to Dr. Messmer. The first one is related to the discussion before lunch. You told us that in 1000 consecutive patients with PTCA, 25 had acute bypass surgery, and that there were 20 urgent and 5 emergency cases. I think this is very interesting. Urgent means within some hours, is that correct? How many patients of the urgent and of the emergency group had myocardial infarction? Do you know that?

Dr. Messmer: No, I can only say that of five patients who were true emergencies, three died. And of the rest of the urgent group, only two died. That is a big difference, and I think that the most important thing is really that the cardiologist can decide very fast whether he is able to reopen the vessel or, what is more important, that he cannot, and does not fiddle around for another hour until it is too late. In most instances nowadays, at least in our experience, it is possible to get at least a marginal flow that can prevent a major infarct.

Dr. Schröder: My second question concerns your very good results after successful thrombolysis and then surgery. I wonder whether this is a selective group, and my question is whether you can find a twin to each patient, in other words, a retrospective case control study. I think with 1000 patients it's probably possible to have more or less a twin to each of them and to look at whether surgery is really superior in patients with the same situation.

Dr. Messmer: It is really a very selective group. Among the first five or six patients, we were not quite sure how long the ischemic time interval should be. And in the beginning we took the 6-h landmark, because we took 6 h for the legs or for the brain, so we thought this would be the same for the myocardium. But then we found out very fast that in ischemic time intervals of less and more than 3 h there was a lot of difference in mortality. So we cut down to 4 h. And, in addition, the patient must be suitable for coronary bypass surgery. So it's probably very difficult to do a randomization and find really similar patients, where you can use one for conservative treatment and the other one for surgical treatment.

Dr. Walter: I would like to congratulate you on the data you have just presented and will take the opportunity to give you some details of the patients we have operated in the last 3 years. Out of a total of 1800 patients we have operated 62 patients between the first 30 min and 3 h of the beginning of symptoms. There was a hospital mortality of 5%. In cooperation with our cardiologists, we are now operating on some patients with evolving myocardial infarction and triple-vessel disease without prior attempts at PTCA or lysis.

Question: Isn't it true that there has been a good deal of surgical experience with primary bypass operation in myocardial infarction – a group in Spokane, Washington, and associates in Iowa, and I think there have been other groups. Isn't that being done actually?

Dr. Walter: These studies were on patients in whom the operation was done much later; after 5 h, 6 h, even days, not in the first 3 h. I think that 6 h is too late. Flameng and his colleagues have recently been using MUGA scans and Thallium 201 scintigraphy and have demonstrated myocardial salvage only in patients revascularized within 4 h – and not if operation was performed later than this.

Dr. Messmer: But I was very much for primary surgery when I was in Zurich, and we were fighting with our cardiologists because they would never give us the patients; but, then, we were considering the time we really need. The patient gets his myocardial infarction at home or at work. So he first has to go to the hospital, and then he has to be studied, because the surgeon cannot operate without the study. Now, I would like to see the surgeon who tells me that he can operate within 30 min – 30 min after what? After acute symptoms? That will never possible.

Question: Having two obviously excellent cardiac surgeons here, perhaps you can also address the question as it relates to the nonthrombolytically treated acute myocardial infarction patient, who develops postinfarction angina at days 2–4. My question is originally because of the early data from Dr. Cooleys' group and others that suggested that if you operated within the first 2 weeks, you had an increased mortality from myocardial infarction, and that you should therefore try to wait 3–4 weeks. My question is: Does your experience now in terms of having treated these early infarctions postthrombolytically made you feel that with the improved techniques patients who develop early postinfarction angina should be managed early, with surgical intervention within the first few days, or should they be tried to be dragged out with medical management for 2–4 weeks before surgery is done?

Dr. Messmer: If a patient has true severe postinfarction angina, which means that he is still at risk, and he still has jeopardized myocardium – i.e., if the anatomy is clear – this is for me a clear indication to go ahead with surgery and not to wait until he has a complete transmural infarct. But there are other patients who have something like an ongoing, slowly evolving infarct. If you can keep them medically, that is, if it goes on for longer than 1 week, it is my experience that the worst time to operate is between 1 and 3 weeks. So either you go really early, or, if you cannot decide at that time, then it's better to wait for 5–6 weeks.

Session V
Rehabilitative Care After Myocardial Revascularization

Chairman: N.K. Wenger

Section V

Intensive Care After Myocardial Revascularization

Long-Term Care and Surveillance of the Patient Following Coronary Angioplasty or Coronary Bypass Surgery

N.K. Wenger

Although coronary angioplasty and coronary bypass surgery can dramatically improve the prognosis, morbidity, and symptomatic status of many patients with atherosclerotic coronary heart disease, neither of these procedures cures the underlying atherosclerosis or significantly alters its progression. Progression of coronary atherosclerosis has been described in 50% of the native arteries within the first decade after coronary bypass surgery; artherosclerosis appears accelerated in saphenous vein grafts. Only limited data are available regarding post-angioplasty atherosclerotic changes, but disease progression in the native circulation is not anticipated to differ. Thus, the long-term care and surveillance of patients following successful coronary angioplasty or coronary bypass surgery should include (a) identification of those individuals at increased risk of recurrent coronary events due to restenosis or closure of the procedure-related arteries or graft vessels or to progression of atherosclerosis in the native circulation, followed by appropriate interventions; (b) modification of conventional coronary risk factors in an attempt to limit progression or induce regression of the obstructive coronary atherosclerotic lesions; (c) restoration and maintenance of residual cardiovascular function; and (d) encouragement of resumption of an active, productive, and satisfying life-style, including return to work when appropriate.

It is estimated that about 175000 coronary angioplasties and an equal number of coronary bypass surgical procedures will be performed in the United States in 1987. Most of these patients will return to the care of their primary physicians, who must be familiar with both the short- and long-term aspects of management, including efforts to prevent progression of the underlying coronary atherosclerosis.

Identification of Patients at Increased Risk of Recurrent Coronary Events

Following Coronary Angioplasty. Restenosis occurs in about 20% – 25% of all patients following successful PTCA, typically within 6 months of the procedure. It remains unclear why restenosis occurs in some patients and not in others, i.e., there are no obvious characteristics that render a patient more prone to restenosis. Typically, the symptoms of restenosis are similar to those that occasioned the angioplasty procedure, most commonly chest pain precipitated by activity; at times, there is sudden onset of chest pain. Patients must be cautioned to report any recurrence of their preangioplasty symptoms; exercise testing, in addition to being performed immediately subsequent to the angioplasty, is characteristically repeated at about 6 months; some centers prefer exercise testing using thallium scintigraphy. Subsequent serial exercise testing at about yearly intervals is recommended to ascertain whether ischemia has recurred, with the testing interval dependent on the extent of atherosclerosis in the non-procedure-related vessels and the adequacy of the angioplasty.

As is the case for patients with other manifestations of atherosclerotic coronary heart disease – angina or myocardial infarction – the characteristics of the ischemic abnormalities at exercise testing determine whether medical management is warranted, or whether coronary arteriography is indicated to identify the need for additional mechanical revascularization. These characteristies include: the time of onset, the duration, and the severity of ischemic ECG changes; the extent of myocardium at potential jeopardy, as documented by thallium scintigraphy; and symptomatic and hemodynamic concomitants of these ischemic abnormalities, e.g., inappropriate heart rate or blood pressure response, angina, arrhythmia at low levels of exercise.

To prevent restenosis at the site of angioplasty, most patients are currently instructed to take daily aspirin and dipyridamole (persantin) at least for the initial 4–6 months. The documentation of efficacy of either antiplatelet and/or anticoagulant therapy remains controversial, and dosage regimens and durations of these adjunct drug therapies vary widely. Additionally, vasodilator drugs such as nitrate or calcium channel blocking preparations are sometimes prescribed for the initial 3–6 months in an attempt to limit the vasospasm that has been postulated as an etiology for restenosis.

It also remains uncertain whether the newer balloon angioplasty techniques, with or without atherectomy catheters, or laser angioplasty techniques will alter the risk of restenosis or influence the need for antiplatelet or anticoagulant therapy.

Following Coronary Bypass Surgery. Recurrence of ischemic symptoms after coronary bypass surgery may be related either to graft closure or to progression of coronary atherosclerosis in the native circulation. Again, the recurrence of symptoms should be investigated, as in patients with angina or those following myocardial infarction; serial exercise testing, with or without thallium scintigraphy, can identify earlier the less symptomatic or the asymptomatic progression of the underlying disease.

In the United States Coronary Artery Surgery Study (CASS) [6, 7], although about two-thirds of patients were asymptomatic at 1 year following their surgery, only about one-half were pain-free at 5 years. A high percentage of these patients had progressive atherosclerosis of the saphenous vein grafts, with the most pronounced graft attrition occurring between 6 and 11 years following surgery. Progressive graft atherosclerosis is far less prominent in internal mammary artery conduits. The management of patients with recurrent ischemic symptoms or with ischemic exercise test abnormalities is as described above for patients following coronary angioplasty.

Additional Assessment of Risk Status and Appropriate Interventions. Since evidence of ventricular dysfunction and the presence of potentially life-threatening ventricular arrhythmias also constitute components of risk, in addition to the patient's ischemic status, evaluation of these two problems is also appropriate. Ventricular function can be examined noninvasively by rest and exercise radionuclide studies, as well as with exercise echocardiography. The roles of positron emission tomography (PET) and magnetic resonance imaging (MRI) have not yet been defined. The status of ventricular function following coronary angioplasty or coronary bypass surgery is typically dependent on the occurrence of prior or procedure-related myocardial infarction, as well as a history of significant systemic arterial hypertension. The adequacy of ventricular function at the initial assessment can further define the appropriate intervals for serial test surveillance. Similarly, potentially life-threatening ventricular arrhythmias seem more ominous in patients with serious ventricular dysfunction and/or recurrent ischemia; particularly for patients with arrhythmia in these selected subgroups, evaluation by ambulatory electrocardiography is appropriate to determine the need for therapy.

As noted above, the pharmacologic prevention of postangioplasty restenosis may involve use of one or more of the cyclooxygenase inhibitors, aspirin or sulfinpyrazone; or the phosphodiesterase inhibitor, dipyridamole; the role of the thromboxane A_2 synthetase inhibitors remains uncertain. In patients with prior myocardial infarction, particulary those who have had incomplete revascularization, consideration should be given to the institution or continuation of β-adrenergic blocking drugs; to date, these are the only pharmacologic compounds that have been shown, in randomized trials, to improve postinfarction survival. However, these studies are inadequate to evaluate benefit in patients with subsequent myocardial revascularization. The potential adverse effects of β-blockade in raising blood lipid levels must be considered in regard to progression of atherosclerosis. The potential role of calcium blocking drugs in preventing restenosis is under investigation; the documentation that diltiazem can prevent recurrent nonfatal infarction in patients with recent non-Q-wave infarction suggests a possible long-term benefit; again, no studies have been reported in this patient subgroup following myocardial revascularization. Further, preliminary data, based on animal studies, suggest that calcium blocking drugs may limit the progression of atherosclerosis. No difference in the occurrence of potentially lethal ventricular arrhythmias has been evident, following either coronary angioplasty or coronary bypass surgery, unless these arrhythmias were precipitated by episodic ischemia. Further investigation is needed to determine the role of prophylactic or therapeutic long-term antiarrhythmic preparations, particularly for patients with incomplete myocardial revascularization.

Modification of Conventional Coronary Risk Factors

Only 60% of saphenous vein grafts remain patent at 10–12 years following coronary bypass surgery, and 45% of the patent grafts have some degree of atherosclerosis (70% of these have at least one-half of the lumen obstructed).

Unfortunately, the performance of coronary bypass surgery or coronary angioplasty does not seem to provide impetus for coronary risk reduction, either as implemented by the patient or as recommended by the treating physician(s). For example, in CASS [6, 7], the preoperative incidences of cigarette smoking, hypercholesterolemia, and obesity were 39%, 32%, and 21%, respectively. Postoperatively, 32% of patients continued cigarette smoking at 1 year, and this percentage persisted to 5 years. The percentage of hypercholesterolemic patients was increased at 5 years, to 40%, as was the percentage of patients with obesity, to 25%.

Modification of conventional coronary risk factors appears appropriate both to limit the progression of atherosclerosis and potentially to induce regression of the atherosclerotic lesions. Several reports identify powerful correlations between persistent systemic arterial hypertension, cigarette smoking, hyperglycemia, and physical inactivity, and the occurrence of saphenous vein graft and coronary arterial atherosclerotic progression. Although an adverse impact of elevated blood lipid levels has not consistently been demonstrated on progression of vein graft occlusion, recent data suggest that significant lowering of serum cholesterol levels can favorably affect saphenous vein graft patency in patients with moderate to severe hypercholesterolemia. The United States Lipid Research Clinics Program and the Blankenhorn et al. colestipol-niacin study [2] recently provided convincing documentation that decreasing serum cholesterol levels in hypercholesterolemic individuals can favorably alter the progression of atherosclerosis in coronary bypass graft vessels. There are no longitudinal studies that describe the relationship of coronary risk factors to coronary angioplasty restenosis; this appears more a thrombotic than an atherosclerosis-related occurrence. Nevertheless, in individuals with documented accelerated atherosclerosis of a severity to warrant coronary angioplasty, limitation of the progression of atherosclerosis in the native circulation appears warranted.

The United States Concensus Conference recommended the institution of broad-based coronary risk reduction, although none of the individual components, to date, has been documented to limit morbidity and mortality. This was because risk reduction, with no evidence of resulting harm, was a rational approach to management and entailed limited expense and inconvenience. The risk modifications recommended include the discontinuation of cigarette smoking and control of elevated serum lipid levels, initially with dietary measures and subsequently with pharmacotherapy. Drugs currently advised include the bile acid sequestrants, nicotinic acid (niacin), fibric acid derivatives, probucol, and the HMG-CoA reductase inhibitors. Control of arterial hypertension is recommended, initially with life-style alterations, including dietary sodium restriction, limitation of excessive alcohol intake, weight reduction if appropriate, and the institution of a regular exercise regimen; these should be followed by pharmacotherapy as needed. Weight control or weight reduction and modest physical activity are additionally recommended to reduce coronary risk status.

The educational approaches to coronary risk reduction include the initial provision of appropriate information, supplemented by persuasion and motivation to adopt healthy behaviors. Training is needed in the skills required to implement these favorable behaviors, and reinforcement of adherence should be provided both by social support and by environmental modification.

Restoration and Maintenance of Residual Cardiovascular Function

In the European Coronary Surgery Study [10], although the patients' exercise capacity improved as a result of surgical intervention, further increase in exercise capacity was achieved by exercise training. The restoration and maintenance of functional capacity can be provided by the usual exercise training regimens for coronary patients, based on specific exercise prescription. The need for supervision varies with the risk status of the patient, but most patients following successful coronary angioplasty or coronary bypass surgery can probably be encouraged to exercise independently on a long-term basis. Control of hypertension, as well as weight reduction, may further improve physical work capacity.

Resumption of an Active Lifestyle, Including Return to Work

Unfortunately, symptomatic improvement and improvement in physiologic functional capacity correlates poorly with improvement in psychosocial status, with return to remunerative employment, or with resumption of the preillness life-style.

In CASS [6, 7], there was no postoperative improvement in employment; other studies describe a 20% – 80% decrease in the employment of previously working patients following coronary bypass surgery. Individuals at high risk for failure to return to work can be characterized by their duration of preoperative unemployment, with unemployment over 6 months rendering less likely the return to work. Older patients and those with increased physical requirements of the job are also less likely to return to work; but commonly the nonmedical features of family, employer, community, and governmental attitudes and policies shape the pattern of unemployment. The advice given by the primary physician also seems importantly to influence the return to work.

In the NHLBI Angioplasty Registry, 84% of patients returned to work. The interval was far shorter than that after coronary bypass surgery, typically 7 versus 73 days. In CASS [6, 7], only 51% of individuals returned to their prior house activity levels.

Therefore, additional components of rehabilitative care include facilitation of resumption of a normal life-style. Exercise training has been described as a valuable intervention to aid patients in renouncing the sick role and in encouraging their return to work; it has also been shown to improve psychosocial status. Counseling should address the resumption of sexual activity and return to prior family and social roles. Important additional components include education and counseling concerning return to leisure and recreational activities. The psychologic components of rehabilitative care are designed to limit the psychosocial consequences of the illness, to enhance compliance with the recommended therapeutic regimens, and to encourage the behavioral modifications needed for secondary prevention.

In summary, a multifactorial approach to the long-term surveillance and management of the patient following coronary angioplasty or coronary bypass surgery is designed to maintain the improvement attained by these procedures. The components of care that can aid in the restoration of the patient to an active, productive, and satisfying life-style have been reviewed.

References

1. Almeida D, Bradford JM, Wenger NK, et al (1983) Return to work after coronary bypass surgery. Circulation 68 [Suppl II]:205 – 213
2. Blankenhorn DH, Nessim SA, Johnson RL, et al (1987) Beneficial effects of combined colestipol-niacin therapy on coronary atherosclerosis and coronary venous bypass grafts. JAMA 257:3233 – 3240
3. Bourassa MG, Enjalbert M, Campeau L, Lesperance J (1984) Progression of atherosclerosis in coronary arteries and bypass grafts: ten years later. Am J Cardiol 53:102C – 107C
4. Bourassa MG, Fisher LD, Campeau L, et al (1985) Long-term fate of bypass grafts: the Coronary Artery Surgery Study (CASS) and Montreal Heart Institute experience. Circulation 72 [Suppl V]:71 – 78
5. Bryson AL, Parisi A, Schechter E, Wolfson S (1973) Life-threatening ventricular arrhythmias induced by exercise. Cessation after coronary bypass surgery. Am J Cardiol 32:995 – 999
6. CASS Principal Investigators and their Associates (1983) Coronary Artery Surgery Study (CASS): a randomized trial of coronary artery bypass surgery. Survival data. Circulation 68:939 – 950
7. CASS Principal Investigators and their Associates (1983) Coronary Artery Surgery Study (CASS): a randomized trial of coronary artery bypass surgery. Quality of life in patients randomly assigned to treatment groups. Circulation 68:951 – 960
8. Cote G, Myler RK, Stertzer SH, et al (1987) Percutaneous transluminal angioplasty of stenotic coronary artery bypass grafts: 5-years' experience. J Am Coll Cardiol 9:8 – 17

9. Eliastam M, Gastel B (1982) Technology assessment forum on coronary artery bypass surgery: economic, ethical, and social issues. Circulation 66 [Suppl III]:1 – 101
10. European Coronary Surgery Study Group (1982) Long-term results of prospective randomized study of coronary artery bypass surgery in stable angina pectoris. Lancet II:1173 – 1180
11. Frye RL, Frommer PL (1982) Consensus development conference on coronary artery bypass surgery: medical scientific aspects. Circulation 65 [Suppl II]:1 – 129
12. Fuster V, Chesebro JJ (1985) Aortocoronary artery vein-graft disease: experimental and clinical approach for the understanding of the role of platelets and platelet inhibitors. Circulation 72 [Suppl V]:65 – 70
13. Grondin CM, Campeau L, Lesperance J, et al (1984) Comparison of late changes in internal mammary artery and saphenous vein grafts in two consecutive series of patients 10 years after operation. Circulation 70 [Suppl I]:208 – 212
14. Holmes DR, van Raden M, Reeder GS, et al (1984) Return to work after coronary angioplasty: a report from the National Heart, Lung and Blood Institute Percutaneous Transluminal Coronary Angioplasty Registry. Am J Cardiol 53:48C – 51C
15. Hultgren HN, Peduzzi P, Detre K, Takato T (1985) The 5-year effect of bypass surgery on relief of angina and exercise performance. Circulation 72 [Suppl V]:79 – 83
16. Jenkins CD, Stanton BA, Savageau JA, et al (1983) Coronary artery bypass surgery. Physical, psychological, soocial, and economic outcomes six months later. J Am Med Assoc 250:782 – 788
17. Kent KM, Bentivoglio LG, Block PC, et al (1984) Long-term efficacy of percutaneous transluminal coronary angioplasty (PTCA): report from the National Heart, Lung, Blood Institute PTCA Registry. Am J Cardiol 63:27C – 31C
18. Levy RI, Brensike JF, Epstein SE, et al (1984) The influence of changes in lipid values induced by cholestryramine and diet on the NHLBI Type II Coronary Intervention Study. Circulation 69:325 – 337
19. Lichstein E (1985) Why do beta-receptor blockers decrease mortality after myocardial infarction? J Am Coll Cardiol 6:973 – 975
20. Molajo AO, Summers GD, Bennett DH (1985) Effect of percutaneous transluminal coronary angioplasty on arrhythmias complicating angina. Br Heart J 54: 375 – 377
21. The NHLBI Type II Coronary Intervention Study (1983) The influence of cholestyramine-induced lipid changes on coronary artery disease progression (Abstract). Circulation 68 [Suppl III]:188
22. Palac RT, Meadows WR, Hwang MH, et al (1982) Risk factors related to progressive narrowing in aortocoronary vein grafts studied 1 and 5 years after surgery. Circulation 66 [Suppl I]:40 – 44
23. U.S. Department of Health, Education, and Welfare, Public Health Service, National Institutes of Health. Proceedings of the Conference on the Decline in the Coronary Heart Disease Mortality, Bethesda 1978. NIH Publication No 79-1610
24. Raichlen JS, Healy B, Achuff SC, Pearson TA (1986) Importance of risk factors in the angiographic progression of coronary artery disease. Am J Cardiol 57:66 – 70
25. Reeder GS (1986) Socioeconomic aspects. In: Vliestra RE, Holmes DR (eds) Percutaneous transluminal coronary angioplasty. Davis, Philadelphia, chapt 16
26. Roberts R, Gibson RS, Boden WE, et al (1986) Prophylactic therapy with diltiazem prevents early reinfarction: a multicentered randomized double-blind trial in patients recovering from non-Q wave infarction (Abstract). J Am Coll Cardiol 7:68

27. Roubin GS, King SB, Douglas JS (1987) Restenosis after percutaneous transluminal coronary angioplasty: the Emory University Hospital experience. Am J Cardiol 60: 39B–43B
28. Singh RN (1984) Progression of coronary atherosclerosis, clues to pathogenesis from serial coronary arteriography. Br Heart J 52:451–461
29. Singh RN, Sosa JA, Green GE (1983) Long-term fate of the internal mammary artery and saphenous vein grafts. J Thorac Cardiovasc Surg 86:359–363
30. Spears JR (1987) Percutaneous transluminal coronary angioplasty restenosis: potential prevention with laser balloon angioplasty. Am J Cardiol 60:61B–64B
31. Topol EJ, Califf RM, George BS, et al (1987) A randomized trial of immediate versus delayed elective angioplasty after intravenous tissue plasminogen activator in acute myocardial infarction. N Engl J Med 317:581–588
32. Walter PJ (1985) Return to work after coronary artery bypass surgery. Psychosocial and economic aspects. Springer, Berlin Heidelberg New York
33. Wenger NK (1986) Rehabilitation of the coronary patient: status 1986. Prog Cardiovasc Dis 29:181–204

The Role of Exercise Testing in Assessment of Myocardial Revascularisation

J. P. Broustet, B. Mora, and H. Douard

In myocardial revascularisation the aims of exercise testing are: (a) to determine a relevant indication for revascularisation; (b) to assess the results of the procedure by comparison to the pre-operative data and in an absolute manner (for example, a patient who has improved the symptom-limited heart rate between 4 and 8 min of exercise duration from 110 to 140 BPM and the ST segment depression from -4 to $-1{,}5$ mm may be considered as having an excellent result although his ability to do manual work has not been recovered); and (c) to identify sufficiently early the recurrence of ischaemia. The need for a pre-operative exercise test is therefore obvious.

The technical considerations here are very important. First of all, every test should be carried out at a proper interval after cessation of anti-anginal drugs. Evaluation of new anti-anginal drugs by means of a symptom-limited exercise test (SLET) demonstrates to what extent the most unfavourable test variables may improve with drugs such as β-blockers, calcium inhibitors, nitroglycerin and nitrates, and their combination. In studying the effects of revascularisation in a cohort of patients by means of SLET, this cohort must be divided into a number of subsets: (a) those who could not have for good or bad reasons an improper preoperative SLET; (b) those who had the preoperative SLET with a false negative or with weakly positive results because drugs were not interrupted; (c) those who return after revascularisation with an improper therapy; and (d) those who even performed a maximum effort without any sign of ischaemia.

The rate of patients unable to carry out a SLET due to cardiac or extracardiac reasons is not very significant. In a sequential cohort of 425 coronary patients, all having significant coronary lesions (one-vessel, 107; two-vessel, 140; three-vessel, 136; left main trunk, 42) the SLET could be performed in 82%. The main contra-indications were found in women; those unable due to age, impairment originating in joints, or muscular weakness made up 48% of revascularised women (Table 1). Another difficulty of exercise testing after revascularisation is evident when a peri-operative myocardial infarction has occurred. Indeed, the bypass may still be patent, and the ST elevation during exercise may conceal ST depression in other areas.

If other areas of myocardium have been revascularized, myocardial scintigraphy is useful. If there was but one bypass in the infarcted area, only coronarograftography is of interest.

Table 1. Contra-indications to exercise testing before 425 consecutive coronary angiographies with significant lesions

	Exercise test		Total
	Done	Not done	
Coronary bypass			
Men	171 (82%)	40 (18%)	211
Women	14 (52%)	13 (48%)	27
PTCA	28 (87%)	4 (13%)	32
Inoperable patients:	35 (68%)	16 (32%)	51
Deliberate abstention:	100 (96%)	4 (4%)	104
Total:	348 (82%)	79 (18%)	425

Table 2. Is PTCA an anti-ischemic agent or only a treatment of any dilatable stenosis?

	n	Before PTCA (%)	After PTCA (%)	Patients under drugs (ββ-nitrates) after PTCA (%)
Exercise ECG	41	33	7	27
Scintigraphy (thallium)	28	54	0	68
Ventriculography (technetium)	31	94	52	0

(From [3])

Table 3. Exercise test data with and without drugs

	n	Kpm	HR max	ST ↓ mm
Group 1 (fibrinolysis + PTCA)	35	6640 ± 3154	145 ± 18	0.54 ± 0.8
Group 2 (control)	34	5439 ± 2900	140 ± 20	0.48 ± 0.88
Group 1 (no drugs)	17	6997 ± 3679	146 ± 17	0.49 ± 0.76
Group 2 (no drugs)	17	5644 ± 3360	144 ± 21	0.48 ± 0.86

In contrast to coronary bypass (CBP), contra-indications to pre-PTCA exercise testing are rare. Also, the facilities for post-PTCA exercise testing are obvious. And although one might expect the literature to provide numerous papers on this subject, this surprisingly is far from the case. The reasons for this are many. First, too many patients have negative exercise tests before PTCA.

This could be due either to non-cessation of drugs or, more probably, to the desire to dilate any dilatable stenosis. The insufficient sensitivity of exercise ECG is not out of question, but if one recalls the excellent prognosis of coronary patients with non-positive or weakly positive exercise tests, the necessity to perform PTCA remains doubtful in many cases.

In spite of these technical and methodological difficulties, the exercise test remains the unique means to assess the results of revascularisation. There are three types of exercise testing: (a) traditional, i.e. effort ECG (x ECG) plus circulatory variables; (b) myocardial scintigraphy with thallium; and (c) exercise ventriculography with technetium 99. Table 2 shows the sensitivity of exercise ECG, thallium scintigraphy and technetium ventriculography before and after PTCA in a study of the NHLBI Registry [3]. The sensitivity of the three methods thus varies. The third has probably less specificity and more sensitivity than the other two. PTCA still more than CBP is too often carried out without a positive exercise test, that is, without any demonstration that the stenosis actually caused reproducible ischaemia. Due to the risk of vasospastic angina, which is a good reason to propose PTCA for any dilatable stenosis, too many patients with a normal exercise ECG receive PTCA. Exercise ventriculography is more sensitive – in fact, perhaps too sensitive. In the NHLBI Registry (Table 2) for example, Rosing and co-workers found only 33% of positive exercise ECGs before PTCA, but 94% of positive exercise ventriculographies. After PTCA 7% of patients had a positive exercise test. However, in the same study 94% of 31 patients had at least one abnormality of kinetics before PTCA, while after the procedure 52% still had an abnormal motion of at least one segment; the thallium scintigraphic perfusion was found positive in only 54% of patients before PTCA versus 0% after PTCA. These data suggest doubts as to the accuracy of the indication. In the same way, Wijns and Serruys [4] controlled their patients after PTCA by means of an exercise test, without interruption of a daily dose of 30–60 mg nifedipine.

In our series, 118 patients in the very acute phase of myocardial infarction were randomised into two groups: group 1 received fibrinolysis and immediate PTCA, and group 2 (control) was given heparin therapy. Of these, 69 patients could have a SLET after the procedure of revascularisation: 35 in group 1 and 34 in group 2. The two groups were comparable in terms of age and location of infarction. Coincidentally, we found in groups 1 and 2 the same number of patients receiving de novo drugs at the time of exercise test. The comparison of SLET results showed no significant differences in exercise capacity and maximum heart rate. The exercise capacity in the control group was good enough to make questionable the interest in PTCA plus fibrinolysis at admission (Table 3).

Because of the excellent situation of many candidates for PTCA, it appears that the main interest of SLET after PTCA is to predict restenosis. Obviously, if the pre-PTCA SLET is not abnormal, there are few possibilities. But when the SLET reveals a strong ischaemia occurring during the test, one may consider that a deterioration of sequential SLET after initial improvement is predictive of restenosis. The patient being his own control, the appearance or reappearance of subtle signs of ischaemia is of interest, whereas the same signs in a diagnostic SLET would not be specific enough to trust. For example, a disappearance of septal Q wave, a reappearance of moderate ST elevation during recovery, or a marked increase of R waves – all these changes having been absent at the first test after angioplasty – herald restenosis. After CBP the same problems arise. Nevertheless, in most cases the degree of ischaemia is more advanced than in candidates for PTCA. Therefore, the pre-operative exercise tests are generally strongly positive.

The practical difficulties are numerous. First, many pre-operative exercise tests are performed with potent anti-anginal drugs. In such cases an improvement of exercise test results after surgery is indeed of value, especially as the anti-anginal drugs have been decreased. But in many instances the ischaemia had been suppressed by a potent association of drugs before surgery, and comparison is therefore difficult. Secondly, the post-operative changes in ECG secondary to pericarditis decrease the amplitude of T waves for 1 – 2 months. Moreover, in 10% – 15% of cases transitory atrial fibrillation requires a therapy by β-blockers or amiodarone, which hinders the interpretation of exercise tests. It seems reasonable to wait for 3 months to assess the results of CBP by means of a comparative SLET. Unfortunately most early occlusions occur during the first 3 months. Thirdly, a peri-operative myocardial infarction is not uncommon after the revascularisation of numerous vessels. This infarction does not preclude that the graft has remained open. In such cases neither exercise ECG nor exercise scintigraphy are able to prove whether the graft is open or closed. And, finally, many patients have been severely impaired for such a long period before revascularisation that their muscles are deconditioned. Here the exercise test must be interrupted for fatigue of legs long before the patient has reached his maximal coronary reserve. The state of physical training is thus a very necessary consideration, and a delay of 2 months after surgery seems a minimum.

There are numerous papers in the literature which provide information concerning the short-term and long-term survey of the results of CBP by means of exercise testing. The greater sensitivity of thallium scintigraphy and of technetium ventriculography is of interest. But it must be kept in mind that the decision to reoperate a patients is a very important one. It depends on a multifactorial analysis using data from the pre-operative exercise test, first coronary angiography, surgical report and technical difficulties encountered, as well as, in the case of certain patients, their life activity and chronic diseases.

References

1. Mukharji J, Kremer SM, Lipscomb K, Blomwvist CG (1985) Early positive exercise test and extensive coronary disease: effect of anti-anginal therapy. Am J Cardiol 55:267 – 270

2. Broustet JP, Series E, Guern P, Vallot F, Pic A (1978) Matching nifedipine and nitroglycerin in the prevention of exercise induced angina. In: Kaltenback M, Lichtlen P, Balcon R, Bussmann W (eds) Coronary heart disease. Thieme, Stuttgart, p 309
3. Rosing DR, van Raden MJ, Mincemoyer RM, Bonow RO, et al (1984) Exercise electrocardiographic and functional responses after percutaneous transluminal coronary angioplasty. Am J Cardiol 53:36C – 41C
4. Wijns W, Serruys PW, Reiber JC, de Feyter PJ, et al (1985) Early detection of restenosis after successful percutaneous transluminal coronary angioplasty by exercise redistribution thallium scintigraphy. Am J Cardiol 357 – 361
5. Saint Pierre A, Mikaeloff P, Roche E, Coll-Mazzei J, Bonnefoy J, et al (1986) Intérêt de la revascularisation complète par pontage aortocoronaire. Appréciation des résultats par épreuve d'effort. Coeur 17:339 – 345

Physical Exercise in Comprehensive Care

J. J. Kellermann

The discussion of physical exercise as a secondary preventive measure may seem rather superfluous since such discussions have been held many times before with rather disappointing results. Newer studies, however, have renewed interest and have increased the challenge in dealing with this subject. The establishment of comprehensive coronary care (CCC), including multiple measures with physical, psychological and pharmacological procedures, together with a new concept of pharmacological and surgical revascularization, have caused a remarkable improvement in the management of coronary heart disease.

To illustrate this further we report here on two studies performed at our Institute in the past 6 years which clearly show the respective modes of intervention of our patient groups who were under constant comprehensive care. In the first study, concluded some 5 years ago, 19.3% of patients did exercise training only, while all the others received additional therapeutic measures. In the second study, 5 years later, 13% exercised, without further intervention, while the proportion who were operated and further rehabilitated increased from 11.7% in the first study to 34% (Table 1). As regards drug distribution, there was a significant reduction in the proportion of patients who received β-blockers in the second study, and there was a slight increase in the number of those who received calcium antagonists (Table 2).

It is obvious that physical training per se cannot be expected as a single measure of CCC to influence a multifactorial disease. In my opinion, irrefutable evidence showing physical training to have an effect on longevity is lacking and will not be available for many years to come, if at all. On the other hand, a number of important physiological and psychological benefits have been found as a result of prolonged physical training programmes in a selected patient population suffering from coronary heart disease. The effect of training is an improvement in cardiocirculatory performance for given work tasks. This includes a decrease in heart rate, systolic blood pressure and the double product and an increase in stroke volume, overall physical work, oxygen pulse and, in some instances, a rise in the angina pectoris threshold heart rate and threshold rate-pressure product.

The beneficial effects of continuous physical training in coronary patients eligible for this kind of programme (which includes patients with impaired ventricular function), are substantial. As regards cardiocirculatory and haemo-

Table 1. Comprehensive coronary care mode of intervention

	Study 1 ($n = 152$)	Study 2 ($n = 253$)
Exercise only	19.3%	13.1%
Exercise + CABG	3.6%	0.4%
Exercise + drugs	69.0%	52.9%
Exercise + CABG + drugs	8.1%	33.6%

Table 2. Comprehensive coronary care drug distribution

	Study 1 ($n = 152$)	Study 2 ($n = 232$)
Beta-Blockers	51.9%	35.3%
Calcium antagonists	27.6%	35.3%
Antiarrhythmic agents	19.7%	17.2%
Nitrates	25.6%	25.0%
Digoxin	3.3%	3.0%

dynamic effects, parameters which have been found to be affected by physical training include increased maximal oxygen output, cardiac output, stroke volume, oxygen extraction, total blood volume, muscular oxidative potential, and mitochondrial enzyme activity in skeletal muscle. Training also decreases, for a given work load, the heart rate, arterial lactic concentration, myocardial oxygen uptake, ventilation, and arterial systolic blood pressure. The arterio-venous oxygen difference remains unchanged in submaximal work, but increases in maximal work. The muscle blood flow decreases in submaximal work but increases in maximal work.

We have also observed numerous other effects. No change was found in left ventricular end-diastolic pressure and volume or ejection fraction after physical training; segmental contractility was found unaffected. It is possible, by physical training, to alter the metabolic properties of human skeletal muscle. It was found that the training effect was not limited to the central circulation only, but that there were also peripheral circulatory alterations as a result of training. One of the most important findings in achieving physiologically effective physical training was the observation that training intensity is directly related to the improvement of function. Physical training is dependent on sufficient intensity, duration and frequency, in order to produce measurable effects and improvement in overall performance. In preparing a suitable training programme, it is

Table 3. Established exercise training effects

Increases	Decreases
VO_2 max.	Heart rate[a]*
PWC*	Systolic blood pressure[a]*
Stroke volume	Rate pressure product[a]*
Oxygen pulse*	Serum lactic acid
A-VO_2 difference	Serum catecholamine levels
ATHR[b]	Total cholesterol*
Target rate pressure product[b]	Triglycerides
EF[b]	
HDL Cholesterol	
Mitochondrial	
Activity in trained selected muscle	

[a] For a given work load.
[b] Occasionally.
* $p<0.001$.

Table 4. Non-established effects on physical training

Not established
Collateral growth
Acceleration of collateral circulation
Alteration of cardiac electrical instability
Effects on fibrinolytic activity, platelet adhesiveness
Tolerance to emotional stress
No effect on
Deteriorated ventricular function
Regression of atherosclerotic process
Effect on mortality
Beneficial in Non-randomized trials (long-term)
Beneficial in randomized trials without statistical significance (short-term)

mandatory to take into consideration the functional capacity of the individual, his age, his sex, and any kind of disability which may interfere with physical activity (Tables 3, 4).

Concerning psychological and socioeconomic effects, physical training programmes of various durations have been reported to show an improvement in emotional stability, general motivation to life and self esteem; and a decrease in fear, anxiety, frustration and drug dependency. They also lead to an early return to work, a greater proportion of return to work especially for CABG patients, and an improvement in the quality of life.

Of late, there is additional evidence, mostly in experimental animals, which shows that daily exercise beneficially affects the susceptibility to sudden cardiac death, and that it increases the threshold for ventricular fibrillation. Moreover, nuclear studies have shown that, at least in selected patients, physical training may improve the left ventricular systolic performance and increase left ventricular ejection fraction. However, in summarizing a large number of studies concerning the left ventricular performance and myocardial perfusion, it must be concluded that their results are equivocal.

Exercise performance in patients with impaired ventricular function does not correlate well with the severity of dysfunction. Patients with ventricular dysfunction can achieve a fairly high work capacity, and physiological variables respond in a similar way, regardless of whether the patient does or does not have impaired function. Furthermore, patients with pump dysfunction can benefit from a supervised physical training programme by improving their functional capacity and, thus, their quality of life. The absolute containdications for exercise therapy in this group of patients with coronary artery disease should, therefore, be identical to those who have normal ventricular function.

In our opinion, special attention should be exercised in patients who have chronotropic incompetence, lack of an elevation or decrease in blood pressure during exercise performance, and in those whose stroke volume is not elevated during even low to moderate work loads. Recommendations as to the implementation of exercise therapy as a therapeutic modality in patients with ventricular impairment must be accepted with caution. The reason for this is that our observations are based on historical, anecdotal trials, most of which included only a modest number of patients. Future research and a prolonged follow-up is needed in order to obtain both a more exact analysis and eventually scientifically based evidence on the benefits and hazards involved. It should be mentioned that there are a number of non-established benefits, namely an effect on collateral growth, acceleration of collateral circulation and a regression of the atherosclerotic process.

Recent analyses of prospective randomized trials concerning physical exercise training as a secondary preventive measure have shown that five of six studies indicated that there may be a benefit from physical training for post-myocardial infarction patients. Unfortunately, all these trials were too short, and the sample size too small. This fact, together with a number of biases concerning drop-out and drop-in rates, make it impossible to reach a clear scientific verdict.

Often there is a lack of a common language or understanding between the physiologist and the clinician. According to our knowledge, to date, physical training should be involved as an integrative part of comprehensive CCC if no contraindication exists. It should definitely be used with prudence and moderation and never on the basis of "a run for your life theory". It is mistaken, in using exercise therapy, that the patient should come to believe that exercise can be considered as a panacea, and that a single intervention will suffice in combatting a multifactoral disease. Ultimately, there is no scientific evidence that exercise therapy, which can easily become an obsession, will prolong the patient's life. Concerning long-term randomized trials involving physical training, it has recently become popular that one should not try to reach hard end points but concentrate rather more on so-called soft end points, such as the quality of survival and not survival per se.

References

1. Scientific Council on Rehabilitation of Cardiac Patients (1983) Myocardial infarction: how to prevent, how to rehabilitate. International Society and Federation of Cardiology
2. Kellermann JJ (1975) Rehabilitation of patients with coronary heart disease. Prog Cardiovasc Dis 18:303–328
3. Wenger NK (ed) (1985) Exercise and the heart. 2nd edn. Davis, Philadelphia
4. Kellermann JJ, Spodick DH (eds) (1986) Left ventricular dysfunction. Karger, Basel (Advances in cardiology, vol 34)
5. Cohen LS, Mock MB, Ringqvist I (eds) (1981) Physical conditioning and cardiovascular rehabilitation. Wiley, New York
6. Pyorala K, Rapaport E, Konig K, Schettler G, Diehm C (eds) (1983) Secondary prevention of coronary heart disease. Workshop of the International Society and Federation of Cardiology. Thieme-Stratton, Stuttgart

Cost-Effectiveness of Noninvasive Surveillance

B. Boskis

The crucial problem that has faced academic medicine as well as cardiologic practice for many years in Argentina is that of cost-efficiency. Today, this same problem, as well as many cost-containment plans, have implications not only for practicing physicians, but for research and academic cardiologists. This has occurred in many countries which, until a short time ago, were free from this concern, as reflected in numerous articles and comments published in prestigious journals. Perhaps the following dilemma, as phrased by Helfant summarizes the concern shared by many of today's cardiologists: "Faced with ever increasing new technologies and the constraints of cost containment, how will the practicing cardiologist provide high quality care without coming into conflict with the new economic realities?" We have expressed this concern in the rehabilitation area, both at the 9th World Congress of Cardiology in Moscow and at the 3rd World Congress of Cardiac Rehabilitation in Caracas.

However we believe this concern over costs should not imply neglect of control and evaluation criteria. Regarding a cost-effectiveness ratio, we propose the following protocols for noninvasive surveillance during rehabilitative care after myocardial revascularization.

Coronary Artery Bypass Grafting Surgery. Postoperative treadmill exercise testing is indicated and performed at 4 – 6 weeks, but is usually submaximal. The target for the indication is to quantify functional capacity and, by comparison, the expected improvement. Besides the time to maximal exercise, we can assess the presence of exertional angina, exercise-induced cardiac arrhythmias, blood pressure, and heart rate responses. Repeat testing may be indicated at 2 months after surgery before return to work and can be performed to near-maximal capacity.

Our second step in evaluating patients after uncomplicated coronary artery revascularization by surgery involves the radionuclide techniques. A small-diameter (5-cm) detector with a converging collimator connected to ECG-gated microprocessors and/or computers, enables automatic real-time calculation of global left ventricular function by measuring the time-activity curve. This ECG-gated scintillation probe device makes it possible to obtain a representative curve of the left ventricular radioactivity content variation throughout the cardiac cycle. Ejection fraction (EF), ejection rate, ejection periods, and diastolic filling phases such as peak filling rate and time to peak filling rate can be measured using the same algorithms used by the gamma camera. These variables can be obtained from the curve, registered beat-to-beat, from the accumulation of hundreds of beats in a predetermined period of time (up to 4 min), with readings performed every 10 min starting at the R peak wave of the ECG.

The good correlation between the EF obtained by gamma camera and the nuclear stethoscope is already a well-determined fact. Values of left ventricular function at rest of 30% seem to be the borderline figure in predicting outcome. Therefore, when the EF value is less than 30%, patients have an adverse prognosis, being to Wiggers decidedly bad, should it reach below 20%. An EF of 30% – 40% falls in a nonspecific zone; one of 45% or more is an acceptable prognosis. If we want a better prognostic stratification in patients with a 40% – 50% EF, we ask for a stress test with gamma camera. A rise to above 5% or fall to 10% or more allows a prognostic stratification of risk. In the experience by Pryor et al., for coronary patients with medically treated stable angina, the EF at rest was the second predictive element that proved best. Again, those patients with an EF between 20% and 35% had a more unfavorable outcome, which is reduced in patients with an EF between 35% and 49%, to become stable in those with 50% or more. Conclusions based on Duke University studies can be extrapolated to patients who already have undergone coronary bypass grafting, a criterion we share.

Exercise Testing after PTCA. In successful PTCA, post treatment exercise testing can be performed with safety during the week after the procedure. In patients with good results and a comprehensive involvement with prevention, and therapeutic and educational components of care, follow-up testing should be performed. Exercise testing at 3 and 6 months evaluates one of the dimensions of quality of life, the functional capacity, or identifies the 20% – 30% of patients who have late restenosis after the procedure.

Radionuclide angiography or the nuclear probe can provide information on functional severity, which is directly related to prognostic evaluation. In patients with atrial fibrillation, it is possible with the nuclear probe, to ascertain the hemodynamic changes associated with the arrhythmia and those caused by the ventricular disease.

Echocardiography after PTCA. The second step for patients undergoing PTCA, either as a single element or together with nuclear techniques is echocardiography. Two-dimensional echocardiography uses advanced technology such as multiple scan heads, new types of phased-array transducers, consistent diagnostic image quality, digital technology, and pharmacological contrast techniques. Rest and exercise imaging and the association with Doppler techniques for flow analysis have expanded the diagnostic power and the capacity to evaluate ventricular structure and function, global contraction and regional wall motion. Thanks to computers, two-dimensional echocardiography is no longer a qualitative image. We can freeze it, store it in memory, recall it, and display it on a monitor for comparative review. The optimal image can be selected and measured for EF, scored for regional function, and quantified to measure changes in wall thickness.

Stress echocardiography is a convenient and cost-effective procedure, and, as Feingenbaum has pointed out, "it is no longer just an investigational procedure." Technology makes it possible to store in memory different cardiac cycles. Computer selection can minimize respiratory interference, and general body movements can be overcome by using supine bicycle exercise. Recalling two complete images synchronized by cursors on ECG, the dual-cine loop allows side-by-side playback for comparative analysis. In many countries throughout the world, including Argentina, it is not always easy to obtain isotopes when needed; therefore, the possibility to image patients during or immediately after exercise, could make stress echocardiography compete as a convenient and cost-effective procedure.

Conclusion. Cardiology and rehabilitation are caught in a conflict between developing technologies and economic realities. In our protocol, the two-dimensional echocardiogram plays an essential part in the diagnosis of clinical problems and functional evaluation. Technology makes it possible to select optimal images and quantitative answers, and this ensures an accurate prognosis. Use of the nuclear probe or radionuclide angiography makes it possible to study systolic as well as diastolic function and also provides valuable and well-confirmed information as to function, evaluation, and prognosis. Therefore, reliable information of the anatomy and the left ventricular function seems to be provided by these techniques; the choice of procedure will depend on the case being studied. Moreover, combined use with exercise testing provides a reasonable, useful, cost-containment protocol with more than enough sensitivity for noninvasive surveillance of cardiac rehabilitation after myocardial revascularization.

Rehabilitative Care After Myocardial Revascularization

H. Sanne

Revascularization in this presentation is used to mean coronary artery bypass grafting (CABG). As a separate presentation on return to work will follow, this topic is not specifically addressed.

Psychological and Social State of the Patient Before Revascularization

Patients who undergo myocardial revascularization are in a certain phase of a chronic disease. We must expect psychological and social consequences because of the patient's earlier experience of the disease, such as suffering from myocardial infarction and disability due to angina pectoris. We also must consider the experience of the disease in the family and at the work place. The psychological and social impact of the illness is related to the social situation of the patient, the type of work, and the degree of support or protection of family, employer, and friends. Of course, the patient's personality and coping capacity is of great significance. Therefore, we can expect that the state after revascularization is influenced both by a long-lasting and life-threatening disease and by the procedures related to revascularization.

Consequences of What?

What does revascularization mean to the patient? What is the intervention? There are preoperative factors, such as the expectations of the patient, which may influence at least the subjective outcome. The mental preparation before the operation may influence the degree of emotional arousal and hospitalization time. There are perioperative factors such as technical operative procedures and anesthesia, possible brain injury, nursing, and care.

Pain relief and improved physical capacity is the most consistent finding after surgery. There can be a considerable variation in readjustment measures after surgery in counselling and instructions, the degree of support, control directiveness, or authority by the doctor, as well as in the assurance and skill of the doctor. The consistency of messages from the staff and also the physical training and other rehabilitation measures may differ. The influence of a social network and social support has not been well studied after coronary artery surgery.

Disability is a term that can be related to a single component, angina pectoris. Revascularization is a biological intervention improving perfusion of the myocardium, giving pain relief and improved physical capacity. Ability is a comprehensive concept, determined by several biological, psychological, and social components. Revascularization gives opportunities for psychological and social adjustment but is obviously not the only prerequisite. When dealing with psychological and social outcomes, we must consider all these determining factors – noncardiac factors that are more closely related to attitudes, feelings, perception of disease, and values of the patient. We are dealing with the person, not only with the heart. The patient is actively involved as a subject, not only an object, of surgery. This is probably the explanation that employability is improved but not always the work status.

What Consequences can be Expected?

The psychological and social outcomes are not limited to resumption of work. It can even be discussed whether return to work is a gain or a poor outcome. The subjective dimension must be included in the evaluation. Satisfaction is an inevitable part of the assessment of psychological and social outcomes (Table 1). The alphabetical classification and order in Table 1 is not scientific; the listing is done to stress how multidimensional the psychological and social outcomes are. The emotional response to revascularization could either be restorative or deteriorative. Behavior can be objectively evaluated as roles and relations, but also subjectively as satisfaction. Cognitive functioning is of interest because of the observed brain injury after surgery, but also as a problem-solving and coping mechanism. Finally, defense reactions can also be included as coping strategies. All these variables are measurable and therefore can be used for scientific evaluation of outcome.

Inconsistency of Investigations

The results of investigations of psychological and social outcomes following coronary artery surgery have been inconsistent. One reason may be differences in selection of patients studied. Different ages influence the results. Socioeconomic factors have been suggested by Gundle (1980) to be the explanation of divergent results. Cultural factors, social systems, social insurance systems, and available work probably influence the readjustment.

The inconsistency of findings may also be due to different assessment techniques. For instance, subjective assessment of the investigator or objective measurement by questionnaires or standardized interviews have been used. We do not have clear and generally accepted definitions of psychological and social concepts. Various aspects and issues are studied. The validity and specificity of

Table 1. Some psychosocial consequences to consider after revascularization

Classification	Functional areas	Variables
Affective		Anxiety Depression Fatigue Self-esteem Self-concept
Behavioral	Roles and relations: At the job as an employee In the family as parent As sexual partner During leisure time In the household	Satisfaction with: Work status Responsibility Sexual activity Everyday activity Social interaction
Cognitive function	Coping strategy	Health preoccupation Health concern Attitudes
	Brain functioning	Memory Concentration
Defense reactions	Personality	Denial Regression Hostility Aggression

outcome variables in various reports differ. Many studies refer to small groups of patients. Adequate control groups are lacking in most studies. The time of investigation in relation to surgery also differs. Historical anamnestic data are unreliable. A considerable emotional arousal can be expected in the days before surgery, and this period may not be suitable to get initial data in a before/after study.

There are many potent factors and moments in care and the care system which can influence psychological and social outcomes without being recognized and considered and without being directly related to the revascularization procedure. Many of these mechanisms are difficult to standardize and measure. In most articles they are not described. It is therefore difficult to attribute the different outcomes that are reported to variations in care and rehabilitation. The fact that an investigator performs a study means an increased interest and may also mean better planning for and management of the patient.

What Psychological and Social Outcome Variables have been Studied?

Folks et al. (1986) studied 96 patients before and 6 months after coronary bypass surgery and used a psychological adjustment to illness scale (PAIS). They found improved sexual function and a significant strengthening of relationships within the patients' nuclear family and in their social activities. There was no change in psychological distress but a negative effect on health concern. Wallwork and Caine (1985) used the Nottingham Health Profile, which is a formal instrument for measuring patients' subjective perceptions of their health state. They examined 30 patients before and 3 and 12 months after coronary surgery. There was a highly significant decrease in all factors, which means higher physical mobility, less pain, better sleep, more energy, less social isolation, and less emotional distress.

Self-perceived health status was reported better in the surgical group compared with the medical group in the Birmingham portion of the Coronary Artery Surgery Study (CASS, [4]), although recreational status of physical activity level did not differ between medical and surgical groups in the total study (Circulation, 1983). Gundle and coworkers (1980) found a decreased sexual activity after compared with before surgery, dealing with a limited cohort of 30 patients. They also reported a constricted social life, low self-esteem and lack of pleasure from close relationships. The findings could be due to a selection of patients with low socioeconomic status. Jenkins et al. (1983) reported in a comparison of before/after coronary artery bypass surgery variables in 318 patients that anxiety, depression, fatigue, and sleep disturbances declined. Vigor and well-being scores rose. Savageau et al. (1982) in the same group of investigators, did not find any difference in before/after variables in considering role functions such as household activities, shopping, car maintenance, or decision making. Social interaction was mainly unchanged. Of these patients 36% felt over-protected, and 50% felt family members were brought closer by surgery. Sexual function and marital satisfaction were unchanged.

Thurer et al. (1980) made a psychodynamic evaluation of 21 patients before and after bypass surgery and noticed a reorientation after operation, with changed priorities in life – valuing human closeness and devaluing work. Subclinical neuropsychological disturbances have been found in some studies, especially early after surgery (Aberg et al. 1984, Smith et al. 1986, Savageau et al. 1982).

A reasonably correct conclusion could be that surgery does not seem to be psychiatrically or socially pathogenic. Emotional disturbances decrease. Sleep, energy, and social interaction are improved. On the other hand, patients may be more "health concerned" and have a lower self-concept after operation. There are inconsistent data concerning return to work, sexual and physical activity, and social life.

Predictors of Outcome

Investigations of determinants of psychological and social outcomes also show inconsistent results. For example, the degree of pain relief is not related to outcome in all studies. Bass (1984) did not find that return to work or psychological state was related to any physical variables before surgery, or to pain relief or the functional capacity after. Significant determinants were preoperative mental state and psychiatric history, preoperative social maladjustment, and neuroticism.

Type A behavior patients had more emotional and social disturbances after operation, which is in agreement with findings of Zyzanski et al. (1981). In a sample of more than 900 patients after CABG, emotional relationship were clearly worse in patients with type A behavior.

Gundle et al. (1980) found that a long preoperative duration of symptoms was related to a poor postoperative adaptation and to a damaged self-concept before operation; the latter was reinforced, rather than repaired, by the experience of surgery. Liddle and coworkers ($n = 565$, 1982) found age, educational level, and preoperative work status to be related to work return. Over 90% returned to work; the authors stated that successful rehabilitation depends on "the impact of the individual physician on the motivation of patients." All patients were advised in advance that work rehabilitation was a principal purpose of the operation, and that disability claims would be supported only if revascularization failed.

In CASS, there was a relationship between psychosocial outcome and success of revascularization, age, and socioeconomic factors (Smith et al. 1983), but the authors concluded that "the patient's own perception of his health appears to be more important" (Smith 1985). Duration of preoperative unemployment and symptoms have prognostic significance according to Boulay and coworkers (1982). Other factors than cardiac ones seemed to be the most important determinants of autcome, such as a passive time on the waiting list and omitted directiveness concerning readjustment. As could be expected, patients with earlier psychiatric history and social maladjustment needed extra support.

Assessment of Different Strategies to Limit Psychosocial Disability

There are no strictly controlled studies evaluating the effectiveness of various approaches to improve psychological and social readjustment after coronary bypass surgery. The inconsistent results of investigations of outcomes may reflect variations in care and rehabilitation. Technically successful operative interventions may fail in the absence of rehabilitation supplementation (Murray and Beller 1983). Bypass surgery represents only a single therapeutic aspect.

Some of the determinants of outcome that have been found are dynamic and may be influenced. Roviaro et al. (1984) studied 48 myocardial infarction and coronary bypass surgery patients who were assigned either to a physical training and educational program, spouse included, or to routine care. The allocation was done on a geographical basis. They reported more positive self-perceptions concerning health, body concept, self-concept, and progress towards goals in the intervention group. They also found better psychosocial functioning, e.g., decreased employment-related stress, more active use and enjoyment of leisure time, and more physical and sexual activity. The effect remained 4 months after the program. Ben Ari et al. (1986) reported a considerably higher rate "good" overall subjective feeling of well-being in an exercise-trained compared with an untrained group of CABG patients. The controls were not randomized and the instrument for evaluation was very coarse.

In a retrospective study of 358 CABG patients, Gutman et al. (1982) found that participation in an outpatient rehabilitation program was significantly related to an improved postoperative work status for men employed before surgery. The investigators raised the question about the role of rehabilitation in altering the patients' perceptions and maintaining work habits that might facilitate work resumption. The authors also suggested that work should be viewed as a process through which interrelated behaviors are developed to support a certain life-style.

Boulay and coworkers (1982) stated that an increased rate of work resumption from 69% in 1968 – 1972 to 90% about 10 years later was related primarily to a shorter period of preoperative unemployment. Liddle and coworkers (1982), who also reported a rate of work resumption over 90%, suggested that the most important factors in effective rehabilitation were the psychological preparation of patients, their families, and the attitude toward rehabilitation expressed by physicians and employers. La Mendola and Pellegrini (1979) state that "quality of life improvement is a function of the patients' postoperative experience and perception of their physical limits, which in turn is likely to influence their decision to work."

Conclusion

The assessment of outcome of myocardial revascularization should not be limited to mortality, morbidity, pain relief, physical capacity, and return to work, but should also include social functioning in other domains, relations, emotions, perceptions, and feelings. There are data in the literature that indicate inadequate psychosocial rehabilitation. Some risk factors for maladjustment have been identified; these are mainly nonmedical. The patients' own perceptions and priorities must be considered.

In care, factors other than the reperfusion seem to be most relevant. Rehabilitative aspects are important – and measures should start – before surgery, for instance, limiting the time of disability and the time out of work. Preparing the patients about the procedures, difficulties, and – which seems to be efficient – the principal objectives for the operation. Patient education aims to prevent and correct misunderstanding and to give basic knowledge about how to handle situations, and how to reorganize one's life. Physical training can be used as a practical instruction to the patients concerning how to use their regained physical capacity, but there are other didactic moments connected with a physical training program as well.

There are no scientific data about which components are necessary and which optional in a comprehensive rehabilitation program; certainly there are cultural and socioeconomic differences. We need further research and evaluation of cost-effectiveness.

References

1. Gundle MJ, Reeves BR, Tate S, Raft D, McLaurin LP (1980) Psychosocial outcome after coronary artery surgery. Am J Psychiatry 137[12]:1591 – 1594
2. Folks DG, Blake DJ, Fleece L, Sokol RS, Freeman AM (1986) Quality of life six months after coronary artery bypass surgery: a preliminary report. South Med J 79[4]:397 – 399
3. Wallwork J, Caine N (1985) A comparison of the quality of life of cardiac transplant patients and coronary artery bypass graft patients before and after surgery. Quality of Life and Cardiovascular Care 2:317 – 331
4. Oberman A, Wayne JB, Kouchoukos NT, Charles ED, Russell RO, Rogers WJ (1982) Employment status after coronary artery bypass surgery. Circulation 65:115 – 133
5. CASS Principal Investigators and their Associates (1983) Coronary artery surgery study (CASS): a randomized trial of artery bypass surgery. Circulation 68:951 – 960
6. Jenkins CD, Stanton B-A, Savageau JA, Denlinger P, Klein MD (1983) Coronary artery bypass surgery. JAMA 250:782 – 788
7. Savageau JA, Stanton B-A, Jenkins CD, Klein MD (1982) Neuropsychological dysfuncion following elective cardiac operation I. J Thorac Cardiovasc Surg 84:585 – 594
8. Savageau JA, Stanton B-A, Jenkins CD, Fraater RWM (1982) Neuropsychological dysfunction following elective cardiac operation II. J Thotac Cardiovasc Surg 84:595 – 600
9. Thurer S, Levine F, Thurer R (1980/1981) The psychodynamic impact of coronary bypass surgery. Int J Psychiatry Med 10[3]:273 – 290
10. Åberg T, Rönnqvist G, Tydén H, Brunnkvist S, Hultman J, Bergström K, Lilja A (1984) Adverse effects on the brain in cardiac operations as assessed by biochemical, psychometric and radiologic methods. J Thorac Cardiovasc Surg 87:99 – 105
11. Smith PLC, Treasure T, Newman SP, Joseph P, Ell PJ, Schneidau A, Harrison MJG (1986) Cerebral consequences of cardiopulmonary bypass. Lancet I:823 – 825
12. Bass C (1984) Psychosocial outcome after coronary artery by-pass surgery. Br J Psychiatry 145:526 – 532
13. Zyzanski SJ, Stanton BA, Jenkins CD, Klein MD (1981) Medical and psychosocial outcomes in survivors of major heart surgery. J Psychosom Res 23:213 – 221
14. Liddle HV, Jensen R, Clayton PD (1982) The rehabilitation of coronary surgical patients. Ann Thorac Surg 34:374 – 382

15. Smith HC, Frye RL, Piehler JM (1983) Does coronary bypass surgery have a favorable influence on the quality of life? Cardiovasc Clin 13:253 – 264
16. Smith HC (1985) Quality of life after coronary artery bypass surgery. Quality of Life and Cardiovascular Care 2:215 – 228
17. Boulay FM, David PP, Bourassa MG (1982) Strategies for improving the work status of patients after coronary artery bypass surgery. Circulation 66:43 – 49
18. Murray GC, Beller GA (1983) Cardiac rehabilitation following coronary artery bypass surgery. Am Heart J 105[2]:1009 – 1017
19. Roviaro S, Holmes DS, Holmsten RD (1984) Influence of a cardiac rehabilitation program on the cardiovascular, psychological, and social functioning of cardiac patients. J Behav Med 7:61 – 81
20. Ben-Ari E, Kellermann JJ, Fisman E-Z, Pines A, Peled B, Drory Y (1986) Benefits of long-term physical training in patients after coronary artery bypass grafting – a 58-month follow-up and comparison with a nontrained group. J Cardiopulm Rehab 6:165 – 170
21. Gutmann MC, Knapp DN, Pollock ML, Schmidt DH, Simon K, Walcott G (1982) Coronary artery bypass patients and work status. Circulation 66:33 – 42
22. LaMendola WF, Pellegrini RV (1979) Quality of life and coronary artery bypass surgery patients. Soc Sci Med 13A:457 – 461

Return to Work After Coronary Artery Bypass Surgery*

P. J. Walter

Introduction

After 20 years of surgical experience in the treatment of ischemic heart disease, the aortocoronary bypass operation can be performed with low early mortality and good long-term results. Although this form of treatment can relieve angina pectoris in a high percentage of patients, postoperative resumption of work is not as high as it might be. Next to other aims of the treatment, this resumption of work represents part of psychosocial reintegration whose economic impact for the individual as well as for the community should not be underestimated. The aim of this study is an analysis of the most important factors for the incidence of return to work. These factors lead us to suggestions on improvement of the rate of return to work after bypass surgery.

The basis for this report are the papers presented at an international symposium, which took place on May 10–11, 1984, in the Herz- und Kreislaufzentrum, Rotenburg, Federal Republic of Germany. The manuscripts were published in the book *Return to Work After Coronary Bypass Surgery – Psychosocial and Economic Aspects* [1].

Results

The rate of return to work after coronary bypass surgery varies among countries from 58% to 91% (Table 1). Changes in employment status from preoperative period to the survey date at different intervals are presented for the United States (Fig. 1), Great Britain (Fig. 2), Switzerland (Fig. 3), and the Federal Republic of Germany (Fig. 4).

A striking discrepancy between functional class (after New York Heart Association), subjective ability to work, and actual postoperative employment rate was found in the Federal Republic of Germany (Fig. 5). Here, postoperative exercise tolerance correlated significantly with the postoperative rate of return to work (Fig. 6).

---

* This work is taken with permission from an article published in *European Heart Journal*, vol. 9 (Supplement).

Table 1. Percentage of return to work after coronary bypass surgery in different countries

Authors	Country	Percentages
Rothlin	Switzerland	58
Vetter	FRG	58
Sergeant	Belgium	63
Gohlke	FRG	65
Hymowitz	Israel	70
Crosby	USA	86/91

From [1]

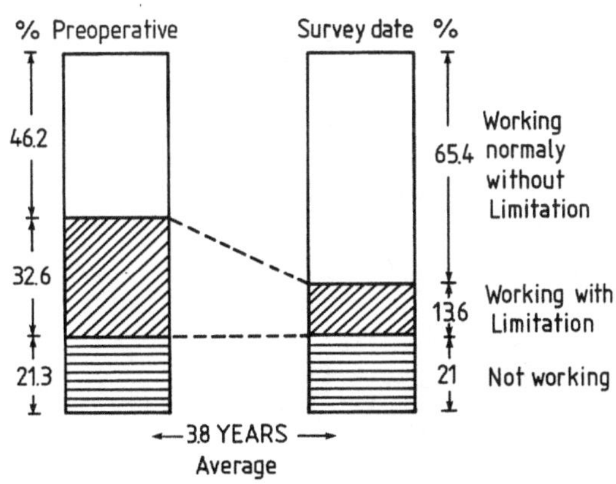

Fig. 1. Pre- and postoperative employment in the United States. Data on men over 55 year of age ($n = 738$). (From Johnson et al., in [1])

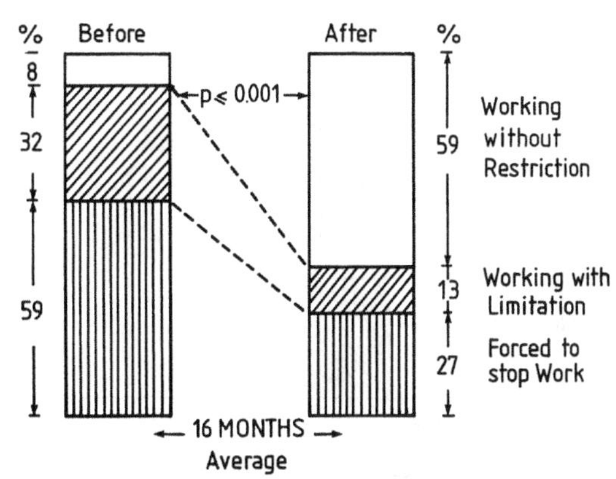

Fig. 2. Pre- and postoperative employment in Great Britain. Data on men ($n = 117$). (From Bentall et al., in [1])

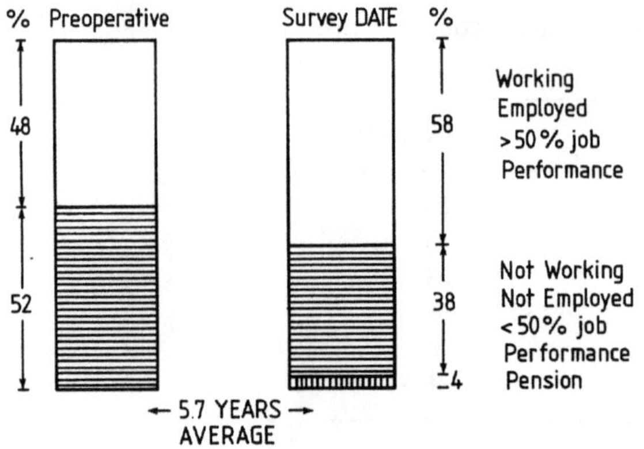

Fig. 3. Pre- and postoperative employment in Switzerland. Data on men ($n = 219$). (From Rothlin et al., in [1])

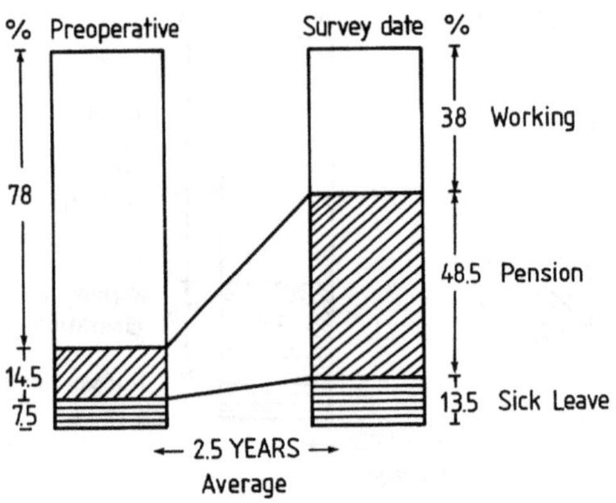

Fig. 4. Pre- and postoperative employment in the Federal Republic of Germany. Data on men ($n = 384$) and women ($n = 27$); mean age 53.6 years. (From [2])

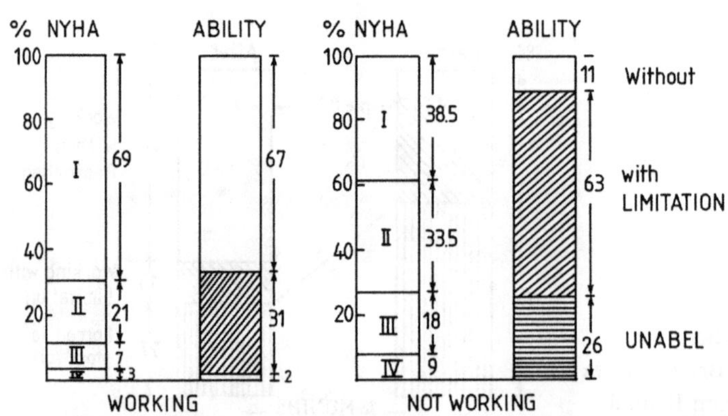

Fig. 5. Discrepancy between functional class (after New York Heart Association, *NYHA*), subjective ability to work, and actual employment status. (From Hacker et al., in [1])

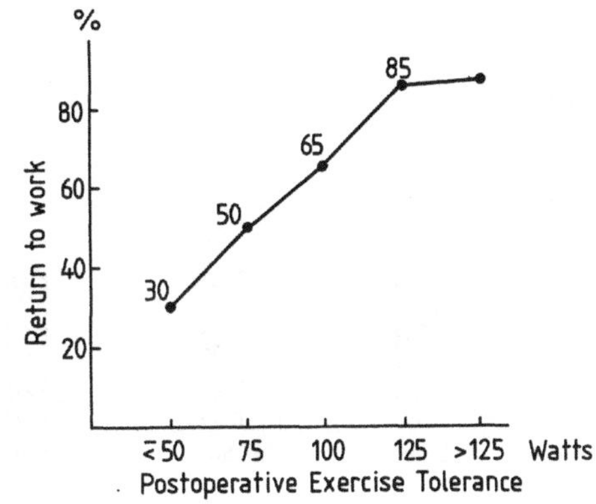

Fig. 6. Postoperative exercise tolerance and return to work ($n = 481$; $p < 0.00001$). (From Gohlke et al., in [1])

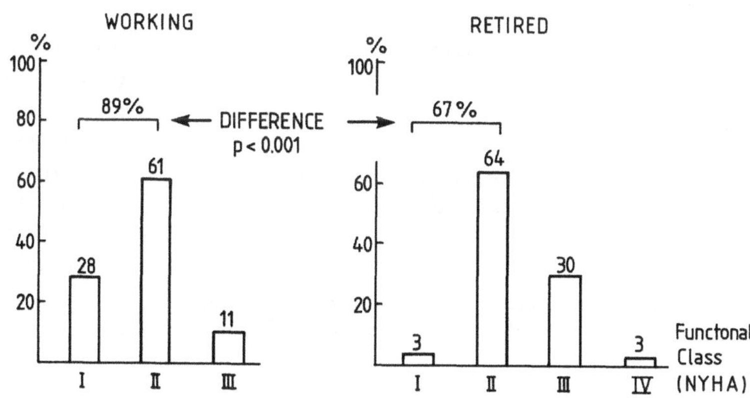

Fig. 7. Functional class (after New York Heart Association, *NYHA*) among postoperatively working ($n = 100$) and retired ($n = 100$) following coronary artery bypass surgery. Data from the Federal Republic of Germany. (From Skupin et al., in [1])

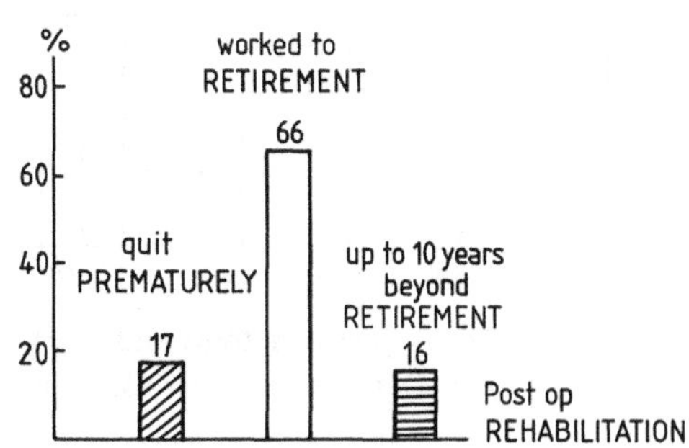

Fig. 8. Working after myocardial revascularization: an avoidable hazard? Data on men ($n = 292$) in the United States. (From Liddle et al., in [1])

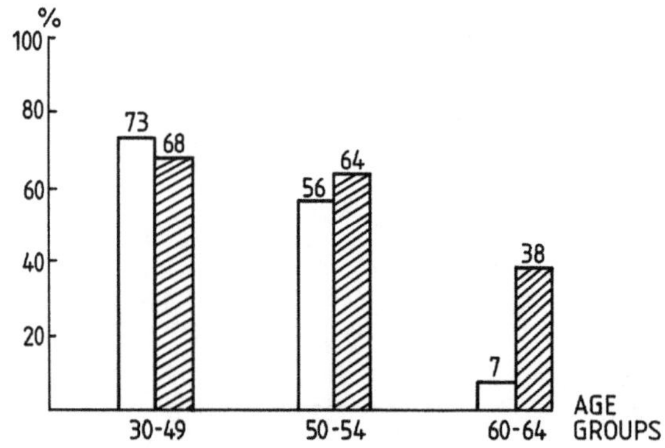

Fig. 9. Age and employment rate after coronary artery bypass graft. Data from the Federal Republic of Germany (*unshaded bars*; from [18]) and the United States (*shaded bars*). (From Johnson et al., in [1]; [2])

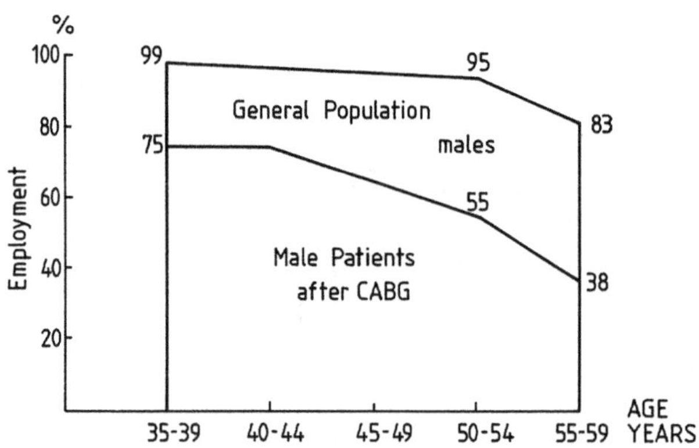

Fig. 10. Age at operation (coronary artery bypass graft, *CABG*) and employment rate, compared to employment rate in general population. Data from Federal Republic of Germany. (From Hacker et al., in [1])

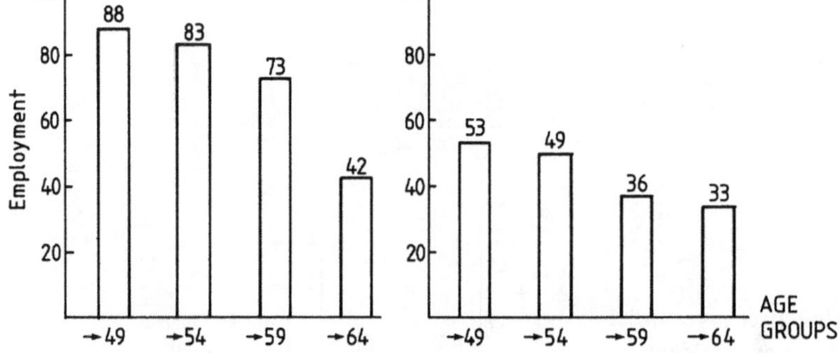

Fig. 11. Relief of angina symptoms and employment rate at 1 year after coronary artery bypass operation. Data on men ($n = 4530$) in the United States. (From Anderson et al., in [1])

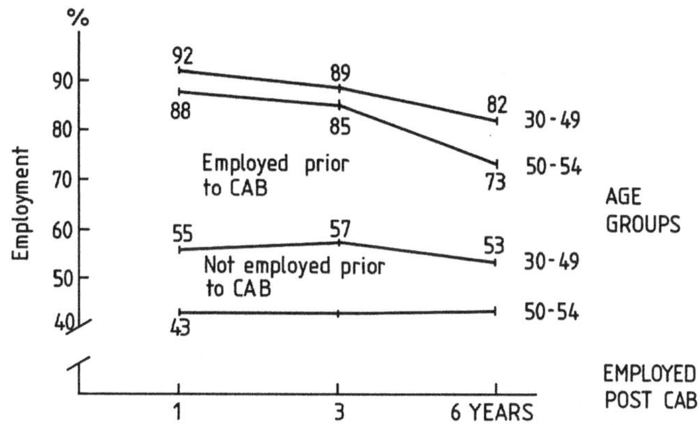

Fig. 12. Effect of working prior to coronary artery bypass operation on postoperative employment rate. Data from the United States. (From Anderson et al., in [1])

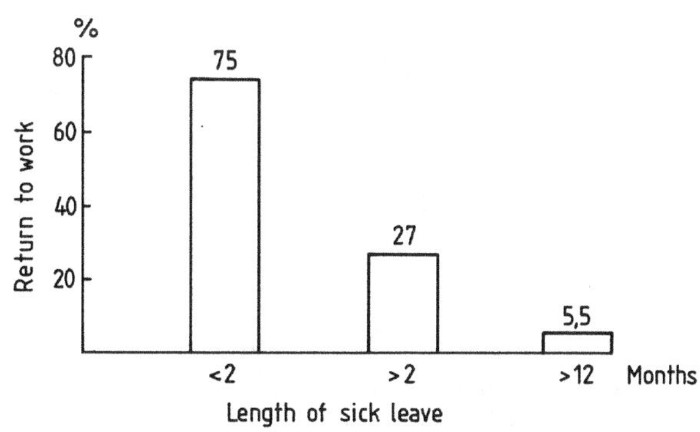

Fig. 13. Length of preoperative sick leave and return to work after coronary artery bypass operation. Data from the Federal Republic of Germany ($n = 111$). (From Carstens et al., in [1])

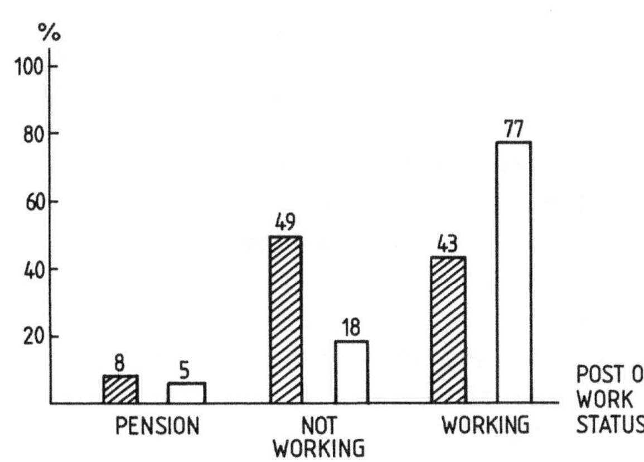

Fig. 14. Preoperative employment status on return to work after coronary artery bypass operation. Data from Switzerland. *Unshaded bars,* employed preoperatively ($n = 105$); *shaded bars,* not employed preoperatively ($n = 114$). (From Rothlin et al., in [1])

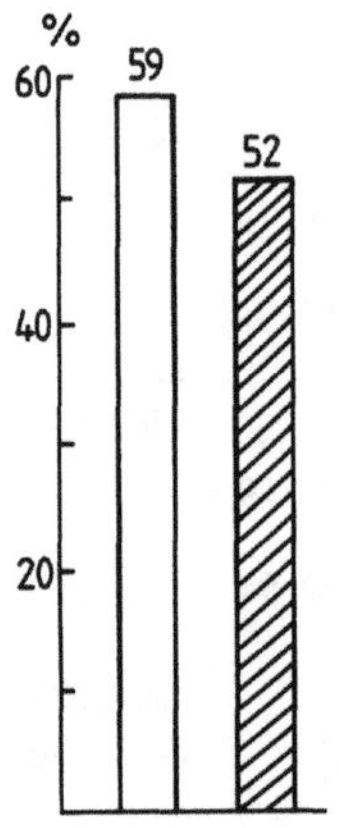

Fig. 15. Physician's advice as reason for failure to return to work among nonworking patients ($n = 542$). *Unshaded bars,* physician's advice: *shaded bars,* cardiac symptoms. (From Wenger et al., in [1])

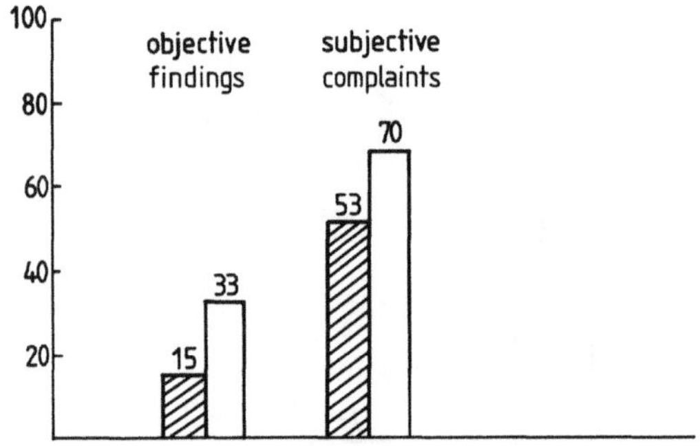

Fig. 16. Psychosomatic problems. *Unshaded bars,* palpitation rhythm disturbances; *shaded bars,* angina pectoris ischemic signs. (From Meffert et al., in [1])

In addition, postoperatively employed patients were in functional class 1 or 2 more often than those not employed postoperatively ($p<0.001$; Fig 7). Postoperative employment to normal retirement age or beyond was also studied in the United States (Fig. 8).

Of all patients, 66% worked up to normal retirement age, and 16% up to 10 years beyond retirement age, while only 17% stopped work before normal retirement age. Several factors have been recognized to predict postoperative resumption of work. One of these is age. In a West German study Walter et al. (Fig. 9) found that 73% of those in the 30 – 49 year-old age group returned to work, compared with only 56% in the 50 – 54 year-old age group and 7% in the 60 – 64 year-old age group, whereas Johnson et al. in the United States found levels of 68%, 64%, and 83%, respectively. The difference in the percentage of patients working in the various age groups compared to the normal population increases with age. This study was done in the Federal Republic of Germany (Fig. 10). If angina was completely or partially relieved postoperatively, more patients up to the age of 59 returned to work than if angina was not relieved. In patients under 19 years of age, the employment rate was 88% in the patients with relief of angina and only 53% if angina was not relieved. In the group aged 50 – 54 years, 83% of patients returned to work if angina was relieved compared with only 49%

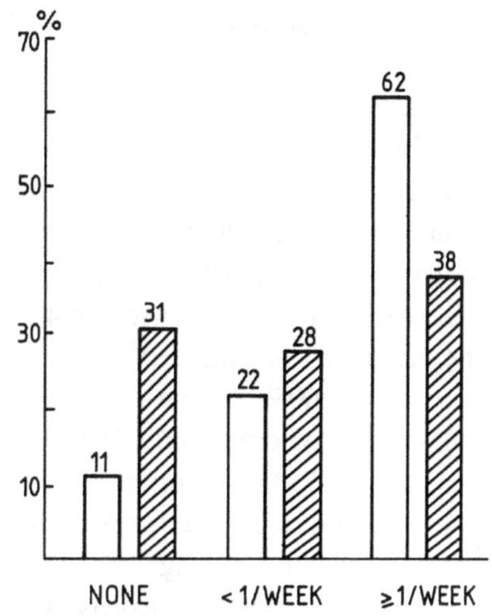

Fig. 17. Comparison of sexual frequency preoperatively (*unshaded bars*) and at 9 months postoperatively (*shaded bars*). (From Kornfeld, in [1])

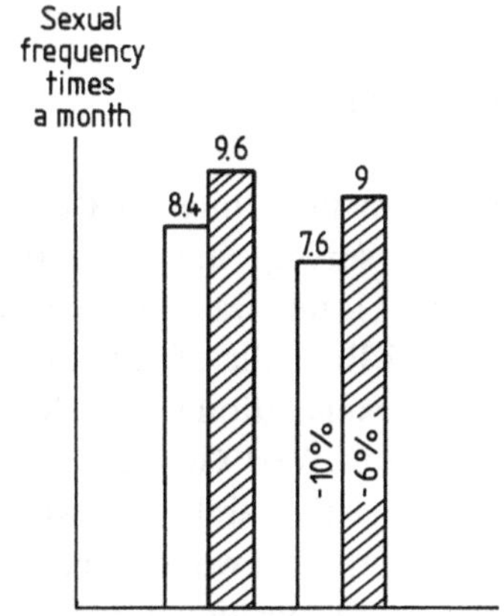

Fig. 18. Frequency of sexual relations preoperatively (*left*) and postoperatively (*right*). Data from Israel (*shaded bars,* from [11]) and the United States (*unshaded bars*). (From Levy et al., in [1])

if angina was not relieved. In patients 55 – 59 years old 73% in the angina-free group and 36% of patients with angina returned to work.

The difference in the 60 – 64 age group was small (Fig. 11). Patients who worked up to the time of their operation were more likely to return to work than patients not employed prior to their operation. This was true in the 40 – 49 year age group and the 50 – 54 year age group and at 1, 3, and 6 years postoperatively (Fig. 12).

Length of preoperative sick leave also correlates with resumption of work. Of those out of work for less than 2 months preoperatively 75% returned to work, compared with only 27% of those out of work for more than 2 months and only 5.5% in those who had not worked for at least a year (Fig. 13). In a Swiss study of 105 patients employed preoperatively, 77 returned to work, 18 were not working, and 5 were retired, whereas of the 114 preoperatively unemployed patients only 43% worked postoperatively, 49% did not work, and 8% were retired (Fig. 14). In a study by Wenger et al. in the United States 95% of patients not working preoperatively sited physicians' advice as an important reason and 52% sited cardiac symptoms as a reason (Fig. 15).

Psychosomatic problems occur frequently after coronary bypass operations. Objective success of an operation does not predict subjective satisfaction. Whereas ischemia was demonstrated in only 15%, as many as 53% of patients complained of chest pain; and whereas in only 33% rhythm disturbances could be demonstrated, 70% complained of palpitations (Fig. 16).

Sexual activity decreases from preoperative to postoperative periods. Preoperatively 11% engaged in no sexual activity at all compaired to 31% postoperatively; 60% of patients had sexual intercourse at least once a week preoperatively, whereas only 38% had sexual intercourse once a week postoperatively (Fig. 17). In comparable studies by Johnson and Fletscher in the United States and Levy in Israel, sexual intercourse took place, respectively, 8.4 and 9.6 times a month on average preoperatively, and this decreased slightly to 7.6 and 9 times a month postoperatively (Fig. 18).

Discussion

While in the United States the incidence of working without limitation after bypass surgery increased from 46% preoperatively to 65% postoperatively (Table 1), this was not true for patients from Switzerland (Fig. 3) and from the Federal Republic of Germany (Fig. 4).

Our explanation for the low incidence of return to work after coronary bypass surgery in West Germany could be a discrepancy between the functional class, the subjective ability to work, and the definitive employment rate. Although 39% of the nonworking group were in class I and 34% in class II, only 11% of this group considered themselves to be able to work without limitation (Fig. 5). On the other hand, a correlation was found between postoperative exercise tolerance and the incidence of return to work in patients who attended a rehabilitation program. The main factors which influenced postoperative work resumption were age, relief of anginal symptoms, and preoperative employment status. If patients were no longer employed or were on sick leave for more than 2 months, the incidence of return to work was negatively affected. The disease itself and the long preoperative period of unemployment seems to produce psychosomatic problems which lead to a discrepancy between objective findings and subjective complaints postoperatively (Fig. 16). These are also reflected in sexual problems manifested by a decrease in sexual activity after surgery (Fig. 17).

These sexual disturbances seem to run parallel with a change in patients' character: a loss of self-esteem, depressive moods, and psychological lability. These psychosomatic problems are probably one of the reasons for the negative advice given by personal physicians to 59% of the patients who failed to return to work (Fig. 15).

Better information and integration of the general practitioner into a team of cardiologists, cardiac surgeons, psychologists, and physical therapists might improve the quality of life after coronary artery bypass surgery of which post-operative employment is an essential part.

Summary

From these studies it can be concluded that the rate of return to work after CABS could be increased, because a relatively high percentage of patients not employed postoperatively are functionally improved. Reduction of the length of preoperative unemployment and better cooperation between cardiologists, cardiac surgeons, rehabilitation physicians and general practitioners might improve the rate of return to work and probably also the quality of life.

References

1. Walter PJ (ed) (1985) Return to work after coronary artery bypass surgery – psychosocial and economic aspects. Springer, Berlin Heidelberg New York
2. Walter PJ et al (1983) Med Klin 78:276–280

Rehabilitation Systems in Different Areas of the World

K. König

The beginnings of cardiac rehabilitation as a new sub-discipline of cardiology go back to 1964, when for the first time a group of specialists discussed the problem of rehabilitation of patients with cardiovasculatory disease on an initiative of the World Health Organization (WHO) [1]. The result was an inventory of up-to-date findings in the field of cardiac rehabilitation; in 1967, a second WHO working group met in Noordwijk in order to enter into practical work [3]. Decisive pioneer work was then provided by the newly founded Working Group on Cardiac Rehabilitation of the International Society and Federation of Cardiology with its founder president Professor Denolin. Soon the activities in Europe were followed by comparable impulses in countries outside Europe, mainly in Israel and the United States. All efforts at standardizing rehabilitative measures resulted at first in a recommendation of how to divide the course of rehabilitation into different stages in chronological order, which has by now been established whole-wide [2]. Phase I includes hospitalization immediately after the acute event; this phase I of rehabilitation lasts until discharge from hospital. This is the start of phase II, which ends with the patient's return to work or with regaining his abilities to cope with everyday life activities. Phase III includes the patient's further life after complete occupational and social reintegration.

In this paper I should like to show how rehabilitation after myocardial infarction or bypass surgery is realized practically in different countries. It is understood that, despite many efforts by the WHO and by the Council of Cardiac Rehabilitation to create a standard, an internationally agreed, standardized procedure could not be achieved because of differing socioeconomic and medicolegal factors in different countries; local traditions also vary from country to country. All this has led to widely differing methods of cardiac rehabilitation, especially as far as phase II and III are concerned. Concerning phase I, that is, rehabilitation in hospital, the organizational concept of so-called early mobilization is more or less standardized and is established in all of those countries in which myocardial infarction plays a role [5, 7]. According to this concept, physical mobilization after uncomplicated infarction begins on the 4th or 5th day after the acute event. Progressive and carefully observed building up of physical activities aims at a discharge from hospital in week 3 or 4. All studies available today agree that early mobilization after myocardial infarction bears no higher risks than late mobilization, often with confinement to bed for many weeks, which formerly was the standard. To be more precise, higher rates of reinfarction and development of aneurysms or a higher mortality rate could not be observed.

Contrary to the course of rehabilitation in phase I, there is no general conformity in the different countries about cardiac rehabilitation in phase II. Today we distinguish between the following four differing methods:

1. Outpatient rehabilitation without an organized structure.
2. Outpatient rehabilitation in specialized units.
3. Inpatient rehabilitation in specialized centres.
4. Rehabilitation in coronary clubs.

Outpatient Rehabilitation Without an Organized Structure

In the United Kingdom, interest in cardiac rehabilitation has grown very slowly [9]. After a short period in hospital during the acute illness, the majority of patients return to the care of their general practitioner. The approach to rehabilitation is usually informal and depends very much on the attitudes of the treating doctor. Exercise testing and programmes of gradually increasing exercise are not routine practice. Instead, the patient is advised to take up again his previous leisure activities, which involve physical exercise, in the belief that he is more likely to bear something that he enjoys. Information an aspects of secondary prevention is usually given by the cardiologist or general practitioner, supplemented by special booklets given routinely to patients in hospital following their infarction. Difficulties can arise in patients with severe rehabilitation problems. They may require more specialized and prolonged psychological and social help than can be given by their physician or general practitioner.

Outpatient Rehabilitation in Specialized Units

This method of organizing cardiac rehabilitation services has gained widespread popularity, and reports of successfully functioning programmes have come from various centres in Israel and the United States [10, 12, 13, 14, 15]. The patient, after early mobilization in hospital, goes to the rehabilitation department as an outpatient several times weekly for a period of weeks or months to take part in a comprehensive care programme that includes medical treatment, graduated exercise, psychological and social helps, and education about ischaemic heart disease. These rehabilitation departments tend to be part of well-equipped university clinics or large regional general hospitals and, as such, offer good facilities for speedy, effective rehabilitation.

The limitation of this kind of service is that it cannot readily be developed in large rural areas with a scattered population, where transport to a large regional hospital is impracticable. Small rural hospitals cannot afford to run rehabilitation departments. In this situation, improved rehabilitation services for those with infarction must be provided by a specialized rehabilitation institute which can admit patients from a wide area for periods of 4 weeks.

Inpatient Rehabilitation in Specialized Centres

Institutional rehabilitation starts immediately when the patient leaves hospital and provides a comprehensive programme lasting 4 weeks and containing the same elements of care as the programme in an outpatient department. There are arguments in favour of rehabilitation being undertaken on an inpatient basis [8]. An exact diagnosis of functional cardiac state can be made. Immediately following infarction it is impossible to perform a thorough investigation of cardiac function in more than a very few patients. Information on this is necessary to prescribe a safe programme for increasing mobilization. This can be done appropriately in the rehabilitation centre using the noninvasive techniques of ergometry, telemetry and long-term ECG monitoring to measure the size of the heart (heart volume) and the coronary reserve and to demonstrate the presence and type of arrhythmias. The results of this investigation together with the case history indicate in a proportion of cases the need for further investigation using the invasive techniques of floating catheterization, coronary angiography and ventriculography, particularly if the possibility of surgery in the further management of the patients is being discussed.

Rehabilitation in Coronary Clubs

So-called coronary clubs have been established as the fourth possibility of organized cardiac rehabilitation in phase II. In the Federal Republic of Germany (FRG) these clubs are nowadays called heart groups; this term implies that not only patients with coronary heart disease can join these groups, but also patients after heart operations of any kinds. Such groups enjoy a growing popularity all over the FRG and here the so-called "Hamburg model" has become a signpost rehabilitative model [11]. The patients are preselected into the groups on the basis of clinical and haemodynamic criteria. They meet once in a week on the premises of a sports club to perform a joint training programme with an observing doctor present. This exercise session is supplemented by relevant discussions, movie showings and diet counselling as well as by a programme for domestic endurance exercises. There is no doubt that this form of ambulant rehabilitation must be considered highly suitable for achieving a life-long motivation of the patient in respect to a healthy life-style.

The model of coronary clubs as a continuation of rehabilitation in phase II certainly has positive aspects: it is cheap and can be organized relatively easy. A more critical view, however, leads to the understanding that the diagnostic practicalities in coronary clubs are far from sufficient to gain an objective picture about functional adaptation processes during physical exercise. Thus, overloads or dangerous rhythm disturbances cannot be monitored on a reliable basis. Rehabilitation in coronary groups already in phase II may be justifiable in low-risk cases but not in high-risk cases. Logically, as a precondition to rehabilitation in coronary groups, the patient should be preselected into such groups before his discharge from hospital. This, again, requires that the acute clinic be equipped with diagnostic facilities and well-trained medical staff of be able to carry out such selection procedures. Up to now, only few clinics are provided with the facilities to gain an objective cardiological assessment by means of ergometer testing, echocardiography and long-term ECG monitoring. Another point of criticism of rehabilitation in coronary groups during phase II relates to the fact that it is hardly realistic to expect positive treatment results when there is only one session per week in which to take necessary measures for an effective health education. Most of the time in these sessions is reserved for the actual training programme; individual care, i.e. dealing with personal problems of the patients, is hardly possible in these groups.

Rehabilitation in phase III basically means a life-long care of patients after myocardial infarction or bypass surgery. The key figure here is, of course, the family practitioner. Apart from this, there are two organizational forms of priority phase III rehabilitation, which have been developed over the past 20 years: (a) repeated inpatient rehabilitation in specialized rehabilitation centres and (b) continuation of rehabilitation in coronary groups. The first form is practised, for instance, in the FRG. After a period of 1 – 3 years the patient returns to the rehabilitation centre for 4 weeks; the initial status of performance and coronary reserve is exactly determined. During the 4-week course further improvement of the patient's performance level is aimed at in individually adapted training therapies. In addition, knowledge of health aspects in life is increased in health education sessions in order to intensify the patient's motivation to an even more health-conscious life-style. The second form of phase III rehabilitation in coronary groups has also become an established system in the FRG; today there are already approximately 1500 coronary groups, and this number is still growing. According to rehabilitation experts in the FRG, effective applicability of coronary group rehabilitation does not lie in phase II, because of the reasons mentioned above, but in phase III of cardiac rehabilitation.

To summarize, it can be stated that the spectrum of organizational forms of cardiac rehabilitation shows significant variations. The scale extends from the simplest form of treatment by the medical doctor, without any means of organization, to the minutely organized form of rehabilitation in highly specialized centres. Considering the enormous differences in cost between the simplest and the highly specialized extremes, it can be understood that the question as to the efficiency of such systems arises again and again. I doubt whether it will ever be possible to find a definite and satisfying answer to this, because rehabilitation is a too complex process, which includes manifold medical and psychological factors. Therefore, an overall, objective quantification of efficiency cannot be achieved; it is only possible to find answers to specific sub-aspects of this whole problem.

As mentioned in the beginning, the wide variations of organizational forms of cardiac rehabilitation in different countries is due to different traditions in the various countries and to their varying socioeconomic structures. On the other hand, it must also be emphazised that the form and the financial burden of rehabilitation depends on the quality of the social system. The fact that in some countries patients return to work earlier than in others does not imply that rehabilitation in those countries is more effective; an early return to work may also be caused by financial pressures. In other words, a cheaper form of rehabilitation is not necessarily a better form of rehabilitation. On the other hand, however, there is no evidence that an expensive rehabilitation guarantees a particularly effective rehabilitation. Therefore, each country, according to its own social system with its own social facilities, should try to institute that organizational form of cardiac rehabilitation which takes into account the medical requirements as well as the findings of psychosocial research in the best possible way.

References

1. WHO (1964) Rehabilitation of patients with cardiovascular disease. WHO, Geneva (WHO technical report, ser no 270)
2. WHO (1968) A programme for the physical rehabilitation of patients with acute myocardial infarction. WHO, Copenhagen
3. Organisation Mondiale de la Santé (1969) La réadaption des malades cardio-vasculaires. Rapport sur un Seminar, Noordwijk on See 1967. Copenhagen (Dokument Euro 0381)
4. Cardiac rehabilitation 1975: report of a working group. J Coll Physicians 9:281 – 346
5. Acker JE (1971) The cardiac rehabilitation unit: experiences with a programme of early activation. Circulation 44 [Suppl 2]:119
6. Acker JE (1977) Pros and cons of organized rehabilitation. Bibl Cardiol 36:114 – 117
7. Bloch A, et al (1974) Early mobilization after myocardial infarction. A controlled study. Arr J Cardiol 34:152 – 157
8. Halhuber ME, König K (1977) Arguments for a comprehensive rehabilitation programme. In: Critical evaluation of cardiac rehabilitation. Bibl Cardiol 36
9. Hutter AM Jr, et al (1973) Early hospital discharge after myocardial infarction. N Engl J Med 288:1141 – 1144
10. Kellermann JJ (1975) Rehabilitation of patients with coronary heart disease. Prog Cardiovasc Dis 17:303 – 328
11. Krasemann EO, Donat K (1981) Zehn Jahre Herzinfarkt-Rehabilitation. Hamburger Modell. Symposium 1981, Boehringer, Mannheim
12. Mulcahy R (1976) The rehabilitation of patients with coronary heart disease. In:

Stocksmeier U (ed) Psychological approach to the rehabilitation of coronary patients. Springer, Berlin Heidelberg New York

13. Rose G (1972) Early mobilization and discharge after myocardial infarction. Modern concepts of cardiovascular disease. 41:59–63
14. Royston GR (1972) Short stay hospital treatment and rapid rehabilitation of cases of myocardial infarction in a district hospital. Br Heart J 34:526–532
15. Wenger NK, et al (1973) Uncomplicated myocardial infarction. Current physician practice in patient management. J Am Med Assoc 224:511–514

Discussion: Session V – Rehabilitative Care After Myocardial Revascularization

Chairman: N.K. Wenger

Dr. Wenger: One of the areas that we will have to examine in future years is whether all these factors are different in patients after PTCA as compared with patients after bypass grafting. I expect the reason why this has not yet been done, is that we do not have good randomized data on comparable patients. We have heard that patients undergoing PTCA are often different in terms of severity of lesions, functional capacity etc. compared to patients undergoing coronary bypass grafting. There are now one or two trials randomizing appropriate patients to either of these interventions. It will be very interesting to see similarities and differences in all the variables in the patients who have successful PTCA or CABG.

Are there any comments or questions about any of the papers presented?

Dr. Kellermann: I should like to congratulate Dr. Walter on his attitude. He is one of the very few surgeons who is interested in questions such as return to work and psychological improvement of his patients. I have to say that in my experience the reasons for the low return to work after CABG is mainly misguidance or lack of guidance. This attitude can be found in Europe, in the United States, and very often in my country, and I consider this to be the number one reason for the failure of a large proportion of patients to return to work after surgery.

I should like to offer an explanation for the discrepancy which was found in one of the papers quoted here by, comparing the New York Heart Association (NYHA) classification and the return to work. It is our experience that when comparing NYHA classification, which is based on symptomatology only, with physical performance under laboratory conditions, one finds that there is at least a 45% discrepancy between the physical work capacity of the patient, as obtained by means of exercise stress testing (preferably spiroergometry), and the functional classification as established by NYHA assessment. I think this is one of the possible explanations, and it is worthwhile analyzing this further. As a consequence of prior studies, we came to the conclusion that NYHA classification, without additional stress testing, cannot be considered a sufficient tool to assess the patient's functional capacity and eligibility to work.

To Dr. König's paper I should like to add that he may recall that 19 years ago we published, for the first time, a paper on the proportion of patients who returned to work after an acute myocardial infarction. Of these patients, 91% returned to work within 3 months, none of whom were in a rehabilitation program, and we concluded from this at the time, that is was the socioeconomic structure of the country which was responsible for the high return to work. While I concur that in selected countries patients after CABG did not return because of the socioeconomic background, I should like to stress again that in most places lack of proper patient education and medical misguidance is to be blamed. In addition to this, the socioeconomic structure has been altered in a number of countries during the years, either negatively or positively, and this too may become an important variable.

Dr. Broustet: I would like to put a question to Dr. König. How do you see the financial problem for outpatient rehabilitation? This is a point on which we have many problems in France, because when patients go to the hospital as outpatients or to a private clinic, they have great difficulties in obtaining their reimbursement from the social security system for the cardiologist or the clinical therapist who cares for patient. How do you solve this in a country like West Germany for outpatients?

Dr. König: We have only the rehabilitation centers and the coronary clubs, not the units; so I cannot give you an answer as to how it works with units. You, Dr. Wenger, have more experience in the United States, as to how it works concerning the costs of such a unit, and who is paying the cost.

Dr. Wenger: In the United States it varies considerably, because each of the separate states has its own jurisdiction as far as reimbursement policies for medical care are concerned, and the degree of insurance coverage, governmental and private, varies widely. So there is no uniformity.

Dr. Kellermann: We did not actually find, during the 25 years that our Institute has been in operation, that the cost per se of a supervised rehabilitation program played a significant role. The Sickness Fund or the patient himself covers the expenses, which are rather low. I personally do not know of any patients who had to drop out of the program due to lack of financial support. The expenses for the social medicine practice in our country are moderate and for the individual service quite low. The Sickness Fund is prepared to cover the rehabilitation programs because of the accumulated experience that when the patient is under supervised comprehensive care, he is very rarely admitted to the hospital, his absence from work is minimal and so are the number of visits to the outpatient clinics of the Sickness Fund. I believe that in considering the cost-benefit balance, the Sickness Fund came to the conclusion that it is worthwhile to pay a few more dollars per month and thereby avoid the higher expenses when patients are not undergoing this kind of supervised care.

Dr. Wenger: Let me return to one of the comments made earlier relating to New York Heart Association functional classification. A study was recently reported in the United States on problems with the NYHA classification, in reference to patients with chronic illness, because the classification of functional status is dependent on the symptomatic status regarding usual or habitual activity. One determines whether the patients are symptomatic with less than usual or habitual activity, usual activity, more than usual activity, or much more than usual activity. What often happens with chronic illness is that the usual level of activity progressively declines, so that what was usual activity 4 or 5 years previously is not usual today. There was good evidence presented that simply asking the patients or their families whether or not they became symptomatic with their usual activity was unwise. If you use objective exercise capacity, as Dr. Kellermann has mentioned, you can define functional status; or if you define specific tasks and resultant symptoms, rather than querying about usual activity, you will obtain a much better comparative evaluation. And at times you will have to question patients about the pace of the activity; patients may limit their symptoms by performing a given activity far more slowly or with intermittent rest periods. One of the major problems with "usual activity" is that usual activity varies markedly from individual to individual and intraindividually as illness progresses.

Dr. Walter: I would like to come back to the subject of return to work. From what I have learned during this meeting in West Germany, we will have made great progess if we can make known to the general practioner that these patients are quite able to return to work after surgery. I can't speak about other countries, but I think that in West Germany the opinion of a great proportion of general practitioners is that, if a patient is operated, he should not return to work, and I think this can be done in West Germany because of the welfare system that exists here. But aside from this, it is of great importance for the quality of life to return to work. And I think we should make more effort to inform general practitioners and the medical world in general that this really is quite possible.

Dr. Wenger: This is really the purpose of this session; the monograph that will derive from this meeting should define for the primary care physicians the "state of the art" in the various procedures that have been discussed yesterday and today. The summary of this session is designed to identify for the primary care physicians what should be done in follow-up of patients who have undergone PTCA and CABG, including the data that you and others have presented on the recommendations for return to work.

Dr. Kellermann: Considering the Federal Republic of Germany, I should like to ask my colleagues from West Germany whether they do not see the link between the general unemployment rate and and the overall return to work after an acute coronary event or CABG.

Dr. König: This question is absolutely to answer with yes. We have a high rate of unemployment, and when the patient is coming from operation and is physically and mentally excellent, we can tell him that he can go back to work. But when three or four other younger people are waiting for his job, one cannot really morally, in a certain sense, advise him to return, and he is, in general, willing to accept this saying, "Yes, I'm now 58 years old; it's enough."

Dr. Wenger: This is fascinating. When I listen to the economists in the United States, they tell us that with the aging population there (and as you know the subgroup in the United States over age 85 is the component of the older population growing most rapidly), sometime within the next half century people will have to work until age 70 or 75. Otherwise there will not be enough working individuals in the economy to support the older nonworking persons. As our population ages in industrialized countries, I expect that we will have an increased duration of work, work at an older age; we may be faced with problems that we do not encounter today, when an escalation of technology transiently has decreased the need for a working force.

Dr. Broustet: You are right in that the problem is with the trade unions. It has for a long time been a goal to reduce the time of working during life. This is something of victory for trade unions, and it is very difficult to convince those people that after a few years we should be back to increasing the time of working. In Paris Holter monitoring studies have been carried out in persons employed in insurance and bank companies. And the mean values of highest heart rate for 24 h in those people with a very sedentary life was 120. And, therefore, if you recall that in 3% on a bicycle the mean value of critical heart rate is 126, this means that most people with a proper therapy are able to work at least in the bank and insurance company. We should not have any unemployment for cardiac reasons.

Dr. Wenger: I believe you are right. Let me try to summarize. We have seen that both the patients and the entire medical system have devoted enormous physical, emotional, and financial resources to the implementation of thrombolysis, angioplasty, and coronary bypass surgery. The aim of long-term care and surveillance is essentially that of an insurance policy, to take care of all of these investments that have been made. I hope that this afternoon we have given some guidance in how to insure these investments. Thank you.

Acknowledgment

This symposium was made possible through the kind support of Bayer AG (Leverkusen) and the Forschungsgesellschaft Rauchen und Gesundheit mbH (Hamburg).

GPSR Compliance
The European Union's (EU) General Product Safety Regulation (GPSR) is a set of rules that requires consumer products to be safe and our obligations to ensure this.

If you have any concerns about our products, you can contact us on

ProductSafety@springernature.com

In case Publisher is established outside the EU, the EU authorized representative is:

Springer Nature Customer Service Center GmbH
Europaplatz 3
69115 Heidelberg, Germany

www.ingramcontent.com/pod-product-compliance
Lightning Source LLC
Chambersburg PA
CBHW061202240926
51846CB00006B/1093
9783642835469